Reshaping
Health
Systems

What Drives Health Care and How You Can Change It

Reshaping
Health
Systems

What Drives Health Care and How You Can Change It

Joshua M. Liao, MD, MSc

Internal Medicine Physician
Department of Medicine
University of Texas Southwestern
Medical Center
Dallas, Texas

Joseph H. Joo, MD, MS

Internal Medicine Physician
Department of Medicine
University of Washington
School of Medicine
Seattle, Washington

Jonathan A. Staloff, MD, MSc

Family Medicine Physician
Department of Family Medicine
University of Washington
School of Medicine
Seattle, Washington

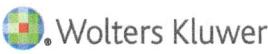 Wolters Kluwer

Philadelphia • Baltimore • New York • London
Buenos Aires • Hong Kong • Sydney • Tokyo

Acquisitions Editor: Joe Cho
Development Editor: Cindy Yoo
Editorial Coordinator: Vinodhini Varadharajalu
Marketing Manager: Kirsten Watrud
Production Project Manager: Justin Wright, Matthew West
Design Coordinator: Stephen Druding
Manufacturing Coordinator: Beth Welsh
Prepress Vendor: S4Carlisle Publishing Services

9 8 7 6 5 4 3 2 1

Printed in the United States of America

Library of Congress Cataloging-in-Publication Data

ISBN-13: 978-1-975221-23-2

Library of Congress Control Number: 2024944430

MPP0924

Dedication

For Geraldine, Abigail, Allison, and Alexander, who despite having little connection to systems factors that drive health care, are nonetheless my unwavering inspiration to work on reshaping and improving it.

Joshua M. Liao, MD, MSc

To my wife for her love, support, and endless patience in the writing of this book, and for always guiding me to think critically about what truly matters in medicine and health care. To my parents for their lifetime of love and encouragement that helped me to believe that any dream could be possible.

Jonathan A. Staloff, MD, MSc

To my parents who gave me the dream to write a book and the support to realize it.

Joseph H. Joo, MD, MS

Endorsements

Interested in changing health care? This book is a great place to start. Using a practical case-based approach that walks readers through common health care scenarios and settings, the authors illustrate something that clinicians and administrators know from their work (that health care delivery is not simple) while offering two things they may not (why it is not simple and what to do about it). Here, Liao, Staloff, and Joo are highly—and among the droves of health systems and care delivery books—uniquely pragmatic. They draw on their real-world experiences to provide perspectives and salient frameworks for much of what we see in health care today, along with actionable approaches for making it better. This book is for practicing clinicians, administrators, and students from all disciplines interested in actually making health care better.

David H. Au, MD, MS[†]
Executive Director of the Center for Care and Payment Innovation
US Department of Veteran Affairs

Efforts to improve US health care must focus on creating a more just system that addresses the health disparities of historically underserved communities. Liao, Staloff, and Joo emphasize this in their book, highlighting equity as a crucial element. They identify key factors shaping health care and propose strategies for change, consistently considering the impact on disparities, access, quality, and costs.

The authors' clinical, scholarly, and leadership experience adds significant value for health care leaders, clinicians, and trainees. The book's main contribution is not just presenting solutions to reshape health care but also emphasizing that these solutions should enhance health equity alongside overall outcomes. It encourages readers to internalize this wisdom and work toward reshaping care within their own clinical environments.

Kavita P. Bhavan, MD, MHS
Chief Innovation Officer
Parkland Health

This book is an essential resource for medical students and residents. It bridges a crucial gap in medical education by comprehensively addressing policy and care delivery topics relevant to health care systems, but typically overlooked in clinical training. The book's structure, divided into understanding systemic factors and exploring actionable solutions, equips future clinicians with the policy knowledge to drive meaningful change in their practices. As a national expert in health policy, I highly recommend this book for its clarity, depth, and practical relevance in transforming health care delivery.

Renee Crichlow, MD
Chair of the Commission on Federal and State Policy
American Academy of Family Physicians

This book is essential reading for any policy-interested clinician and a must-read for anyone aiming to improve health care in the United States. It highlights the challenges that plague health care in this country and proposes effective solutions, educating clinicians on policy and health system structures influencing care delivery while providing practical tools for making changes in clinical settings. Each topic is introduced with a continuous patient narrative, emphasizing the relevance of different policy and systems factors to clinical practice.

Yalda Jabbarpour, MD
Director
Robert Graham Center for Policy Studies in Family Medicine and Primary Care

---

[†]*The views expressed are those of the authors and do not reflect the official policy of the Department of the Army, Department of the Navy, Department of the Air Force, Department of Defense, Department of Veterans Affairs, or the US Government.*

If you want to be a good clinician in the modern health care system, it is no longer enough to know which medications to prescribe or tests to order; you must also know how to help patients navigate complicated systems of care to promote their health. If you want to be a *great* clinician, you also need skills to improve those systems of care. This book masterfully covers both knowledge and skills, buoying complex concepts by constantly tying them to the experiences of a patient and a clinician. If every health professional reads this book, care in the United States would immeasurably improve.

Christopher Moriates, MD
Executive Director
Costs of Care

Troves of books and articles have been written about the failings of health care delivery systems and the necessary interventions to transform them. Most offer only partial explanations of the challenges and one-size-fits-all solutions. In this important new book, Liao, Staloff, and Joo take a human-centered approach, looking at all of the complex systems factors in health care through the experiences of patients and the clinicians seeking to serve them. The authors offer a simple yet comprehensive tool kit for creating productive change to support the needs of people giving and receiving care, all organized around a chapter-by-chapter learning system. This book is a must-have resource for students, teachers, and leaders interested in how to make health care safer, of higher quality, and, ultimately, better.

Read G. Pierce, MD
Chief Quality, Safety, and Transformation Officer
Denver Health

Foreword

A patient presents with symptoms.

But what actually ails them?

To make that determination, the clinician must arrive at a diagnosis and then recommend a treatment plan.

Similarly, in our modern health care system, symptoms of dysfunction abound. Our costs are high, and our outcomes are uneven. Care is often inaccessible and frequently delivered by an array of people and organizations with competing interests and misaligned priorities. And yet, when faced with these facts, too often we fail to align on a common diagnosis that might enable us to pursue an approach toward improving the system.

A defining reason for this stubborn inaction is modern health care's leadership crisis. People in leadership positions, who have the ability to effect change, are often unable to reconcile the trade-offs required to build and run systems that rein in costs while improving patient outcomes. Blame is often assigned to administrators and executives; while many of them are culpable, it is also true that too many clinicians who occupy positions from which they might effect change remain oblivious to how the larger and often hidden structures of the system in which they function impact care delivery. Indeed, many clinicians show little interest in acquiring knowledge that is not purely clinical in nature or lack salient foundational resources to translate health systems interests into knowledge and skill. But this is a missed opportunity: as much as we need nonclinical leaders who speak the language of medicine, we need a class of clinicians who speak the language of health systems and can make decisions that lie at the intersection of pathophysiology and care delivery.

Which is where this book comes in. Inside these pages, Drs Liao, Staloff, and Joo use their experience and viewpoints as clinicians to undertake a case-based approach to understanding what ails our health care system. Then, having made their diagnosis, they offer "systems solutions" that other clinicians can use to plan, implement, and evaluate changes inside clinical environments.

"How you define a problem determines how you solve the problem," one of my mentors used to say. By looking at health care from the viewpoint of a single patient, the authors define the system's inadequacies not in abstract terms, but rather around the framework of a real patient story described in actual sites of care and designed to enhance an understanding of different clinical scenarios.

By taking this approach, the authors embrace opportunities for improvement through a comprehensive understanding of how the delivery system is organized around the inflection points in the patient journey. As much as this is an informative guide to the way our health system works, it is also a call to action.

I believe readers will come away—as I did—both informed and inspired.

Sachin H. Jain, MD, MBA
President and CEO
SCAN Group and Health Plan
Long Beach, California

Preface

This book is a labor of love. As practicing clinicians, we were driven to write this book by our different experiences with health systems leadership, research, policy, and education.

Our intention was to design a book that would be useful to clinicians and trainees at all levels; relevant for self-study or structured curricular teaching; and consumable whether read cover to cover or as needed for reference in practice or educational settings. Given our collective experiences, achieving these goals was high priority for several reasons. First, health systems topics are excluded from much of medical education, creating an overall dearth of useful resources.

Second, existing resources are often fragmented across different disciplines. In particular, some health systems–relevant knowledge is found in the quality improvement literature, while other types are found in policy, operational, or implementation literature. Clinicians and trainees are faced with a challenging task: to piece together information on their own from disparate disciplines and fields into useful, applied knowledge. Third, the few available resources framed explicitly on health systems are often theory-driven and conceptual, far from the real-world and lived experiences of clinicians and trainees. A practical, unified health systems resource was needed.

We chose the case-based format intentionally to mirror the way clinicians train, think, and work. The goal was to frame the content in a structure that is intuitive, enjoyable, and accessible, connecting the often complex and hidden factors driving health care to the real-world clinical experiences that result from them.

The book is divided into two parts. In Part I, "Factors That Drive Health Care," readers follow the journey of a patient as they navigate their medical care across clinicians and care settings. Each chapter first presents a set of problems that the patient encounters—problems that can be traced back to systems factors influencing how our health care is structured, delivered, or experienced. Each chapter then illuminates salient points for each systems factor by describing its history, evolution, and/or core components. In each chapter, Takeaways sections encourage synthesis; Implications sections review how each systems factor can influence access, quality, cost, and equity of care; and Multiple-choice questions assess and consolidate learning.

In Part II, "Solutions to Change Health Care," readers follow the journey of a clinician from Part I. This switch in perspective enables readers to view systems factors—and in turn, consider systems solutions—through the lens of a clinician who desires to enact changes to address problems and improve care delivery. Across chapters, readers are led through a life cycle of approaching a problem; identifying a problem and solutions; planning and implementing solutions; and evaluating solutions. Throughout, readers are introduced to concepts, tools, and strategies from fields such as quality improvement, change management, design thinking, and implementation science. Like Part I, Part II contains Takeaways and Multiple-choice questions. Distinct from Part I, Part II includes examples of real-world applications. The two parts complement and build off each other.

No resource is comprehensive, and every book requires trade-offs. Entire volumes could be dedicated to a number of systems factors or solutions; our book omits certain details for space and usability. Some topics are also poised to change and evolve after the writing of this book.

This book was a labor of love and a product of experience. May that experience inform yours, illuminating factors driving health care and offering ways to improve it.

About the Authors

The authors are local, regional, and national health systems leaders with expertise in policy and practice change. This expertise is grounded in the depth of their collective experiences: in addition to their clinical practices, they have worked on health systems issues through administrative leadership, rigorous evaluation and research, and service on groups advising local, regional, and national decision-makers.

Joshua M. Liao, MD, MSc, is an internal medicine physician and faculty at the University of Texas Southwestern Medical Center where his work lies at the nexus of health systems policy, care delivery, evaluation, and research. He serves as the chief of the Division of General Internal Medicine, director of the Program on Policy Evaluation and Learning, and director of research methods in the Clinical and Translational Science Program.

Dr Liao is an international leader in health systems, policy, and care delivery. He advises the US Congress and Department of Health and Human Services through service on the Medicare Payment Advisory Commission and the Physician-Focused Payment Model Technical Advisory Committee—the first person in history to be simultaneously appointed to both expert groups. He has also served on numerous national advisories and committees through groups such as the National Academy of Medicine and the American College of Physicians. He obtained his medical degree from Baylor College of Medicine and internal medicine residency at Brigham and Women's Hospital, where he was a clinical fellow at the Harvard Medical School. He obtained advanced policy and research training from the University of Pennsylvania, where he is an adjunct senior fellow in the Leonard Davis Institute of Health Economics in the Wharton School.

Jonathan A. Staloff, MD, MSc, is a family medicine physician and faculty at the University of Washington (UW). There, he also serves as the medical director of Population Health for Value Management, supporting value-based care initiatives across the UW Medicine enterprise. Dr Staloff is a health services researcher focused on primary care–related issues, including payment reform, telemedicine, and behavioral health integration; he also serves as an associate editor for *Healthcare: The Journal of Delivery Science and Innovation*.

Dr Staloff has been actively engaged in primary care policy, cochairing the Washington Advisory Committee on Primary Care and serving on the American Academy of Family Physicians Commission on Federal and State Policy. He attended medical school and completed a Master of Science in Population Medicine at Brown University, family medicine residency at UW, and an advanced fellowship in health systems research through the US Department of Veterans Affairs.

Joseph H. Joo, MD, MS, is an internal medicine physician and faculty at the University of Washington, where he also serves as the director of the Program on Policy Evaluation and Learning in the Pacific Northwest (PROPEL-PNW). Through the Program, Dr Joo directs a leading policy unit that applies scholarly and policy expertise and content knowledge in evaluation and scholarship to partner with decision-makers on pressing policy topics. PROPEL-PNW serves as the formal evaluation partner to the Washington Health Care Authority, the largest purchaser of health care services in the state.

Dr Joo conducts research with emphasis on health systems topics, including population health interventions, to improve care transitions. He completed medical school at Texas A&M University and internal medicine residency with Distinction in Care Transformation at Dell Medical School at the University of Texas at Austin. Dr Joo obtained his Master of Science in Health Services from the University of Washington.

Contents

Contents

Part I

Factors That Drive Health Care

Ambulatory Care

Clinical Case

Jessica is a 67-year-old woman having her very first visit with her new primary care clinician, Dr Jackson. Jessica is accompanied by her husband, Daniel, and comes in with recent laboratory results from her previous clinician, whom she could no longer see because her clinic stopped accepting Jessica's insurance, which she receives through Medicare and Medicaid as someone who is dually eligible for both.

In clinic, her vitals are normal. Jessica shares that she has a longstanding diagnosis of type 2 diabetes, and that her most recent hemoglobin A_{1c} assessed 4 months ago was elevated. She is also concerned about left knee pain, and her husband wants to talk about changes in Jessica's memory.

The primary care clinician has 30 minutes allotted to see Jessica, who was unfortunately 10 minutes late because of delays connecting with the transportation service provided by Medicaid to bring her to the clinic. The primary care clinician shares that, regrettably, they may not have the time to address all concerns today and suggests focusing instead on highest priority items. Together, the primary care clinician and Jessica decide to focus on reconciling medications, addressing diabetes care, and evaluating knee pain, setting aside other concerns for a future visit.

This situation is common for an initial visit in a primary care practice. In this case, the patient has a preexisting chronic condition, for which disease management is not at guideline-based goals. She has a musculoskeletal complaint and a possibly new or developing memory problem that merit evaluation. Decisions made by primary care clinicians in these situations are often driven not just by clinical considerations but also considerations driven by health systems factors (eg, how to triage priorities and focus areas during a visit).

Many primary care clinicians see approximately 20 to 25 patients per day and will have fewer than 20 minutes to spend with each patient. Like the patient in this case, many individuals seeking primary care have a combination of new or established medical problems and preventive health needs that merit attention. In addition to directly interacting with patients during visits, primary care clinicians have other demands of their time, including the following:

- Responding to electronic messages and phone calls from patients and their caregivers
- Reviewing and delivering diagnostic test results
- Communicating with a range of other clinicians (eg, medical or surgical subspecialists, physical and occupational therapists, social workers, and behavioral health specialists) in order to coordinate care
- Reaching out to patients who recently visited the hospital or emergency room and require primary care follow-up
- Speaking with insurance companies to receive approval for diagnostic testing or therapeutic treatments
- Participating in or leading population health, quality improvement, or health equity–focused initiatives

Along with limitations on the time allocated for patient visits, these demands often compel primary care clinicians to triage issues to either address in a given visit or save for follow-up at a later time. This reality is driven in part by systems factors such as the reimbursement system for outpatient care.

SYSTEMS FACTOR: REIMBURSEMENT SYSTEM FOR OUTPATIENT CARE

While there are a variety of health care reimbursement methods in the United States, fee-for-service serves as a foundational method for outpatient care. As the name suggests, under fee-for-service, clinicians and their organizations receive payment for each reimbursable service they provide. Because more services lead to more payment, this system can create the incentive for outpatient clinicians and medical care organizations to increase the number of patients seen in clinic, which can functionally restrict the time available and number of issues that can be addressed per visit.

Both the amount of reimbursement and type of reimbursable services vary by payer, but Medicare policy is widely used as a benchmark or starting point for other payers, such as commercial insurance companies. Therefore, it is important to understand the history of Medicare's outpatient reimbursement system.

1965 to 1992: Customary, Prevailing, and Reasonable

Medicare has reimbursed clinicians on a fee-for-service basis since the program's inception in 1965. Initially, this approach was implemented in a "customary, prevailing, and reasonable" manner. Medicare defined customary charge as the median of what a clinician charged for a given service over a predetermined period of time—that is, the typical amount at which clinicians priced their services. Medicare defined prevailing charge as a percentage (initially 90%, later 75%) of average customary charges across clinicians in a geographic area. Reasonable charge was defined as the lowest of three types of charges: a clinician's actual charge, the clinician's customary charge, or the prevailing charge in the area of the clinician's practice. Ultimately, Medicare reimbursed clinicians based on reasonable charges. Several features defined this customary, prevailing, and reasonable reimbursement method:

Payment based on charges. The customary, prevailing, and reasonable method paid clinicians based on what they chose to charge. Because charges could vary widely, this approach created the potential for high charges to lead to large reimbursement amounts.

Payment that varied across clinicians and geographies. By reimbursing clinicians based on either actual charges, customary charges, or prevailing charges, the customary, prevailing, and reasonable method created the possibility of variation. In particular, the lowest of the three charge types— and, in turn, reimbursement—could vary across different services, clinicians, and geographies.

Ultimately, the customary, prevailing, and reasonable method contributed to increases in health care spending over time. By the 1980s, these issues prompted policymakers to reform the reimbursement method. The result was the creation of the Medicare Physician Fee Schedule.

1992 to Present: The Relative Value Unit and Medicare Physician Fee Schedule

Implemented in 1992, the fee schedule was largely inspired by work led by William Hsiao and published in 1988. The study examined services and procedures of four specialties: family medicine, general surgery, internal medicine, and thoracic and cardiovascular surgery. Researchers assigned resource-based relative values to different services based on the estimated resources required to provide them—that is, assigning value to each service based on what it required of clinicians to provide it. These relative values were based on several inputs, including physician work, opportunity cost of specialty training, and relative practice costs for each specialty.

Researchers then simulated potential changes in reimbursement by applying this resource-based relative value scale to Medicare data under the stipulation that overall Medicare spending remain the same. Under this simulation, initially procedure-heavy specialties experienced reimbursement decreases (eg, 40% decrease for ophthalmologists), while other specialties initially experienced increases (eg, 60% increase for family medicine clinicians).

Medicare adopted a modified version of this relative value scale in creating its physician fee schedule. The fee schedule catalogued services using a set of codes called Current Procedural Terminology (CPT) codes. Each code was assigned a relative value, counted in relative value units (RVUs), intended to represent the effort and resources required to provide a given service. While Medicare has adjusted methods for calculating RVUs over time, the general approach has remained consistent. Under the current approach, the RVU consists of three components:

Work. The work RVU accounts for approximately 55% of the RVU and is intended to include the time and intensity required to complete a service. The time component consists of the time spent before (eg, training and preparation), during, and after delivering the service itself. Intensity is meant to capture the degree of technical skill, physical effort, clinical judgment, or stress related to the service being provided.

Practice expense. The practice expense RVU accounts for approximately 41% of the RVU. It is meant to capture the resources needed to provide a service, such as the labor of clinician staff and equipment.

Malpractice. This component accounts for approximately 4% of the RVU and is intended to account for a physician's required malpractice insurance expenses.

RVUs are converted to reimbursement dollars via two additional steps: applying a geographic adjustment that accounts for cost of living and wages as well as a conversion factor that translates RVU into dollar units (Figure 1.1).

Ultimately, the RVU system is based on a straightforward concept: payment should be service specific and predicated on clinician effort, practice expense, and malpractice. While time has led to changes in codes (what codes are created, discontinued, or modified) and RVUs (how much clinicians are paid for different codes), as well as alternative reimbursement methods (eg, Medicare Advantage, value-based payment models), the RVU-based fee schedule method remains firmly in place within Medicare at present.

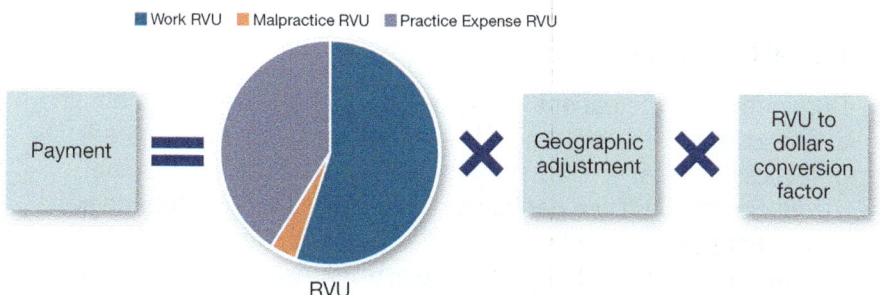

Figure 1.1 RVU Calculation. RVU, relative value unit. (Source: Johnson SE, Newton WP. Resource-based relative value units: a primer for academic family physicians. *Fam Med.* 2002;34(3):172-176.)

While other payers have based their outpatient care reimbursement approach on Medicare's, it is important to note that reimbursement amounts differ across payers. Commercial payers have historically reimbursed clinicians, on average, 40% more than Medicare for physician services, while Medicaid reimbursement rates are on average 30% less than Medicare rates.

Back to the Clinical Case

The patient in this case has a number of medical concerns, including type 2 diabetes, knee pain, and memory challenges. Each of these concerns is important for her health, longevity, and quality of life, and each merits attention. However, each concern also potentially requires a number of immediate, follow-up, and ongoing steps to coordinate care. Because of the dynamics created by fee-for-service reimbursement, it is infeasible for a clinician to address all facets of each issue facing the patient. Instead, the prevailing fee-for-service reimbursement method in outpatient care can place time and scope constraints on this patient's visit with her primary care clinician.

TAKEAWAYS

- Historically, the predominant form of reimbursement in US health care has been fee-for-service, a system in which clinicians receive a payment for each eligible service provided.
- One potential consequence of a fee-for-service reimbursement system for outpatient care is incentives to increase reimbursement by restricting patient visits to short periods of time in order to see larger numbers of patients.

Clinical Case Continued

During the visit, the patient's primary care clinician attempts to obtain a more comprehensive medical history and reconcile an accurate list of Jessica's medications. In asking for refills, Jessica takes out several medication bottles from her bag. Unfortunately, she did not bring all her medications and is unable to recall the dosages of the others at home.

Without access to Jessica's prior electronic health records (EHRs), her primary care clinician decides to refill certain prescriptions based on the medication bottles brought by Jessica to the visit. Her primary care clinician decides to hold off on prescribing other medications, which are not urgently needed, and arranges for Jessica to call the office to provide information that will allow these prescriptions to be filled accurately. Jessica signs a consent form so that the office can directly request and receive a transfer of her prior records.

This scenario—the inability for a clinician to access a patient's prior clinical records—exemplifies the challenges of health care data interoperability. Interoperability is the capability of different organizations to access, exchange, and integrate care records in a coordinated, timely manner.

Interoperability requires the electronic accessing and sharing of health information, broadly conceived as health information exchange (HIE). In turn, the ability to exchange health information is predicated on information technology systems for storing and analyzing health information—collectively termed health information technology (HIT). Practically, HIT and HIE occur in clinical settings via EHRs, systems that enable clinicians to document and store patient health records electronically, rather than on paper.

Since the transition from paper records to electronic records, interoperability continues to improve among care organizations. In 2021, approximately 62% of hospitals engaged in sending, receiving, querying, and integrating EHRs, an increase from approximately 41% of hospitals doing so in 2017. During this 4-year span, there were also increases in the availability and usage of EHR information received from outside organizations at the point of patient care.

Despite this progress, data interoperability remains a major systems challenge in health care. Poor interoperability can impede or delay clinical decisions, create patient safety concerns (eg, erroneous testing or treatment), or duplicate care, with different clinicians making diagnostic or therapeutic decisions without the knowledge of other clinicians' decisions. In these ways, data interoperability is a systems factor that can continue to affect the ability to achieve desired health outcomes.

SYSTEMS FACTOR: DATA INTEROPERABILITY

Data interoperability is vital for clinicians to coordinate the delivery of effective and efficient care across organizations. Traditionally, patients have had to complete documentation—generally, a health or medical record release form—for their clinicians to request and receive either mailed or faxed copies of records from other clinicians.

With technologic advancements, more clinicians and medical care organizations have shifted toward EHRs for storing and transmitting patient health records. During the 1960s, EHRs were mostly utilized by government entities and a limited number of medical care organizations. In the 1990s, when computers and the internet began to be introduced, EHRs were mostly implemented at academic medical centers for claims processing and document capture.

In 2004, efforts to achieve interoperability received a boost with the creation of the Office of the National Coordinator for Health Information Technology (ONC). The ONC was created to lead the implementation of HIE and HIT at the national level. Later, with the passage of the Health Information Technology for Economic and Clinical Health (HITECH) Act in 2009, the ONC adopted a new charge to promote adoption and meaningful use of HIT.

HITECH encouraged the adoption of EHRs and improved privacy and security of medical records. A portion of the budget allocated for the HITECH Act was used to fund an EHR Incentive Program through Medicare and Medicaid called Meaningful Use. The Meaningful Use program sought to encourage adoption of EHRs by initially providing financial incentives to eligible clinicians, groups, and hospitals that utilized "certified" EHR technology—with certified being defined by storage of data in an established and structured format consistent with predetermined criteria.

While it initially provided financial incentives to eligible clinicians and organizations, Meaningful Use eventually shifted toward penalizing clinicians who failed to meet program criteria. There were three basic program components, each of which was implemented in phases: use of a certified EHR in a meaningful manner (eg, to prescribe medications), electronic exchange of health information to improve quality of care, and use of certified EHR technology to submit clinical quality measures.

Over time, different aspects of the Meaningful Use program were phased out, sunset, or transitioned into other programs. For instance, in 2015, Meaningful Use was transitioned to become one of the four components of what was then a new national payment program, the Merit-Based Incentive Payment System. Behind these changes, EHR adoption increased rapidly, growing from adoption at approximately 10% of hospitals in 2008 to approximately 95% by 2017.

Data interoperability was advanced again in December 2016, when the 21st Century Cures Act was signed into law to address persistent interoperability gaps. This act called on the Department of Health and Human Services, in conjunction with ONC and Centers for Medicare and Medicaid Services, to publish the ONC Final Rule in March 2020. The rule was designed to achieve several things.

First, it sought to prevent information blocking practices as strategies to limit data interoperability. Second, the rule was intended to promote patient access to their own records at no additional costs, and exchange of medical records via automated services between clinicians and hospitals. Third, the rule aimed to minimize the costs of achieving data interoperability via EHRs by standardizing medical records transfers. By December 2022, significant progress toward interoperability had been achieved through the adoption of application programming interfaces, which are set of rules or a common language that enable different applications to communicate with each other.

Application programming interfaces act as third-party intermediary layers that process transfer of medical records between organizations. Through use of application programming interfaces, patients can share diagnostic information with their clinicians in real time (eg, blood sugar levels) and clinicians may be able to review active medication lists from another health organization's EHR system.

Overall, EHR adoption can support the goals of HIT, HIE, and, ultimately, data interoperability. For instance, EHR use can potentially lead to greater care standardization (eg, via documentation and ordering processes), reduced charting errors (eg, by reducing errors from misinterpretation of handwritten orders and notes), increased accessibility (eg, allowing multiple members of the care team to access and retrieve records simultaneously), and easier data access and sharing between clinicians and organizations. Although several EHR vendors hold the vast majority of market share, the presence of a given vendor at different clinics does not necessarily mean that those clinics can share medical records. Reasons cited for this challenge include privacy concerns and costs of achieving interoperability.

Importantly, despite a number of policies and programs such as those described, not all care organizations have adopted EHRs as an avenue for achieving data interoperability. In 2017, there were about 5% of hospitals that did not use EHRs. Fax machines are still very much in use by many medical care organizations; one poll in 2018 found that nearly half of physicians who use EHRs still also use paper notes, scanning, and faxing to work around EHR limitations. Even in an era marked by widespread EHR adoption, it can also be common for clinicians and patients to use other electronic workarounds in which patients bring or use printouts or electronic records on their smartphones, tablets, or laptops.

Back to the Clinical Case

In this case, the patient unfortunately did not bring a comprehensive medication list, and the clinician did not have access to medical records generated from the care she received previously through another clinician. The lack of interoperability contributed to a suboptimal approach to prescription refills, as well as the need for the patient and clinician to take extra steps to obtain the patient's records.

TAKEAWAYS

- EHRs have been poised to improve data interoperability, the capability of organizations to access, exchange, and integrate care records.
- A number of policies and programs have sought to encourage data interoperability for patients and clinicians, in part through EHR adoption.
- Despite such policies and programs, not all care organizations have adopted EHRs as an avenue for achieving data interoperability.

Clinical Case Continued

After discussing a plan for medication refills, Jessica and her primary care clinician spend the remainder of their visit on two additional issues. First, Jessica shares about her worsening left knee pain. She states that she was diagnosed a number of years ago with knee osteoarthritis for which she has received multiple steroid injections. Unfortunately, her most recent injection did not bring relief for more than a few weeks. Due to the severity of her pain, her primary care clinician refers her to an outside orthopedic surgeon. Second, Jessica and her primary care clinician discuss her diabetes control, deciding together that an endocrinology consultation would also be beneficial, given Jessica's prior difficulties with blood sugars.

Two months later, Jessica returns to her primary care clinician's clinic for follow-up. She reports that the endocrinologist, Dr Taylor, prescribed insulin and requested laboratory tests, including several that duplicated tests that had recently been ordered for Jessica. Jessica asks whether she should complete the laboratory tests ordered by the endocrinologist, and who would be managing her diabetes medications and laboratory tests going forward.

Jessica also shares that on the recommendation of Dr Lee, the orthopedic surgeon, she recently completed preoperative evaluation and is now looking for dates to schedule a knee replacement surgery. Jessica asks her primary care clinician, who is hearing about this for the first time, whether this plan makes sense.

This case exemplifies the importance of care coordination between clinicians. The Agency for Healthcare Research and Quality defines care coordination as "deliberately organizing patient care activities and sharing information among all of the participants concerned with a patient's care to achieve safer and more effective care." An important systems factor, care coordination can potentially affect care effectiveness and safety, the quality of communication, and the ability to enact whole-person and value-aligned care plans. Care coordination has become increasingly critical given many patients' multiple care needs and the ever-increasing complexity of the US health care system. Medicare patients, for instance, see a median of 5 specialists per year, and patients with multiple chronic conditions see as many as 16 specialists per year.

SYSTEMS FACTOR: CARE COORDINATION

It is difficult to argue against clinicians working together on patient care by intentionally sharing information and organizing necessary services—that is, working together to provide coordinated care. The potential benefits are only likely to increase given the aging US population, as patients' health conditions, medical team members, and needed services increase in number. Indeed, patients with chronic conditions who perceive their care to be well coordinated have higher satisfaction with their clinicians as well as their overall care.

Conversely, poor care coordination can fragment care in ways that result in duplicate testing, medical errors, and delayed care. Primary care clinicians and specialists each report that they receive insufficient and untimely information from one another when providing care for shared patients. One-third of patients in the United States who see multiple clinicians share that needed results or medical records were not available at the time of visits or that clinicians duplicated tests. In addition, patients who experience highly fragmented care have increased rates of preventable hospitalizations, receive twice as many diagnostic tests, and experience a total cost of care more than 75% higher than patients with similar disease burden, but low levels of care fragmentation. Nationally, costs related to poor care coordination in the United States were estimated to be more than $27 billion in 2019.

Patient-Centered Medical Home

While relevant to all outpatient care, care coordination is arguably best rooted within primary care. In 1967, the American Academy of Pediatrics introduced the notion of a "medical home," which they first referred to as a place where a child would receive care that is accessible, family-centered, coordinated, comprehensive, continuous, compassionate, and culturally effective.

Over time, different medical specialties iterated on the concept of the medical home, culminating in 2007 when the American Academy of Family Physicians, American College of Physicians, American Academy of Pediatrics, and American Osteopathic Association—groups collectively representing more than 300 000 physicians, and part of the voice of US primary care—outlined a set of joint principles for the patient-centered medical home (PCMH; Figure 1.2). Care coordination was one such principle underlying a PCMH, which was defined as "a health care setting that facilitates partnerships between individual patients, and their personal physicians, and when appropriate, the patient's family."

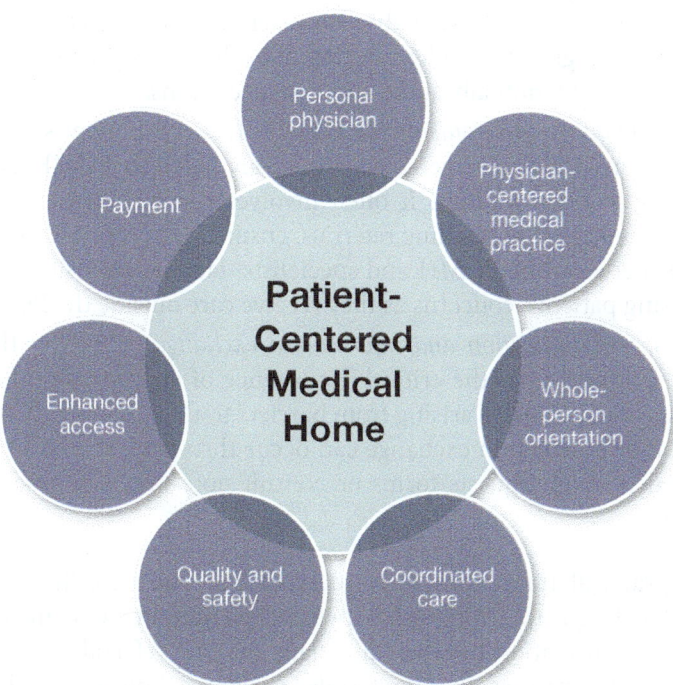

Figure 1.2 The 2007 Joint Principles of the Patient-Centered Medical Home. (Source: American Academy of Family Physicians, American Academy of Pediatrics, American College of Physicians, American Osteopathic Association. Joint principles of the patient-centered medical home [Internet]. March 7, 2007. https://www.aafp.org/dam/AAFP/documents/practice_management/pcmh/initiatives/PCMHJoint.pdf)

PCMH has proven to be one of the most consequential and significant frameworks for promoting coordinated care, among other things, in US health care. One reason is that PCMH has created a conceptual canopy under which more specific, care coordination–focused models of care have been developed.

The PCMH framework has given rise to care models such as the Care Coordination Model—an approach that uses observed best practices and successful relationships between outpatient clinicians and facilities to articulate desired components of care coordination. According to the model, effective care coordination has the following characteristics:

PCMH accountability for care coordination. This component involves clinicians comprising the PCMH taking on the responsibility of coordinating across a team of clinicians so that patients receive high-quality care.

Clear expectations among clinicians. This component acknowledges that clear expectations can affect the quality of care patients receive across different clinicians or health organizations within and outside the PCMH. Consequently, successful PCMHs directly reach out to these clinicians or organizations to grow an understanding of each other's practice styles, and sometimes write mutually agreed upon expectations.

Logistical support for care outside the PCMH. This component speaks to the need for proactive management of referrals between PCMH and other clinicians or organizations. It often involves the PCMH having a team member dedicated to tracking referrals, ensuring appropriate information transfer between the PCMH and specialists, facilitating visits, or directly addressing patients' concerns as they receive care outside the PCMH.

Established communication and information exchange pathways. This component acknowledges the critical importance of appropriate information exchange and problems arising from barriers to that exchange. Communication and information exchange can occur through a shared EHR, standardized referral requests forms or consult notes, or web-based referral systems.

Another practical framework for understanding care coordination in the outpatient setting is to distinguish between consultation and comanagement as types of coordination between clinicians making referrals (referring clinicians) and clinicians receiving referrals (receiving clinicians; Table 1.1). In some situations, consultation is needed because the referring clinician requests that the receiving clinician provide input, that is, to consult on some aspect of a patient's care. In this shorter term type of coordination dynamic, the receiving clinician makes a recommendation on how to approach the patient's care, but the referring clinician retains primary responsibility for shared

Table 1.1 Care Coordination Through Consultation and Comanagement

	Consultation	Comanagement
Description	Shorter term relationship between a patient and clinicians involved in referrals (referring and receiving), where the receiving clinician is asked by the referring clinician to use their expertise to answer a specific question	Longer term relationship between the patient and referring and receiving clinicians, where both clinicians share ongoing responsibility for managing the relevant medical condition(s) Principal roles assumed by either the referring clinician (comanagement with shared care) or receiving clinician (comanagement with principal care)
Role of the referring clinician	Asking a clear and specific question of the receiving clinician, and receiving and acting on appropriate components of the receiving clinician's recommendation	Indicating the condition(s) or services that would benefit from comanagement with the receiving clinician Together with the receiving clinician, determining specific expectations around communication and management of the different aspects of care (eg, diagnostic tests, therapeutic treatments, need for additional referrals)
Role of receiving clinician	Ensuring the referral question is understood and responding with specific recommendations Recommendations can include guidance about whether a situation merits comanagement instead of consultation, as well as if/then scenarios for future consultation.	Ensuring the comanagement request is understood Together with the referring clinician, determining specific expectations around communication and management of different aspects of care (eg, diagnostic tests, therapeutic treatments, need for additional referrals) Can provide guidance about whether a situation merits consultation instead of comanagement
Responsibility for clinical decisions	While informed by receiving clinician recommendations, responsibility resides primarily with the referring (eg, primary care) clinician in conjunction with the patient via shared decision-making.	Responsibility resides with both referring and receiving clinicians, the specifics of which would ideally be clearly articulated and agreed upon.

Source: American College of Physicians. Beyond the referral: principles of effective, ongoing primary and specialty care collaboration: an American college of physicians position paper; 2022.

decision-making with the patient and for implementing a care plan. Consultation type of care coordination can involve a face-to-face visit between the receiving clinician and the patient; or can be an e-consult, where the receiving and referring clinicians communicate asynchronously through the EHR and no direct visit takes place between the patient and the receiving clinician.

In other situations, coordination can be operationalized via comanagement. Under this approach, a referring clinician still initiates a request for the receiving clinician to participate in some aspect of a patient's care. Compared to consultation, the distinction of comanagement is that it will likely involve a longer term relationship where both the referring and receiving clinicians share ongoing responsibility for managing the relevant medication conditions. In a comanagement approach, groups such as the American College of Physicians have outlined that principal roles can be assumed by either the referring clinician (referred to as comanagement with shared care) or by the receiving clinician (referred to as comanagement with principal care).

In each approach to comanagement, the responsibility for care decisions is shared among the patient as well as the referring and receiving clinicians, with the specifics of how this responsibility is shared ideally being agreed upon in advance.

Patient-Centered Medical Neighborhood

The PCMH framework has evolved with time, broadening to encompass more clinical settings (eg, long-term care, hospitals, and emergency rooms) and community-based organizations that contribute to health (eg, schools and employers, social services organizations). This wider scope has been defined as the medical neighborhood, which can be understood as the collection of partnerships between clinical and community organizations to provide the medical and social supports needed to promote patient and population health (Figure 1.3).

Back to the Clinical Case

In this case, the patient's care has potentially been threatened in several ways due to suboptimal coordination between her clinicians. The lack of comanagement between the primary care clinician and endocrinologist about her ongoing diabetes management could have exposed the patient to the risk of duplicated diabetes laboratory tests and the additional time, discomfort, and resources involved. The lack of effective communication around surgical consultation could have confused the patient or caused her to lose confidence about the respective roles of her primary care physician and surgeon.

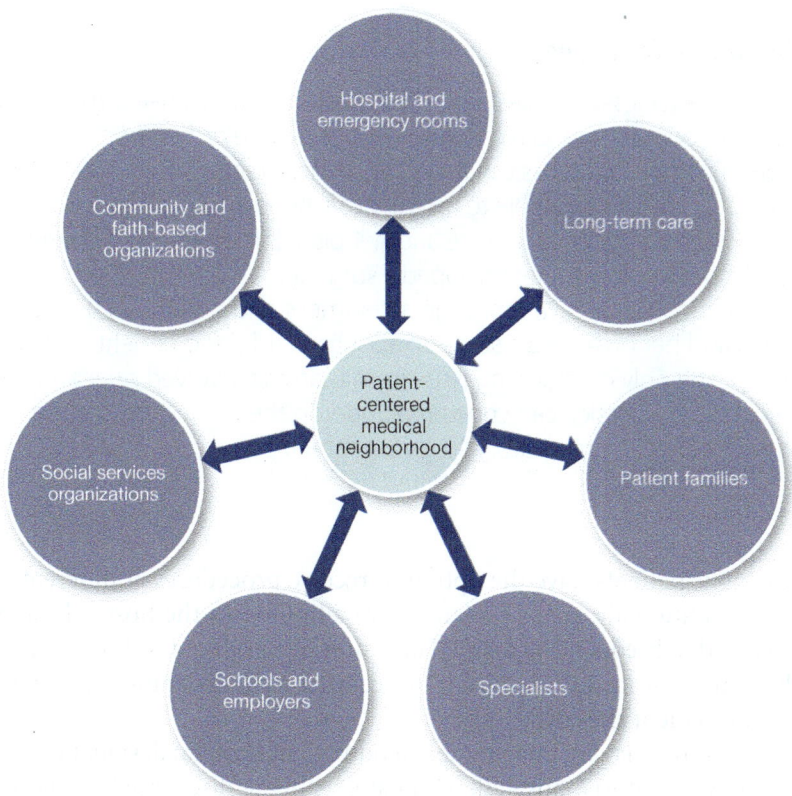

Figure 1.3 The Patient-Centered Medical Neighborhood. (Source: Primary Care Collaborative. Medical neighborhood [Internet]. https://www.pcpcc.org/content/medical-neighborhood)

TAKEAWAYS

- Care coordination is critical for promoting good outcomes, but its absence can lead to redundant testing, medical errors, and reduced patient satisfaction.
- Care coordination is a pillar of primary care and can be conceptualized via frameworks such as the PCMH and the medical neighborhood.
- Principles from the PCMH framework can be extended to models describing ideal components of coordinated care, such as the Care Coordination Model, and constructs for consultation and comanagement as coordination approaches between referring and receiving clinicians.

Clinical Case Continued

In response to Jessica's question about a potential total knee arthroplasty (TKA), her primary care clinician attempts to call the orthopedic surgeon's office to discuss this aspect of Jessica's care. Unfortunately, he is operating and unavailable to take the call. As an alternative, Jessica and her primary care clinician pursue another plan of having records faxed from Jessica's visit with her orthopedic surgeon.

The records reveal a thorough assessment and discussion between Jessica and her orthopedic surgeon about the risks and benefits of knee surgery. The only outstanding issue from that visit involved selecting the site of surgery: Jessica can choose to undergo the procedure in either the hospital or an ambulatory surgical center (ASC).

Increasingly, patients have the option to receive procedures at different sites of care. Traditionally, many patients were admitted to the hospital for procedures and subsequent recovery. For a number of decades, however, there has been interest in shifting certain procedures away from inpatient settings toward outpatient sites of service.

Procedures that are done under an outpatient hospital designation occur within or adjacent to a hospital, with patients being discharged on the same day or shortly thereafter. Procedures can also be done in stand-alone facilities consisting of operating rooms and postanesthesia recovery units, known as ASCs.

The ability to shift where procedures are performed may be particularly useful for lower risk procedures that do not require overnight stays or intensive postoperative recovery. Given the potential implications on patient experience as well as safety, quality, and cost-efficiency, site of service is an increasingly important systems factor that can affect how individuals receive procedural care.

SYSTEMS FACTOR: SITE OF SERVICE FOR PROCEDURES

In the United States, interest in outpatient procedures grew during the 1960s. Evaluations of an outpatient procedures at that time demonstrated the feasibility of a "program of anesthesia for outpatient surgery without compromising patient safety," reporting approximately $28 000 and 1000 hospitalization days saved across more than 800 patients through use of properly equipped and staffed outpatient hospital units. Of these patients, fewer than 1% were reported to have been admitted postoperatively for anesthetic complications. The first in-and-out (or same-day) surgeries were performed in 1967 and the first US ambulatory surgery facility was opened in 1970.

Subsequently in 1982, the Centers for Medicare and Medicaid Services (known at the time as the US Health Care Financing Administration) established the first standards for ambulatory surgical services, announcing the ASC Covered Procedures List and began to approve payments for those procedures. In 2018, Centers for Medicare and Medicaid Services began removing CPT codes from Medicare Inpatient Procedure Only List, a list created initially in 2000 to identify procedures requiring inpatient stay to be eligible for Medicare reimbursement. More recently, the agency has expressed interest to eventually phase out the nearly 1800 CPT codes from the Medicare Inpatient Procedure Only List and add procedures to the ASC Covered Procedures List. Beyond Medicare, other payers have adopted policies permitting or encouraging some procedures to be performed under outpatient designations or at outpatient sites (eg, Medicaid managed care organizations encouraging certain procedures at ASCs).

Over time, advances in medical technology and anesthesia techniques have permitted a growing number of procedures to be performed beyond the inpatient setting. These include procedures such as lens and cataract procedures, incision or fusion of joints (destruction of joint lesion), and cholecystectomies, among others. Such procedures generally pose a comparatively lower risk of compromising patients' airways, breathing or cardiac physiology, and do not routinely require overnight hospital admission.

This issue of site of service is particularly salient to, and well exemplified through, procedures such as TKA. Generally an elective surgery, TKA has been subject to many of the changes described earlier. The Centers for Medicare and Medicaid Services removed TKA from the Medicare Inpatient Procedure Only List in 2018, allowing the procedure to be performed in the outpatient hospitals. In 2020, the Centers for Medicare and Medicaid Services added TKA to the ASC Covered Procedures List.

Given that Medicare is the primary payer for more than 60% for total joint arthroplasty procedures, which include TKAs, these policy changes had significant impact. Prior to the policy changes in 2017, nearly no Medicare TKAs (save 0.2% of cases due to rare exceptions) were performed in outpatient hospitals, where costs have been estimated as approximately 30% lower and complication rates are comparable to surgeries done in inpatient settings. By the second quarter of 2019, more than 36% were reported to be performed in the outpatient hospitals. The share of TKAs performed at ASCs is predicted to increase over time from approximately 13% in 2020 to 18% in 2028.

Back to the Clinical Case

In this case, the patient has several options for where to receive her elective TKA. The ASC option can be appealing to the patient because of convenience (eg, rapid discharge, proximity to home) and clinicians and the health care system because of cost-efficiency. Had the patient required a different type of procedure, such as cardiothoracic surgery, or had additional complex health needs, an ASC may not be a suitable option due to the potential need for escalation of care or additional monitoring.

TAKEAWAYS

- There has been decades of interest in addressing site of service for procedures.
- Given a series of policy changes and scientific advancements, a number of procedures can now be performed either in outpatient hospitals or ASCs.
- Performing procedures in these non–inpatient sites of services may have patient experience and cost-efficiency benefits.

Clinical Case Continued

Jessica decides to undergo surgery at a nearby ASC. Her surgery goes well and she is discharged home the same day with 1 week of pain medications and plans for a follow-up visit. Her orthopedic surgeon tells Jessica to reach out if she develops fever, severe new joint pain, or rash.

Ten days later, Jessica has run out of prescription pain medications and is having significant knee pain. She also develops a new rash. It's a Friday at 5:45 PM and the primary care clinician and orthopedic surgeon's offices are both closed. Jessica is concerned by her knee pain and rash and would like to discuss them with a clinician.

This situation—being unable to reach outpatient clinician(s) due to hours of operation—is difficult but common. The patient in this case might have residual operative site pain that can be managed with a short-term refill on pain medications, or an urgent issue requiring medical attention such as a septic joint. But short of going to the emergency room or urgent care, patients may have difficulty navigating the health care system and reaching a clinician outside of daytime, weekday clinic hours of operation.

Expanding hours of operation to include after-hours care during evenings and/or weekends can save time and money for patients and the health care system. Expanded hours could help patients receive care from clinicians who know them well and prevent time-consuming and potentially expensive urgent care or emergency room visits. In these ways, clinic hours of operation is a systems factor impacting ambulatory care.

SYSTEMS FACTOR: HOURS OF OPERATION

It would be infeasible for many outpatient care sites to maintain operations around the clock. However, clinicians and organizations have implemented strategies to address health concerns that arise outside of the traditional weekday, 9:00 AM to 5:00 PM hours of operation.

There are a number of approaches to expanding hours of operation after-hours. Small solo community practices, for instance, sometimes implement an approach where the primary care clinician is available by phone at all times and opens the physical office for patients after-hours on a case-by-case basis. This facilitates interpersonal continuity between the patient and their personal clinician, but may be difficult to operationalize long term.

Larger practices have several potential options. First, multiple clinicians within a given practice can share after-hours responsibilities, allowing for patient continuity with the practice, if not their personal clinician specifically. Second, practices can organize into practice networks, which could then implement a series of solutions that cover the needs of patients seen across participating practices, such as 24-hour phone and/or in-person coverage, as well as nurse triage lines. Third, some practices, particularly those that are part of larger integrated health systems, could implement freestanding after-hours clinics rather than after-hours coverage at existing clinics.

In addition to after-hours solutions provided through clinicians, payers can also implement approaches to address after-hours care needs. These solutions include around-the-clock nurse call lines, where patients can speak with a registered nurse about medical or behavioral health symptoms any time and receive recommendations on how to address their concerns at home or receive the advice to be triaged to emergency care.

Collectively, these clinician- and payer-driven approaches are important efforts to improve access to care via after-hours services. Despite them, however, availability outside of traditional weekday hours of operation remains limited in the United States compared to other countries. Increasingly, retail clinics have emerged as another option for seeking care elsewhere.

These clinics are staffed by clinicians and colocated and affiliated with retail companies or pharmacies. Because of their location in retail locations, these clinics are often open on weekday evenings and weekends and accept patients on a walk-in basis. They are lower cost options than other settings, such as emergency rooms. For some minor conditions, such as ear infections and bronchitis, retail clinics have performed similarly to traditional clinics with respect to certain quality-of-care measures (eg, appropriate antibiotic prescribing).

Although there is overlap between the services provided at retail clinics and other outpatient care sites, there are also differences. The vast majority (90%) of visits to retail clinics are for basic preventive services or certain acute minor conditions, such as upper respiratory infection, sinusitis, sore throat, urinary tract infection, and conjunctivitis. In contrast, these issues comprised only the minority of primary care visits (18%) and emergency room visits (10%).

Back to the Clinical Case

This patient's situation exemplifies the challenges of hours of operation as a health systems factor. She has a medical problem that leads her to seek medical attention from either her surgeon or primary care clinician. Her concerns might be as simple as needing a refill of her pain medication or may require urgent medical evaluation for a serious postoperative complication. In either case, access to and timeliness of care beyond usual hours of operation is critical.

TAKEAWAYS

- Traditionally, hours of operation in outpatient care settings have been limited to weekday, daytime hours.
- The absence of expanded or after-hours care can create difficulties for patients who develop care needs outside of traditional hours of operation.
- Clinicians, payers, and retailers have implemented different approaches to provide after-hours or expanded hours of care.

Implications

The systems factors discussed in this chapter can pose implications for health care access. It can be limited directly by hours of operation and the inability for patients to receive care from their regular clinicians outside of weekday, daytime periods. Fewer than one-third of US primary care practices offer after-hours care, compared to the vast majority of offices in other developed countries. In addition, access can be limited by uneven distribution of clinics and outpatient care sites. For instance, sites for primary and other outpatient care, as well as ASCs, are not evenly distributed across geographic communities and areas.

The prevailing outpatient reimbursement system can also potentially affect access, both by affecting patient-clinician interactions and the clinical workforce. As described earlier, clinicians may be subject to time and patient volume pressures, and the need to triage defers certain patient care needs. An adequate workforce is also a necessary precondition for ensuring that patients can access health care. However, an RVU-based system has led to uneven reimbursement for procedural versus nonprocedural care, contributing to differential reimbursement across specialties and threatening parts of the clinical workforce.

For instance, there are reasons to worry about the adequacy of the primary care workforce. Primary care comprises up to 50% of all office visits in the United States and is associated with a number of desirable health outcomes. However, primary care only accounts for 5% to 7% of US health care spending—far lower than the 14% observed in other developed countries. Despite national increases in the concentration of US physicians in the past decade, the primary care physician concentration has decreased over the same period. By some estimates, the United States may face a shortage of up to 124 000 physicians by 2034, with primary care accounting for almost 40% of that shortage—the largest of any group.

In outpatient care, systems factors can also impact health care quality and costs. In the ideal state, strong care coordination can promote whole-person care, safety, and streamlined communication. Ideally, reimbursement aimed at promoting health would also emphasize good outcomes and experiences as outputs of health care, not just expense and resource inputs needed to deliver services. But until very recently, the fee schedule did not reimburse activities needed to coordinate care across the different services provided by different clinicians, leaving this as uncompensated work for clinicians to do when they were not providing reimbursable services.

Unfortunately, one of the unintended consequences of dynamics related to several factors—fee-for-service reimbursement, data interoperability challenges, and historical underemphasis on care coordination in payment and delivery systems—has been care fragmentation.

A fragmented system is a costly one, both from human and financial perspectives. For instance, diagnostic tests can be duplicated due to data interoperability challenges and inability for clinicians to share access to patient records. Fragmentation can be inadvertently reinforced by outpatient care reimbursement systems that reimburse clinicians for each service provided, regardless of whether it duplicates or contradicts other parts of a patient's care plan or goals. Redundancies can expose patients to added discomfort, exposures (eg, radiation from medical imaging), errors, and cost (in terms of time and money), while also adding to health care costs.

Although indirectly, these quality and cost implications can also stoke workforce challenges. Clinicians can be worn down by the real or perceived need to see large numbers of patients, prioritize and defer needs that require more time, rely on patients or go through separate processes for accessing patient records from other care sites, use uncompensated time to coordinate care for patients, and/or manage the additional utilization and spending that can arise from care fragmentation.

Finally, systems factors in outpatient care pose important equity implications. Within the prevailing outpatient reimbursement system, disparate rates across payers—that is, differences in how much clinicians are paid for providing care to individuals with different types of insurance—can also perpetuate inequity. For example, reimbursement rates are so much lower for Medicaid, as opposed to other insurance sources, that some clinicians do not accept new Medicaid patients in their clinics. Individuals with lower incomes and from minority communities make up substantial shares of those insured through Medicaid insurance.

Traditional outpatient hours of operation present potential challenges for all patients—fewer than one-third of US primary care practices offer after-hours care. But this problem can disproportionately affect certain groups, such as individuals living in rural areas or insured through Medicaid, who can be least likely to have access to after-hours primary care. And while retail clinics can potentially offset some of these challenges, these sites are geographically concentrated in certain areas and disproportionately located in those with White and higher income populations. Similar dynamics have been observed for ASCs, which can be disproportionately located in wealthier communities and underutilized by certain groups, such as racial minorities.

Multiple-Choice Questions

1. What are the three components of the RVU?
   A. Customary, prevailing, and reasonable
   B. Work, practice expense, and malpractice
   C. Specialty, time, and geography
   D. Insurance type, patient complexity, and specialty

2. Which of the following is *not* one of the three major components of the Meaningful Use program as part of the HITECH Act?
   A. Using certified EHRs
   B. Exchanging electronic health information
   C. Adopting application programming interfaces
   D. Submitting clinical quality measures

3. Samuel is a 58-year-old with a history of coronary artery disease and stable depression who sees his primary care clinician. The patient says that he's been having some worsening chest pain when walking up the stairs. The primary care clinician suggests the patient see his longstanding cardiologist, who the primary care clinician referred the patient to when he was first diagnosed with coronary artery disease. Which of the following expectations for the primary care clinician and cardiologist would be consistent with a comanagement relationship?

   A. The primary care clinician asks the cardiologist to provide recommendations on whether an angiogram is indicated for this patient, and to perform the angiogram if recommended. After this recommendation and procedure, the primary care clinician will resume complete management of the patient's coronary disease.

   B. The primary care clinician asks the cardiologist to manage the patient's coronary artery disease moving forward, after setting clear expectations about communication on any changes as part of shared responsibility for the patient's cardiac care plan.

   C. The primary care clinician tries to avoid the patient having to schedule an in-person visit and decides to send an e-consult to the cardiologist. In the e-consult message, the primary care clinician asks whether any medication changes are recommended, with the expectation that the cardiologist would indicate whether an in-person visit is more appropriate.

   D. Because coronary artery disease is such a large component of this patient's overall care, the primary care clinician asks the cardiologist to manage the patient's coronary artery disease and the patient's noncardiac conditions including his depression.

4. Which of the following has become an alternative site of service for procedures that have been historically performed only in inpatient hospital settings?

   A. ASC
   B. Emergency room
   C. Physician office
   D. All the above

5. Retail clinics, which are colocated and affiliated with retail companies or pharmacies, provide an alternative for after-hours care. What types of services are most commonly delivered at retail clinics?

   A. Chronic disease management for multiple chronic conditions
   B. Care for minor conditions, such as acute otitis media or strep throat
   C. Basic preventive services, such as vaccines and laboratory screenings
   D. B and C

Answers

1. The correct answer is B. The three components of the RVU are work, practice expense, and malpractice.

2. The correct answer is C. Adopting application programming interfaces is not one of the three major components of the Meaningful Use program as part of the HITECH Act.

3. The correct answer is B. In this example, the primary care clinician (the referring clinician), the cardiologist (the receiving clinician), and the patient are in a longer term relationship where both the referring and receiving clinicians share ongoing responsibility for managing the relevant medical condition. The primary care clinician and the cardiologist determine specific expectations around communication and different aspects of the patient's care.

4. The correct answer is A. ASCs have become alternative sites of service for procedures that have been historically performed only in inpatient settings.

5. The correct answer is D. Care for minor conditions (such as acute otitis media or strep throat) and basic preventive services (such as vaccines and laboratory screenings) are most commonly delivered at retail clinics.

Bibliography

Adler-Milstein J, Jha AK. HITECH Act drove large gains in hospital electronic health record adoption. *Health Aff (Millwood)*. 2017;36(8):1416-1422.

Agency for Healthcare Research and Quality. Care coordination. https://www.ahrq.gov/ncepcr/care/coordination.html

AMA CPT International. CPT implementation guide: component 12 RBRVS. https://cpt-international.ama-assn.org/cpt-implementation-guide-component-12-rbrvs

Ambulatory Surgery Center Association. Reducing Medicare costs by migrating volume from HOPDSs to ASCs. Advancing Surgical Care. https://www.advancingsurgicalcare.com/advancingsurgicalcare/reducinghealthcarecosts/costsavings/reducing-medicare-costs

American Academy of Family Physicians, American Academy of Pediatrics, American College of Physicians, American Osteopathic Association. Joint principles of the patient-centered medical home. Published March 7, 2007. https://www.aafp.org/dam/AAFP/documents/practice_management/pcmh/initiatives/PCMHJoint.pdf

American College of Physicians. Beyond the referral: principles of effective, ongoing primary and specialty care collaboration. Position Paper. American College of Physicians; 2022. https://assets.acponline.org/acp_policy/policies/beyond_the_referral_position_paper_2022.pdf

Anumula N, Sanelli PC. Meaningful use. *AJNR Am J Neuroradiol*. 2012;33(8):1455-1457.

Barnes CL, Iorio R, Zhang X, Haas DA. An examination of the adoption of outpatient total knee arthroplasty since 2018. *J Arthroplasty*. 2020;35(6S):S24-S27.

Basu S, Berkowitz SA, Phillips RL, Bitton A, Landon BE, Phillips RS. Association of primary care physician supply with population mortality in the United States, 2005-2015. *JAMA Intern Med*. 2019;179(4):506-514.

Belden J, Plaisant C, Johnson TR, et al. Inspired EHRs: designing for clinicians. http://inspired-ehrs.org/

Bodenheimer T. Coordinating care—a perilous journey through the health care system. *N Engl J Med*. 2008;358(10):1064-1071.

Centers for Medicare and Medicaid Services. Certified EHR technology. https://www.cms.gov/Regulations-and-Guidance/Legislation/EHRIncentivePrograms/Certification

Centers for Medicare and Medicaid Services. Fact sheet CY 2022 Medicare hospital outpatient prospective payment system and Ambulatory Surgical Center Payment System Final Rule (CMS-1753FC). https://www.cms.gov/newsroom/fact-sheets/cy-2022-medicare-hospital-outpatient-prospective-payment-system-and-ambulatory-surgical-center-0

Chatterjee A, Amen TB, Khormaee S. Trends in geographic disparities in access to ambulatory surgery centers in New York, 2010 to 2018. *JAMA Health Forum*. 2022;3(10):e223608.

Clarke JL, Bourn S, Skoufalos A, Beck EH, Castillo DJ. An innovative approach to health care delivery for patients with chronic conditions. *Popul Health Manag*. 2017;20(1):23-30.

Cohen DD, Dillon JB. Anesthesia for outpatient surgery. *JAMA*. 1966;196(13):1114-1116.

Definitive Healthcare. 10 most common inpatient EHR systems by market share. https://www.definitivehc.com/blog/most-common-inpatient-ehr-systems

Drees J. EHR market share 2021: 10 things to know about major players Epic, Cerner, Meditech & Allscripts. Becker's Hospital Review. https://www.beckershospitalreview.com/ehrs/ehr-market-share-2021-10-things-to-know-about-major-players-epic-cerner-meditech-allscripts.html

Evans RS. Electronic health records: then, now, and in the future. *Yearb Med Inform*. 2016;25(suppl 1):S48-S61.

FitzGerald M, Gunja MZ, Tikkanen R. Primary care in high-income countries: how the United States compares. Commonwealth Fund. Published March 15, 2022. https://www.commonwealthfund.org/publications/issue-briefs/2022/mar/primary-care-high-income-countries-how-united-states-compares#3

Fleming NS, Culler SD, McCorkle R, Becker ER, Ballard DJ. The financial and nonfinancial costs of implementing electronic health records in primary care practices. *Health Aff (Millwood)*. 2011;30(3):481-489.

Frandsen BR, Joynt KE, Rebitzer JB, Jha AK. Care fragmentation, quality, and costs among chronically ill patients. *Am J Manag Care*. 2015;21(5):355-362.

Friedman A, Howard J, Shaw EK, Cohen DJ, Shahidi L, Ferrante JM. Facilitators and barriers to care coordination in patient-centered medical homes (PCMHs) from coordinators' perspectives. *J Am Board Fam Med*. 2016;29(1):90-101.

Guth M, Haldar S, Rudowitz R, Artiga S. Medicaid and racial health equity. Published March 17, 2022. Kaiser Family Foundation. https://www.kff.org/medicaid/issue-brief/medicaid-and-racial-health-equity/

Hariri S, Bozic KJ, Lavernia C, Prestipino A, Rubash HE. Medicare physician reimbursement: past, present, and future. *J Bone Joint Surg Am*. 2007;89(11):2536-2546.

Health IT Buzz. Achieving a major milestone: health IT developers certify to cures update. Published February 10, 2023. https://www.healthit.gov/buzz-blog/health-it/achieving-a-major-milestone-health-it-developers-certify-to-cures-update/

HealthIT.gov. Health information exchange. 2019. https://www.healthit.gov/topic/health-it-and-health-information-exchange-basics/health-information-exchange

HealthIT.gov. Interoperability and methods of exchange among hospitals in 2021. https://www.healthit.gov/data/data-briefs/interoperability-and-methods-exchange-among-hospitals-2021

HealthIT.gov. Non-federal acute care hospital electronic health record adoption. https://www.healthit.gov/data/quickstats/non-federal-acute-care-hospital-electronic-health-record-adoption

HealthIT.gov. What is meaningful use? 2013. https://www.healthit.gov/faq/what-meaningful-use

Hedley-Whyte J, Milamed DR. The evolution of sites of surgery. *Ulster Med J*. 2006; 75(1):46-53.

Helbing C, Latta VB, Keene RE. Hospital outpatient services under Medicare, 1987. *Health Care Financ Rev*. 1990;11(4):147-158.

HHS.gov. Hitech Act enforcement interim final rule. https://www.hhs.gov/hipaa/for-professionals/special-topics/hitech-act-enforcement-interim-final-rule/

Hoff T, Prout K. Comparing retail clinics with other sites of care: a systematic review of cost, quality, and patient satisfaction. *Med Care*. 2019;57(9):734-741.

Holgash K, Heberlein M. Physician acceptance of new Medicaid patients. Medicaid and CHIP Payment and Access Commission; 2019. https://www.macpac.gov/wp-content/up-loads/2019/01/Physician-Acceptance-of-New-Medicaid-Patients.pdf

Hsiao WC, Braun P, Dunn D, Becker ER, DeNicola M, Ketcham TR. Results and policy implications of the resource-based relative-value study. *N Engl J Med*. 1988;319(13):881-888.

Huang A, Ryu JJ, Dervin G. Cost savings of outpatient versus standard inpatient total knee arthroplasty. *Can J Surg*. 2017;60(1):57-62.

IHS Markit Ltd. The complexities of physician supply and demand: projections from 2019 to 2034. AAMC; 2021. https://digirepo.nlm.nih.gov/master/borndig/9918417887306676/9918417887306676.pdf

Jabbarpour Y, Greiner A, Jetty A, et al. Investing in primary care: a state level analysis. Patient-Centered Primary Care Collaborative and Robert Graham Center; 2019. https://www.pcpcc.org/sites/default/files/resources/pcmh_evidence_report_2019_0.pdf

Janeway MG, Sanchez SE, Chen Q, et al. Association of race, health insurance status, and household income with location and outcomes of ambulatory surgery among adult patients in 2 US states. *JAMA Surg*. 2020;155(12):1123-1131.

Johnson SE, Newton WP. Resource-based relative value units: a primer for academic family physicians. *Fam Med*. 2002;34(3):172-176.

Kern LM, Safford MM, Slavin MJ, et al. Patients' and providers' views on causes and consequences of healthcare fragmentation in the ambulatory setting: a qualitative study. *J Gen Intern Med*. 2019;34:899-907.

Larochelle JL, Feldman DE, Levesque JF. The primary-specialty care interface in chronic diseases: patient and practice characteristics associated with co-management. *Healthc Policy*. 2014;10(2):52-63.

Lin S, Brasel KJ, Chakraborty O, Glied SA. Association between Medicaid expansion and the use of outpatient general surgical care among US adults in multiple states. *JAMA Surg*. 2020;155(11):1058-1066.

Lopez CD, Boddapati V, Neuwirth AL, Shah RP, Cooper HJ, Geller JA. Hospital and surgeon Medicare reimbursement trends for total joint arthroplasty. *Arthroplast Today.* 2020;6(3):437-444.

Lopez E, Neuman T, Jacobson G, Levitt L. How much more than Medicare do private insurers pay? A review of the literature. Kaiser Family Foundation. Published April 15, 2020. https://www.kff.org/medicare/issue-brief/how-much-more-than-medicare-do-private-insurers-pay-a-review-of-the-literature/

Machado SR, Jayawardana S, Mossialos E, Vaduganathan M. Physician density by specialty type in urban and rural counties in the US, 2010 to 2017. *JAMA Netw Open.* 2021;4(1):e2033994.

Mann C, Striar A. How differences in Medicaid, Medicare, and Commercial health insurance payment rates impact access, health equity, and cost. Commonwealth Fund. Published August 17, 2022. https://www.commonwealthfund.org/blog/2022/how-differences-medicaid-medicare-and-commercial-health-insurance-payment-rates-impact

Medicare program: list of covered surgical procedures for certain ambulatory surgical services. Health Care Financing Administration. Proposed notice. *Fed Regist.* 1982;47(56):12591-12593.

Molina Healthcare. Nurse Advice Line. https://www.molinahealthcare.com/members/wa/en-US/hp/medicaid/apple-health/overvw/coverd/nurseadvice.aspx

Mosalpuria K, Wilson FA, Siahpush M. Disparities in access to after-hours care in the U.S.: a national study. *J Health Dispar Res Pract.* 2021;14(1):1. https://digitalscholarship.unlv.edu/jhdrp/vol14/iss1/1

National Center for Health Statistics. National Ambulatory Medical Care Survey: 2019 National Summary Tables. https://www.cdc.gov/nchs/data/ahcd/namcs_summary/2019-namcs-web-tables-508.pdf

Neprash HT, Everhart A, McAlpine D, Smith LB, Sheridan B, Cross DA. Measuring primary care exam length using electronic health record data. *Med Care.* 2021;59(1):62-66.

Office of the National Coordinator for Health Information Technology. About APIs: HHS API educational tool eLearning. https://www.healthit.gov/api-education-module/story_html5.html

Office of the National Coordinator for Health Information Technology. HEALTH IT: advancing America's health care. https://www.healthit.gov/sites/default/files/pdf/health-information-technology-fact-sheet.pdf

Office of the National Coordinator for Health Information Technology. The ONC Cures Act final rule. https://www.healthit.gov/sites/default/files/page2/2020-03/TheONCCuresAct-FinalRule.pdf

O'Malley AS, Samuel D, Bond AM, Carrier E. After-hours care and its coordination with primary care in the U.S. *J Gen Intern Med.* 2012;27(11):1406-1415.

Parasrampuria S, Henry J. *Hospitals' Use of Electronic Health Records Data, 2015-2017, no.46.* Office of the National Coordinator for Health Information Technology; 2019.

Primary Care Collaborative. History: major milestones for primary care and the medical home. https://www.pcpcc.org/content/history-0

Primary Care Collaborative. Medical neighborhood. https://www.pcpcc.org/content/medical-neighborhood

Pylypchuk Y, Johnson C. New EHR certification requirements and their association with duplicate tests and images. *J Am Med Inform Assoc.* 2022;29(8):1391-1399.

RAND Corporation. The evolving role of retail clinics. RAND Corporation; 2016. https://www.rand.org/pubs/research_briefs/RB9491-2.html

Rankin KA, Freedman IG, Rubin LE, Grauer JN. Centers for Medicare & Medicaid Services' 2018 removal of total knee arthroplasty from the inpatient-only list led to broad changes in hospital length of stays. *J Am Acad Orthop Surg.* 2021;29(24):1061-1067.

Reisman M. EHRs: the challenge of making electronic data usable and interoperable. *P T.* 2017;42(9):572-575.

Richter DL, Diduch DR. Cost comparison of outpatient versus inpatient unicompartmental knee arthroplasty. *Orthop J Sports Med.* 2017;5(3):2325967117694352.

Schoen C, Osborn R, Huynh PT, et al. Taking the pulse of health care systems: experiences of patients with health problems in six countries. *Health Aff (Millwood).* 2005;24(suppl 1):W5-W525.

School of Medicine. Why your doctor's office still depends on a fax machine. https://med.stanford.edu/school/leadership/dean/precision-health-in-the-news/why-your-doctors-office-still-depends-on-fax.html

Shrank WH, Rogstad TL, Parekh N. Waste in the US health care system: estimated costs and potential for savings. *JAMA.* 2019;322(15):1501-1509.

Starfield B. *Primary Care: Balancing Health Needs, Services and Technology.* Oxford University Press; 1998.

Steiner CA, Karaca Z, Moore BJ, Imshaug MC, Pickens G. Statistical Brief #223: Surgeries in hospital-based ambulatory surgery and hospital inpatient settings, 2014. In: *Healthcare Cost and Utilization Project (HCUP) Statistical Briefs.* Published May 2017. Updated July 20, 2020. Agency for Healthcare Research and Quality (US); 2006. https://www.ncbi.nlm.nih.gov/books/NBK442035/

The Physicians Foundation. *2020 Survey of America's Physicians COVID-19 Impact Edition.* Published August 2020. https://physiciansfoundation.org/wp-content/uploads/2020/08/20-1278-Merritt-Hawkins-2020-Physicians-Foundation-Survey.6.pdf

Vogelzang R. Medicare and physician payment: history and current implementation of the resource-based relative value scale (RBRVS). *Semin Intervent Radiol.* 1995;12(03):254-259.

Wagner EH, Sandhu N, Coleman K, Phillips KE, Sugarman JR. Improving care coordination in primary care. *Med Care.* 52(11 suppl 4):S33-S38.

Wang MC, Mosen D, Shuster E, Bellows J. Association of patient-reported care coordination with patient satisfaction. *J Ambul Care Manage.* 2015;38(1):69-76.

Yian EH, Schmiesing AM, Kwong BD, Prentice HA, Patel SP. Procedure cost comparison of outpatient and inpatient shoulder arthroplasty and lower-extremity arthroplasty within a managed-care organization. *Perm J.* 2022;26(4):6-13.

2

Emergency Care

Clinical Case

Jessica goes to a retail clinic where they tell her to monitor her symptoms and if they worsen, to go to the emergency room (ER). By the evening, Jessica has worsening pain in her recently operated knee. It is red, warm to touch, and significantly more swollen than before. Her husband, Daniel, is concerned, as he notices Jessica is also dizzy and feverish. He decides to call 9-1-1.

Within 10 minutes of speaking to the 9-1-1 call center, emergency medical technicians (EMTs) and a paramedic arrive at Jessica's home by ground ambulance. They perform their initial assessments, obtain a brief history of her recent total knee arthroplasty (TKA), and note the swelling, redness, and tenderness of her knee. Her vitals show that she has a fever, slightly low blood pressure, and elevated respiratory rate and heart rate.

The EMTs and paramedic determine that Jessica requires urgent further evaluation; she and her husband are transported to a nearby ER by ground ambulance.

In the setting of her recent knee surgery, the patient's vital signs and examination findings are concerning for a significant infection from a postsurgical complication. This case represents a common scenario in which patients and their loved ones call 9-1-1 for assessment of worrisome signs and symptoms. There are an estimated 240 million 9-1-1 calls in the United States each year, with more than 600 000 per day on average. Overall, most calls involve phone triage without the need to provide emergency medical services (EMS) by dispatching EMTs and paramedics to assess patients further. When dispatches do occur, they can involve groups funded by local fire districts, police departments, and other government agencies, as well as private equity firms or publicly traded companies.

EMS represents an important part of the US health care system. The absence of such services would leave patients more vulnerable to poor outcomes due to urgent or potentially emergent medical conditions. EMS must be provided in a timely manner and meet the needs of different patients in different localities with different signs and symptoms. In these ways, the EMS is a systems factor that shapes how Americans receive health care.

SYSTEMS FACTOR: EMERGENCY MEDICAL SERVICES

Emergence of Emergency Medical Services and Emergency Medical Services Philosophies

Following World War II, EMS in the United States was sparse and consisted of little more than first aid services. By the mid-1960s, there were growing concerns that emergent conditions such as traumatic injuries were "the neglected disease of modern society." Accidents were the leading cause of death among US citizens younger than 37 years old and the fourth leading cause of death across all ages. Few communities possessed regulations on EMS standards and personnel formally trained in first aid services such as cardiopulmonary resuscitation.

These circumstances changed with increasing public awareness about the quality of care for emergent conditions. A 1966 report by the National Academy of Sciences and National Research Council highlighted the lack of attention paid to "the problem of accidental death and injury." Subsequently, policymakers made a push for developing better EMS in the United States, including expansion of medical ambulances and calls to support services for emergency medical care.

In 1973, Congress enacted the EMS Systems Act, which created a new grant program to accelerate development of EMS. More than $300 million was appropriated toward EMS personnel training, equipment, and research. While the Act identified ideal components of the EMS system at the federal level, the grant program ultimately emphasized the development of an EMS system driven by specific needs at the state, regional, and local levels.

During the 1970s, two major philosophies of EMS emerged. The first, a "stay and stabilize" philosophy, focused heavily on dispatching physicians to the scene and bringing medical services with them to patients. This philosophy reflected the Franco-German model of EMS, which became widely implemented in Europe over time. This implementation resulted in many patients being treated at the scene and comparatively fewer patients being transported to hospitals or other facilities for additional care. Under this approach patients ultimately requiring transport generally bypass the ER and are directly admitted to the hospital by physicians initially dispatched to the scene.

In contrast, the "scoop and run" philosophy was based on the idea of using trained personnel, such as paramedics and EMTs, to bring patients to the hospital rapidly with fewer prehospital interventions. Under this philsophy, which was exemplified in the Anglo-American model of EMS, became implemented over time in the United States.

Components of the Emergency Medical Services System

EMS is defined as a system that "responds to emergencies in need of highly skilled prehospital clinicians." The system encompasses a wide range of services that can be largely categorized into three main components:

- Response to 9-1-1 call
- On-scene care
- Care in transit

Response to 9-1-1 call. Most 9-1-1 calls do not result in EMS personnel being dispatched to the scene. Studies have shown that within cities, nearly 80% of calls are deemed to be due to nonemergent needs. When dispatch does occur, EMS can be sent to the scene via either ground or air ambulances. Given the higher costs of operation, air ambulances are typically reserved for the most critical patient conditions such as surgical emergencies, conditions requiring emergency coronary intervention, and acute strokes. Fewer than 3% of total ambulance transports were estimated to be through air ambulances in 2020.

The majority of patients are transported to ERs by ground ambulances. While there is much variation among states and local governments, ground ambulance provider organizations are largely operated by and categorized into five ownership structures:

- Private equity firms or publicly traded companies
- Facilities (eg, almost exclusively hospitals)
- Nonprofit organizations (non–facility based)
- Independent private companies
- Public sector entities (eg, fire districts, police departments)

Groups owned by public sector entities—mostly fire districts, police departments, and other local government organizations—provide the majority (>60% in 2020) of ground ambulance transportations in the United States. In comparison, groups owned by private equity firms or publicly traded companies, such as the American Medical Response and Acadian Ambulance Service, provide approximately one-third (about 30% in 2020) of ground ambulance transports.

The organization and business practices of ground ambulance providers vary widely in communities throughout the United States. For instance, EMT and paramedic staffing for ground ambulances varies greatly by geography, with a president of the International Association of EMS Chiefs describing the variance in this way: "in Dallas, TX, it's the Dallas Fire Department; in Boston, MA, it's the Boston EMS, a third service department; in Wellman, IA it's the Wellman Volunteer Ambulance; in San Mateo County, CA it's American Medical Response; in Newark, NJ, it's University Hospital." Some local governments impose levies or taxes to support EMS services through fire districts, whereas other local governments choose to contract with private organizations.

Depending on the nature and location of a 9-1-1 call, ground ambulance provider organizations will dispatch an advanced life support (ALS) or basic life support (BLS) ambulance to the scene. Organizations dispatch these ambulances via one of two response systems: (1) an all-ALS response system that sends ALS ambulances to the scene for patients both acutely ill and deemed to be less acutely ill and (2) a tiered response system that utilizes both ALS and BLS ambulances, dispatching ALS ambulances only for patients assessed to be more acutely ill and BLS ambulances for patients deemed to be less acutely ill.

On-scene care and care in transit. While ALS and BLS ambulances are both designed for prehospital interventions, the ambulances differ in the capabilities of personnel and minimum necessary equipment. Because ALS ambulances are typically staffed with paramedics plus EMTs, they must be equipped with medications, airway kits, and cardiac monitors. BLS ambulances, on the other hand, are typically staffed with only EMTs and must be equipped for noninvasive interventions.

Although they often work in tandem, EMTs and paramedics differ in their training duration and skillset. EMTs are trained to assess critical illnesses, provide first aid, and perform basic life-saving measures; paramedics receive advanced training to administer intravenous (IV) medications, monitor electrocardiograms, and perform procedures such as tracheotomies. Studies are ongoing to better understand the comparative advantages of ALS versus BLS ambulances in different clinical situations.

Back to the Clinical Case

In this case, the concerns that the patient's husband expressed on the 9-1-1 call led to activation of EMS with potential for ALS ambulance being dispatched to their residence. Given on-scene assessment by the EMS personnel, ALS services were indeed provided to the patient in transit to the ER.

Given the nature of the patient's concerns, and the time and hour of the day services were needed, the EMS system was a system factor that played a key role in her receiving timely care.

TAKEAWAYS

- In the United States, the EMS system is based on a "scoop and run" philosophy and the Anglo-American model that aims to bring patients to the ER rapidly with fewer prehospital interventions.
- The majority of patients requiring EMS are transported by ground ambulances.
- Ground ambulance provider organizations and their business practices widely vary with respect to local communities throughout the United States.
- Ground ambulance EMS can involve either ALS ambulances, which must be staffed with EMTs plus paramedics and equipped with medications, airway kits, and cardiac monitors, or BLS ambulances, which are staffed with EMTs and equipped for noninvasive interventions.
- EMTs can provide first aid and perform basic life-saving measures; whereas paramedics are further trained to be able to monitor electrocardiograms and perform advanced procedures.

Clinical Case Continued

When they arrive at the ER triage desk, Jessica and her husband realize they have left Jessica's identification and insurance information at home. The EMTs provide the triage nurse with Jessica's clinical history, and vital signs taken by the triage nurse are similar to those taken initially on the scene by the EMTs.

The nurse tells Jessica to take a seat in the waiting room and that she'll be brought to an examination room to see a physician shortly. Jessica and her husband are relieved they'll receive medical attention despite lacking proof of identification and insurance.

In this situation, the patient is brought to the ER out of concern for a potential medical emergency and is offered medical services despite being unable to provide evidence that she can pay for them. The patient and her husband's surprise at being offered emergency care is rooted in an understanding that access to medical services depends on an ability to pay for them, often demonstrated by proof of health insurance. This dynamic—guaranteed access to certain aspects of emergency care under protections that do not exist for other types of nonemergent care—is a systems factor that affects how many Americans receive health care.

SYSTEMS FACTOR: ACCESS TO EMERGENCY CARE

Because they are open around the clock, accept patients for any medical condition, and serve as an entry point to hospital services, ERs play a key role in health care access in the United States. In fact, this role is so critical that ERs have a legal obligation to provide care to any person experiencing an emergency medical condition, regardless of their income, insurance status, race, or citizenship status.

This obligation was set forth in a landmark piece of federal legislation, the Emergency Medical Treatment and Active Labor Act (EMTALA), passed in 1986. Although not every person who seeks care in an ER may be experiencing an emergency condition, the history of EMTALA nonetheless provides critical lessons about access to emergency care in the United States.

Early 1980s: "Patient Dumping" and Calls for Reforming Emergency Care Access

In the early 1980s, researchers, clinicians, patients, and policymakers noticed an increasing trend in hospital transfers throughout the United States, often from the ERs of private hospitals to those of public hospitals. Patient transfers increased from 70 per month in 1982 to more than 200 per month in 1983 in Dallas; fewer than 200 per year in 1981 to more than 900 per year in Washington, DC in 1985; and fewer than 1500 per year in 1982 to more than 5500 per year in 1984 in Chicago. There was increasing concern that the rise in transfers was not necessarily due to medical reasons but rather increases in what became referred to as "patient dumping," a practice defined as "the denial of or limitation in the provision of medical services to a patient for economic reasons and the referral of that patient elsewhere."

In a notable 1986 study, researchers studied 467 patients who were transferred from different ERs to a public county hospital ER and then subsequently admitted. This study found that 89% of the transferred patients studied were Black or Hispanic; that 87% of these patients were transferred because they were uninsured or underinsured; and that only 6% of transferred patients had documentation of consent for transfer. Nearly one in four transferred patients were in an unstable condition before transfer, and the patients admitted to the county hospital's inpatient medicine service via transfer were more than twice as likely to die during their admission than patients on the inpatient medicine service who were not transferred. Researchers concluded that patients transferred to the public county hospital were most often transferred for economic rather than medical reasons, despite the fact that many of them were in an unstable or a critical condition during transfer.

Patient dumping occurred despite multiple existing efforts to discourage discriminatory practices. The Hill-Burton Act was landmark legislation passed in 1946 that funded a rapid expansion of hospitals in the United States after World War II, and, as a function of such funding, sought to influence the practices of US hospitals. The Act prohibited hospitals from excluding patients from receiving care due to insurance status. In addition, the Joint Commission on Accreditation of Hospitals, the largest hospital accreditation body in the country, specifically prohibited the practice of patient dumping and required that hospitals provide emergency care. The 1982 guidelines from the American College of Emergency Physicians stated that "emergency care must be available to all such patients without regard to their ability to pay" and "evaluation, management, and treatment of the patient with a life- or limb-threatening condition must be appropriate and timely."

However, despite these well-intentioned efforts, a combination of noncompliance, insufficient enforcement, and increasing public attention and concerns about patient dumping led in the mid-1980s to growing interest in legislative action to protect patient access to emergency care.

1986 to Present: The Emergency Medical Treatment and Active Labor Act

The result of that concern was the passage of EMTALA in 1986. The Act persists to this day, protecting patient access by requiring that all hospitals who participate in the Medicare program adhere to the following three core provisions:

Medical screening examination
Requirements to stabilize or transfer
Patients who need specialized services

Medical screening examination. EMTALA requires hospitals that possess the capacity to deliver emergency services to perform an appropriate "medical screening examination," within their capability, for any patient who comes to the ER. The goal of this examination is to determine whether patients have an "emergency medical condition"—an acute medical condition—that, if unaddressed, can place a patient's health in jeopardy, result in serious impairment to bodily function, serious organ damage, or dysfunction to a body part. For pregnant patients, emergency medical condition includes when a patient's unborn child's health is at risk, if the patient is having contractions and there is not enough time to get to another hospital before delivery, or if transferring the patient would put the patient or their unborn child's health at risk.

An appropriate medical screening examination includes a history and physical, laboratory or imaging tests, and specialist consults needed to effectively rule in or out an emergency medical condition. For pregnant patients, the examination includes a cervical examination and monitoring of fetal heart and evaluation of the pregnant patient's health tones; for patients with psychiatric complaints, it includes evaluation for suicide risk.

In addition to requiring medical screening examination, EMTALA prohibits delaying this examination or subsequent care in order to determine that patient's insurance status or ability to pay. This protection applies to any person who presents to the ER requesting a medical screening examination, regardless of income, insurance status, race, or citizenship status.

Over time, there was evolution in the understanding of when a medical facility had an obligation to a patient through EMTALA. Originally, it was thought that the EMTALA requirement to provide medical screening examinations applied only to hospitals with dedicated ERs; however, it is now understood that any hospital with a capacity to perform emergency services has this obligation to patients. Further, a patient is considered to have their access to emergency care protected by EMTALA if they are on the hospital's campus, which is defined to include all structures within 250 yd of the hospital itself. In addition, hospital-owned ambulances and satellite clinics also fall under EMTALA obligations to perform medical screening examinations.

Requirements to stabilize or transfer. This provision of EMTALA becomes relevant if the medical facility determines that a patient has an emergency medical condition. Under these circumstances, the Act requires the hospital, often in its ER, to stabilize or facilitate an appropriate transfer of the patient to a different facility.

According to EMTALA, a patient is considered stabilized if one can reasonably judge that "no material deterioration" would occur during or because of a transfer to another medical facility, or from discharging the patient to their home or the community. The care needed to stabilize a patient may take hours or even several days. If the emergency medical condition has not been stabilized, a patient cannot be legally transferred or discharged unless that patient specifically requests transfer or discharge and has been informed of the risks, or if a physician has signed a certificate stating that the benefits of being treated at a different facility outweigh the risks.

EMTALA also defines an appropriate transfer as one meeting the following:

- The transferring medical facility provided medical treatment within its abilities to minimize risk to a patient's health (or in the case of a patient in labor, the health of the patient and fetus).
- The receiving medical facility has space and personnel available and agreed to accept the patient transfer.
- The transferring medical facility sends all medical records related to the emergency medical condition and the contact information of a relevant on-call physician to the receiving medical facility.
- The patient is transported to the accepting facility by qualified medical personnel.

Patients who need specialized services. EMTALA contains a provision that protects patient access to medical facilities' specialized services that otherwise may not be commonly available at all facilities, for example, burn units or neonatal intensive care units. Since such services are specialized and less common, EMTALA requires facilities with specialized services and requisite capacity (eg, bed space) to accept appropriate transfer requests.

Violation or noncompliance with EMTALA can lead to three types of penalties. First, the US Department of Health and Human Services (HHS) can fine a facility or an individual clinician for each violation of EMTALA. Since a medical facility or clinician can violate the Act in multiple ways, HHS can impose multiple fines for a single patient encounter. HHS can fine up to approximately $60 000 per violation for hospitals with fewer than 100 beds, $120 000 per violation for hospitals with more than 100 beds, and $120 000 per violation for clinicians.

Between 2002 and 2015, the HHS issued more than $6 million in penalties for EMTALA violations, more than 95% of which were of hospitals rather than individual clinicians, and most of which were due to failure to perform a medical screening examination and stabilize a patient. In these cases, patients were turned away from hospitals 16% of the time due to insurance or financial reasons—a substantial decrease from patterns in the 1980s before EMTALA.

Second, EMTALA violations can lead to clinicians or hospitals being excluded from Medicare and Medicaid. This consequence is quite rare, occurring among 2% of hospitals found to be in violation of EMTALA from onset of the legislation through 1994 (notably, half of these hospitals were later reinstated). No hospitals were excluded due to EMTALA violations between 2002 and 2015. Third, separate from HHS action, individual patients can file a civil lawsuit against clinicians or hospitals for any damages as a result of their failure to comply with EMTALA.

EMTALA represents an important way to assess and encourage behavior that supports access to emergency care and hold medical facilities accountable when they fall short. Part of why EMTALA has been impactful is that it has been actually enforced. For example, over the course of the 10-year period between 2005 and 2014, more than 40% of hospitals which provided care to Medicare or Medicaid patients were investigated for a possible EMTALA violation. ERs that are investigated or cited for an EMTALA violation are required to take corrective measures on an aggressive 23- to 90-day timeline to avoid serious penalties. Measures usually focus on recruiting and sustaining improved staffing levels to ensure that facilities have sufficient capacity to prevent any future violations.

However, annual investigations for EMTALA violations decreased by 40% in this time period, and confirmed violations decreased by 35%, suggestive of medical facilities improving overall compliance with the law over time. Recent research estimates that confirmed EMTALA violations between 2005 and 2014, such as for patient dumping, occurred at rates as low as 1.3 per 1 million ER visits. Although there is a lack of reliable data on the rate of patient dumping prior to EMTALA, it is believed to be far less frequent afterward—a belief reflective of EMTALA's place as landmark legislation and factor protecting access to emergency care.

Back to the Clinical Case

This patient's case exemplifies the impact of EMTALA in multiple ways. First, the ER where the patient presented for care has an obligation to do a medical screening examination regardless of the patient's income, insurance status, race, or citizenship status. Under EMTALA, the patient's examination cannot be delayed to determine her insurance status or ability to pay. EMTALA also provides reassurances for patients where concern for an emergency medical condition, such as a severe septic joint, could require additional services for stabilization and/or appropriate transfer.

TAKEAWAYS

- Rising transfers from private to public hospitals raised concerns for patients being denied access to emergency care based on insurance status and race (patient dumping).
- These concerns, along with ineffectual prior efforts to prevent patient dumping, led to the passage of the EMTALA.
- As landmark legislation aimed at protecting access to emergency care, EMTALA contains provisions that require medical facilities to

perform a medical screening examination to assess for presence or absence of an emergency medical condition, stabilize a patient before facilitating appropriate transfers, and accept transfers if possessing specialized capabilities and capacity.
- EMTALA is enforced by the HHS, which can levy fines or exclude violators completely from the Medicare and Medicaid program; patients can also file civil lawsuits for damages related to EMTALA violations.

Clinical Case Continued

Jessica and her husband are brought to an examination room where they meet Dr Clark, an ER clinician. Based on history gathered from the EMTs and paramedic, repeat vital signs from ER triage staff, and physical examination findings, the ER clinician suspects that Jessica may have a knee infection. He orders blood work and *x-rays* and obtains a sample of synovial fluid from Jessica's knee for analysis. With these results pending, he orders acetaminophen, IV fluids, and antibiotics for Jessica.

By the time the medications are administered, it's 2:00 AM and the time has come for the ER clinician to hand off to a colleague. The outgoing ER clinician summarizes Jessica's history and explains the concern for knee infection amid pending tests. The incoming ER clinician confirms her understanding of Jessica's care plan and introduces herself to Jessica.

This case represents a typical occurrence in an ER, where a clinician's shift concludes and he must hand off the care of patients to another clinician starting her shift. With the patient coming to the ER late into the evening, her care is transferred overnight via a patient handoff.

ERs are one of the few sites of care that are open 24 hours a day, 365 days a year, driven in part by requirements by federal authorities in 1969 for hospitals to establish 24-hour emergency services in order to maintain their tax exemption status. As a result of around-the-clock hours of operation, ER clinicians commonly work in shifts. The length of ER shifts can vary; they are 8 to 12 hours in length in many cases, but some rural ERs can operate through clinicians on 24-hour shifts. In turn, shift work approaches create the need for clinicians to hand off patients at various hours of the day.

Patient handoffs are an inevitable by-product of shift work. The ubiquity of handoffs necessitates approaches to promote communication and support safe, high-quality care. In this way, patient handoffs are a key systems factor that impacts care that patients receive in ERs.

SYSTEMS FACTOR: PATIENT HANDOFFS

Definition and Method of Handoffs

Handoffs refer to the "transfer and acceptance of patient care responsibility achieved through effective communication" and involves an approach to "passing patient-specific information … for the purpose of ensuring the continuity and safety of patient care."

The method of handoffs tends to vary depending on the clinicians and the established practices of medical care organizations. During ER shift change, clinicians are known to hand off patients "verbally, with handwritten notes, at the bedside, by telephone, by audiotape, nonverbally, using electronic reports, computer printouts, and memory."

Patient Handoff Risks and Guidelines

Unfortunately, the communication required for patient handoffs can create potential risks of harm. In particular, varying methods can cause communication gaps between clinicians and lead to inaccurate, incomplete, or misinterpreted information. These gaps and related risks can be compounded by the high frequency of handoffs occurring in ER and other settings. To this end, scholars have compared handoffs to the game of telephone with respect to their "inherent potential for errors."

Studies have shown that miscommunication is involved in nearly 80% of serious medical errors and 30% of all malpractice claims in the United States. With increasing evidence behind the potential harms of miscommunication during patient handoffs, The Joint Commission announced a new National Patient Safety Goal in 2006 to address handoff communication and subsequently established guidelines for medical care organizations. To provide guidance to medical care organizations to improve patient handoffs, The Joint Commission describes a set of guidelines that can be summarized as the following:

- To demonstrate leadership's commitment to successful handoffs and other aspects of safety culture
- To standardize critical content to be communicated by the sender (clinician providing information about the patient) during a handoff—both verbally and in written form—and to standardize tools and methods to communicate to receiver (clinician receiving the information and assuming care of the patient)

- To conduct face-to-face handoffs between sender and receiver in locations free from interruptions and include multidisciplinary team members, patients, and family as appropriate
- To standardize training on how to conduct a successful handoff, both from the perspectives of the sender and the receiver
- To use electronic health record (EHR) capabilities and other technologies, such as apps, portals, and telehealth, to enhance handoffs
- To monitor the success of interventions to improve handoff communication and use the lessons to drive improvement
- To sustain and spread best practices in handoffs, and make high-quality handoffs a cultural priority

Patient Handoff Tools

A number of tools have emerged to address potential pitfalls of handoff communication in ERs and other settings. SOUND was first developed as a tool to standardize the verbal and written format of handoffs in pediatric ERs. In a study implementing SOUND among staff physicians, residents, and nurses over the course of 10 months, SOUND was shown to increase the completeness of handoffs by nearly 40% in ERs. A complete handoff was defined as successful transmission of at least four of the five components of SOUND. The components of SOUND are as follows:

- Synthesis: Diagnosis or differential diagnosis
- Objective data: Relevant examination findings, laboratories, studies
- Upcoming tasks: To-do list
- Nursing input: Additional information/updates from nursing team
- Double check: Read back and/or clarifying questions

The PSYCH tool was introduced to guide clinicians to identify key information needed for verbal and written handoffs in psychiatric ERs. In a 12-week study analyzing residents who train in an on-call system and present morning handoffs, the use of PSYCH was shown to decrease the number of omissions of key patient information during handoffs. In addition, on the scale from 1 (not clear) to 4 (very clear), the study showed an increase in the clarity of expectations between clinicians from 2.79 to 3.83. The components of PSYCH are as follows:

- Patient information/background: Age, race, sex, psychiatric history, substance history

- Situation leading to the hospital: How, why, and brief statement of events leading to the hospital visit
- Your assessment: Brief statement to describe patient status
- Clinical information: Pertinent medical history, history of violence, awaiting results, medication clarification
- Hindrance to discharge: Collateral, outpatient linkage, placement/housing, awaiting inpatient bed, transfer status

Originally developed by the US Navy for the purposes of submarine communication, SBAR has subsequently been adapted for use in health care settings by Kaiser Permanente as an approach for structuring conversations between physicians and nurses. Although not explicitly designed for patient handoffs, SBAR has been studied for the purposes of patient handoffs in a range of clinical settings, including in ERs. In a systematic review studying the use of the SBAR for patient handoffs, the tool was shown to increase the number of patients reaching target international normalized ratio values, decrease the rate of patient falls, and also decrease the rate of in-hospital mortality. More specifically in the ER setting, one study involving 180 patients found that the incidence of adverse events was lower (8.9% vs 23.3%) among patients for whom SBAR was used compared to patients for whom SBAR was not used for patient handoffs. The components of SBAR are as follows:

- Situation: A concise statement of the problem
- Background: Pertinent and brief information related to the situation
- Assessment: Analysis and considerations of options
- Recommendation: Action requested and/or recommended

The 5P tool was first used to ensure that all essential patient information was transferred between clinicians during verbal and written patient handoffs in the hospital setting. The tool has since been adapted to other settings, including ERs. In a case study, after implementing the 5P tool for handoffs as part of a patient safety initiative across the hospital and ER settings, a medical care organization reported a 23% decrease in in-hospital mortality from 2003 to 2008. Furthermore, the study also reported a decrease in the rate of patient falls with injuries by 52% from 2003 to 2009 as well as a decrease in central line–associated bloodstream infections by 89% from 2002 to 2009. The components of the 5P are as follows:

- Patient: Who is to be handed off?
- Plan: What is to happen next?

- Purpose: What is the desired end state?
- Problems: What is known to be different, unusual, or complicating about this patient?
- Precautions: What could be expected to be different, unusual, or complicating about this patient?

The SIGNOUT tool was developed originally to standardize verbal handoffs. Although not directly studied in the context of ER handoffs, SIGNOUT has been shown in hospital settings to decrease medical errors associated with verbal handoffs. In a study implementing the SIGNOUT tool in inpatient pediatric units for handoffs among residents over the course of 3 months, the use of SIGNOUT was associated with decrease in medical errors from 33.8 to 18.3 per 100 patient admissions and preventable adverse events decreased from 3.3 to 1.5 per 100 patient admissions. The components of SIGNOUT are as follows:

- Sick or DNR (do not resuscitate): Highlight sick or unstable patients, identify do-not resuscitate or do-not-intubate patients
- Identifying data: Name, age, gender, diagnosis
- General hospital course
- New events of day
- Overall health status/clinical condition
- Upcoming possibilities with plan, rationale
- Tasks to complete overnight with plan, rationale

Finally, the I-PASS tool was introduced as a way to provide structure to verbal patient handoffs in the hospital setting and is frequently utilized across residency programs. In a study implementing I-PASS across nine pediatric hospitals between 2011 and 2013, its use was associated with a 23% decrease in medical errors and a 30% decrease in preventable patient adverse events among pediatric residents. Subsequent studies of I-PASS have also shown greater clinician satisfaction with handoff organization, unchanged or shorter handoff times (reflecting improved efficiency of handoffs), and fewer handoff interruptions (reflecting greater attention to handoffs). The components of I-PASS are as follows:

- Illness severity: Stable, watcher, unstable
- Patient summary: Summary statement, events leading up to admission, hospital course, ongoing assessment, plan
- Action list: To-do list, timeline, and ownership

■ Situation awareness and contingency planning: Know what's going on, plan for what might happen

■ Synthesis by receiver: Receiver summarizes what was heard, asks questions, restates key action/to-do items.

Back to the Clinical Case

The outgoing ER clinician hands off patient care to the incoming ER clinician using I-PASS to provide the following information:

Illness severity. Notes that the patient is a "watcher," meaning unsure of clinical trajectory and at risk for deterioration; requires close monitoring and may require further interventions overnight

Patient summary. Summarizes the patient as a 67-year-old woman with a history of recent left knee surgery who came to the ER with signs and symptoms concerning for an infection of her knee surgery

Action list. Describes the follow-up on pending blood cultures, x-ray, and synovial fluid analysis

Situational awareness. Notes that if patient's vital signs or clinical condition worsens, could consider broadening antibiotics and giving additional fluids out of concern for bacteremia

Synthesis by receiver. The outgoing ER clinician asks the incoming clinician to confirm when empiric antibiotics were given and whether orthopedics has been consulted in patient's care

TAKEAWAYS

• Patient handoffs refer to the transfer and acceptance of patient care responsibilities between clinicians.

• The method of handoffs tends to vary depending on the clinicians and the established practices of medical care organizations.

• The communication required for patient handoffs can create potential risks of harm and necessitate standardized approaches to promote effective communication.

• A number of tools, including SOUND, PSYCH, SBAR, 5P, SIGNOUT, and I-PASS, have been adapted or designed for use in patient handoffs to support clinician communication and have been shown to decrease the omission of key patient information and the incidence of patient adverse events.

Clinical Case Continued

After receiving IV fluids and acetaminophen, Jessica shares that her dizziness has improved and she is no longer feeling feverish. The ER clinician examines Jessica and notes that she is no longer diaphoretic, but still has limited range of motion and tenderness at her knee. Jessica's laboratory test results return: Her knee x-rays showed no notable findings, but her white blood cell count, erythrocyte sedimentation rate, and C-reactive protein are elevated. Despite Jessica's clinical improvement, based on her laboratory results and vital signs, which continue to show elevated heart and respiratory rates, the ER clinician consults orthopedic surgery out of concern for knee infection related to her surgery.

While awaiting a call back from the orthopedic surgery team, the ER clinician reviews a dashboard of current ER patients. She sees that Jessica has been in the ER for 8 hours, while other patients have been in the ER for as short as 7 minutes and as long as 15 hours. The ER clinician also observes that there are 15 patients needing to be clinically assessed, with wait times ranging from 30 minutes to 3 hours.

The orthopedic team says that their consulting clinician who is in the operating room will see Jessica as soon as the current case is complete. The laboratory notifies the ER clinician that the final results of the joint synovial fluid analysis will require 1 to 2 hours. Worried about the amount of time Jessica has already been in the ER, the increasing number of patients in the waiting room, and the uncertainty of when the orthopedic surgeon will be able to leave the operating room, the ER clinician places an order to admit Jessica for hospital observation.

This situation is typical for an ER, which at any given time has a range of patients with different medical conditions of varying urgency or acuity. In that context, ER clinicians must balance the needs of patients currently being evaluated, those being treated, those awaiting next steps in their evaluation or treatment plans, and patients in the waiting room needing to be seen.

As a result, ER clinicians such as the one involved in this patient's care must pay close attention to the time patients spend in the ER, how their care is progressing, and how patients ultimately flow through an ER. In turn, a series of flow management approaches and time-based metrics have emerged as part of emergency care. Such flow management processes and time-based metrics are important systems factors for understanding the unique position that ERs hold in the US health care system.

SYSTEMS FACTOR: FLOW MANAGEMENT AND TIME-BASED METRICS

Due to uncertainty and variation in the volume and needs among patients seeking emergency care, ERs benefit from systems that guide the flow of patients and metrics that assess performance. Flow management and time-based metrics are particularly important because of patient demand for ER services (challenges with crowded ERs are widespread, with 90% of ERs routinely reporting crowded conditions) and the potential consequences of time inefficiencies (delays in care, medical errors, reduced number of patients able to receive care).

Flow Management

Once patients arrive in the ER, the first step in managing overall patient flow is to triage which patients will be seen and when. To that end, ERs have developed triage systems that stratify patients based on the initial impression of a patient's illness severity. One commonly used triage method is the Emergency Severity Index, a system in which patients are assigned a number 1 through 5 based on their perceived illness severity (1 being most critically ill and 5 being least critically ill), and ER resources are allocated with priority to those thought to be most critically ill.

Illness severity can inform how to assess patients and optimize patient flow. In a 2016 report focused on improving crowding in ERs in the United States, the American College of Emergency Physicians outlined a number of strategies to manage patient flow through the ER. The report categorized strategies based on focus on managing patient influx (who comes to the ER and when), managing patient throughput (how patients are processed, evaluated, and managed while in the ER), or managing patient output (how patients are prepared for ER discharge).

Approaches for managing patient influx include the following:

Listing wait times. ERs can post the wait times that patients can expect to experience before being roomed and seen by a clinician. Wait times can be posted online, through smart phones, or in waiting rooms themselves. This approach is intended to inform patients who need medical attention but who have lower acuity conditions, so they can possibly come to the ER for evaluation at a less busy time.

Creating ER appointments. By creating scheduled, predetermined appointments, ERs are able to assess and treat patients with nonlife-threatening emergencies at times of day that are less busy and allow for patients to wait at home instead of in a busy ER. Similar to posting waiting times, creating ER appointments aims to address flow among patients with lower acuity and nonemergent conditions.

The American College of Emergency Physicians report also included suggestions for managing patient throughput. These included the following:

Incorporating registration and triage management approaches. The ER registration process creates a potential bottleneck for patients. Traditionally, patients wait in several sequential lines upon arrival in the ER, one for registration, one for triage, and one for medical screening. ERs can work to streamline this process by having patients wait in a single line where all of these processes will occur simultaneously.

For common symptoms or complaints that prompt patients to go to the ER (eg, chest pain or cough), ERs can implement evidence-based order sets that nurses can initiate. This empowers nurses to order certain preset medications and tests so that when a patient is roomed in an ER bed, physicians and other practitioners will have available results to use in their decision-making. In addition, ERs can place a physician, nurse practitioner, or physician assistant in the triage environment to initiate testing and management for all patients before they receive a dedicated ER bed.

Creating separate patient tracks. ERs can implement different tracks for patients admitted to the ER. In particular, patients can be stratified depending on level of acuity or presenting issues into tracks that involve different ER workflows, assigned ER clinicians, and designated physical spaces.

One track system that can be used in ERs is the "Fast Track." In this approach, patients who are considered to have a lower acuity condition are placed on a special track where they receive care from clinicians who are assigned solely to seeing "Fast Track" patients—an arrangement that enables patients in this track to be seen and managed more quickly. Approximately 10% to 30% of patients qualify for such Fast Tracks, and this approach has been shown to reduce ER wait times and length of stay.

Implementing innovative staffing approaches. ERs can implement new staffing approaches to streamline care processes and improve on time-based metrics. For instance, the return of imaging studies often delays decision-making and treatment plans in the ER. ERs can address this issue by having ER imaging studies read and interpreted by a dedicated ER radiologist, rather than having ER studies go into a general reading list and queue alongside other hospital or outpatient studies.

Another staffing approach can focus on documentation, which can take up a large proportion of ER clinicians' time (some studies estimate

22%-32%). ERs can hire medical scribes—individuals trained in medical documentation who help clinicians write their care notes—to free up clinician time to provide care for patients rather than document care.

In addition, ERs can hire nurses or social workers for dedicated ER care coordination positions. Care coordinators can help streamline services for people who frequently use the ER or who have health-related social needs but might not be experiencing a medical emergency. For instance, care coordinators can help facilitate admission and transportation to overnight shelters for patients visiting the ER who are experiencing housing instability. Employing care coordinators can reduce length of stay in the ER for certain situations, thereby increasing patient throughput.

Another staffing approach ERs can employ to increase patient throughput would be hiring physician assistants and nurse practitioners. The overall wage of these highly trained clinicians is less than that of a physician, and these clinicians can increase the overall capacity of an ER to evaluate and treat patients. This is an approach that been increasingly adopted. From 1993 to 2009, the percentage of ER visits that involved the care of a physician assistant or nurse practitioner increased from 4% to nearly 15%.

Finally, the report from the American College of Emergency Physicians included strategies for managing patient output. These included the following:

Boarding patients in hospital ward hallways. Though suboptimal for patients, this approach can address situations when a patient requires hospital admission but a hospital room is not yet available. Under this approach, patients can be functionally hospitalized but remain physically in a hallway or other boarding space in a hospital ward, rather than remaining in the ER. By boarding patients to inpatient hallways rather than in ER space, ERs can turn over rooms and use them to evaluate new patients. Although certainly unideal, approximately 85% of patients report they would prefer hallway boarding to ER boarding, and this approach has been found to reduce ER length of stay by up to 25%.

Creating discharge lounge areas. This approach can address delays in discharges for patients that are deemed medically ready for discharge and awaiting discharge information and supplies (eg, discharge medications and instructions). Under this approach, ERs can move patients out of ER rooms into dedicated spaces, such as discharge lounges, to await discharge information and supplies. This method can allow ERs to more quickly turn over rooms and use them to evaluate new patients.

Modifying admission processes. Sometimes delays occur in the admission process due to pending diagnostic tests or because admitting clinicians have not yet seen the patient in the ER. ERs can modify admission processes in ways that can streamline the process of admitting patients from the ER to the hospital. For instance, while patients needing admission are evaluated by hospital clinicians or still have diagnostic tests pending, ERs can work in parallel to institute standing orders that expedite the admission process. Ultimately, modifying admission processes can reduce the time between when the ER decides to admit a patient and when patients are actually moved to hospital rooms.

Time-Based Metrics

To ensure that flow management processes produce efficient care, ERs are subject to time-based metrics that seek to measure emergency care performance. Important time-based metrics focus on wait times and patients' decisions to leave without being seen. The two can be related: Wait times can influence whether a patient decides to stay in the waiting room, leave the ER without being seen, or return to a particular ER in the future. One study found that more than half of people are willing to wait just 2 hours in an ER before leaving without being seen. Among patients who have chosen to leave an ER in the past without being seen, more than three-quarters said they left because of long wait times.

Groups such as the Centers for Medicare and Medicaid Services and the Agency for Healthcare Research and Quality have developed and implemented a range of time-based metrics for ERs, including the following (Figure 2.1):

- Arrival time to departure time for admitted patients: This measures the median amount of time it takes from a patient's arrival in the ER to their leaving the ER for hospital admission.
- Arrival time to departure time for discharged patients: This measures the median amount of time it takes from a patient's arrival in the ER to them being discharged from the ER, for a patient who is not admitted to the hospital.
- Decision to admit to departure time: This measures the median time it takes from a clinician deciding that a patient in the ER needs to be admitted to that patient actually leaving the ER and being admitted.
- ER wait times: This measures the time from a patient's arrival in the ER waiting room to the time they've been evaluated by a qualified medical professional.
- Patient left before being seen: Although not directly a time-based metric, this focuses on the percentage of patients who leave the ER waiting room without ever having a diagnostic evaluation by a medical professional, which in many cases is related to dissatisfaction with wait times.

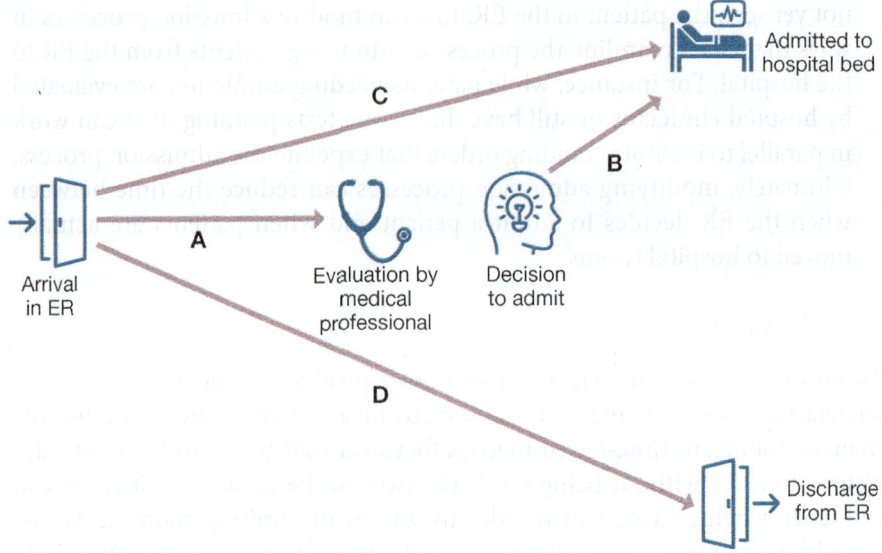

Figure 2.1 Time-Based Metrics in the ER. A refers to ER wait times; B to decision to admit to departure time; C refers to the arrival time to departure time for admitted patients; and D the arrival time to departure time for discharged patients. ER, emergency room.

ERs are required to report on certain time-based metrics. In turn, many ERs have implemented data dashboards that incorporate and trend time-based metrics, including those assessed by the Centers for Medicare and Medicaid Services. ERs can also incorporate additional metrics deemed important by their leadership and thought to promote performance, such as number of patients in the ER, number of patients waiting to be seen stratified by severity of their reason for coming to the ER, and number of patients in the ER for more than 6 hours, among others.

Back to the Clinical Case

In our patient's case, the ER clinician determines that hospital observation is warranted given the concern for a possible infection. Although the patient has not yet been evaluated by orthopedic surgery and some diagnostic tests are still outstanding, a combination of clinical concerns and desire to optimize patient flow management prompts the ER clinician to initiate the hospital observation process. Given that the patient has already arrived and undergone evaluation in the ER, the most relevant flow management approaches in her case may relate to managing patient output. For instance, the ER clinician might consider transitioning the patient to inpatient boarding or admitting her with modified admission processes to facilitate her flow from the ER to hospital observation.

TAKEAWAYS

- Uncertainty and variation in patient volume require ERs to assess the time patients spend in the ER, how their care is progressing, and how patients ultimately flow through the ER.
- Strategies to manage patient flow through the ER can be categorized by focusing on managing patient influx, managing patient throughput, or managing patient output.
- ERs track and report on time-based metrics such as wait times and patients' decisions to leave the ER without being seen.

Implications

The systems factors in this chapter have implications for patients' access to emergency care. Ideally, patients would have access to emergency care in their community through an EMS system, and consistent, reliable, and timely care upon arrival at a medical facility dependent on the severity of their medical condition. However, access can be limited in certain circumstances, depending on multiple factors, including patients' geographic location, the ownership structures of their local ground ambulance provider organizations, and the volume of patients seeking care at certain times in surrounding ERs. EMS in rural communities are known to cover larger coverage areas, with ground ambulances in turn needing to cover more difficult terrain and weather conditions. This situation of navigating larger and more difficult-to-navigate areas can be associated with longer response times from when a patient calls 9-1-1 to when the ground ambulance arrives at their location, and longer transport times from picking up a patient to arriving at the hospital.

For instance, while the average national EMS response time is estimated to be 7 minutes, this increases to more than 14 minutes in some rural areas, with 1 in 10 EMS encounters in rural areas having a wait time of longer than 30 minutes. Studies have also shown that, on average, EMS teams in rural areas spend more time at the scene of an emergency and have longer transport times to an ER than do EMS teams in urban areas. Longer response and transport times can be particularly important for time-sensitive emergency medical conditions such as trauma, myocardial infarctions, or cerebrovascular accidents.

Once a patient arrives to an ER, access can be influenced by whether there are policies in place to protect a patient's right to receive emergency care. As described earlier, EMTALA was passed in response to calls for legislation to curb ER patient dumping behaviors that were insufficiently addressed by preceding efforts. Through EMTALA, patients can file civil lawsuits for damages related to violations, and the HHS can exclude violating medical facilities entirely from the Medicare and Medicaid program. Recent estimates of EMTALA violations have been low and decreasing, suggesting that patients have had greater access to medical screening examination and stabilization or transfer for emergency medical conditions.

Even though patients have the protected right to a medical screening examination and stabilization or transfer for emergency medical conditions, a key component of access is the timeliness and expedience of care delivered within the ER. Because the ER is such a commonly utilized care setting, with 146 million annual ER visits even before the COVID-19 pandemic, the potential for delays in care due to overcrowding persists. The implementation of time-based metrics addressing the influx, throughput, and output of patients can impact the accessibility and timeliness of care in the ER.

The systems factors discussed in this chapter have implications for quality of care. Miscommunication between clinicians during patient handoffs can put patients at higher risk of adverse events and, in turn, can negatively affect the quality of care in ERs. As part of ongoing efforts to improve handoffs, the Accreditation Council for Graduate Medical Education has identified handoffs as a required competency for trainees and now requires residency programs to develop formal handoff curriculums. Similarly, the incorporation of time-based metrics is directly related to the goal of improving care quality. ER crowding can lead to delays in receipt of medical care, such as delayed administration of antibiotics for infections, poor pain control, increased medical errors, and increased hospital mortality.

The systems factors also have implications for health care costs. The variance in ground ambulance provider organizations' ownership structures (whether they're operated by fire districts, hospitals, or private equity firms) can have a direct impact on costs. Studies have shown that being transported by ground ambulance operated by private equity firms leads to higher charges and patient cost sharing compared to being transported by ground ambulance from public sector entities.

Since the enactment of EMTALA and evolution toward ERs operating around the clock, patients have increasingly sought ERs for nonurgent care in the United States, defined as care that if delayed by several hours would not likely result in a poor health outcome. Nearly 40% of ER visits have been estimated to be for nonurgent conditions. This comes at a cost to the health care system and to individuals, as the average ER visit costs 12 times more than being treated at an outpatient office. Nonurgent visits have been estimated to cost more than $30 billion to the health care system annually.

Lastly, systems factors discussed in this chapter have important equity implications, starting with the response time within the EMS system. For instance, EMS response times to patients experiencing cardiac emergencies, a life-or-death emergency where timely care is essential to the likelihood of a good outcome, are more than 5 minutes longer for patients in the poorest neighborhoods compared to response times to patients in the wealthiest neighborhoods. Equity is relevant to legislation such as EMTALA as well. It's been reported that even after the law's implementation, when patient dumping does occur, the patients most often affected are either experiencing homelessness, undocumented immigrants, uninsured, or otherwise unable to pay for treatment.

Since ERs are always open and have a statutory responsibility to provide emergency care regardless of a person's ability to pay, they have become a regular site of nonurgent health care delivery for underserved populations. In fact, people from lower socioeconomic status backgrounds have been found to seek care in ERs for nonurgent visits at higher rates than other groups.

Multiple-Choice Questions

1. A 24-year-old man is found to be in acute respiratory distress and his family member calls 9-1-1. In the United States, who is likely to perform the emergency airway procedure on the scene?

   A. EMT
   B. Nurse
   C. Paramedic
   D. Physician

2. Which of the following statements about the EMTALA is false?

   A. ERs are required to perform a timely medical screening examination to determine whether a patient has an emergency medical condition for any patient regardless of income, insurance status, race, or citizenship status.
   B. When patients do have an emergency medical condition, ERs are required to stabilize the patient, and if needed, facilitate an appropriate transfer.
   C. Medical facilities that have special capabilities (eg, burn units), are required to accept transferring patients if they have the capacity.
   D. EMTALA only applies to hospitals and ERs if the patient is inside the physical structure of the facility.

3. Which of the following methods is *not* a potential tool clinicians can use to promote communication during patient handoffs?

   A. I-PASS
   B. SOUND
   C. SBAR
   D. EMTALA

4. A 2016 report from the American College of Emergency Physicians outlined strategies for managing ER influx, throughput, and patient output in order to improve ER crowding and timely delivery of emergency care. Which of the following approaches are aimed at improving ER throughput?
   A. Stratified patient tracks
   B. ER appointments
   C. Modified admission protocols
   D. Posting wait times

Answers

1. The correct answer is C. Paramedics receive advanced training to administer IV medications, monitor electrocardiograms, and perform procedures such as tracheotomies.

2. The correct answer is D. A patient's access to emergency care is protected by EMTALA if they are on the hospital's campus, which is defined to include all structures within 250 yd of the hospital itself. In addition, hospital-owned ambulances and satellite clinics also fall under EMTALA obligations to perform medical screening examinations.

3. The correct answer is D. The EMTALA protects patient access to ERs by requiring that all hospitals that participate in the Medicare program adhere to the three core provisions: medical screening examination, requirements to stabilize or transfer, and patients who need specialized services.

4. The correct answer is A. ERs can implement different tracks for patients admitted to the ER. In particular, patients can be stratified depending on level of acuity or presenting issues into tracks that involve different ER workflows, assigned ER clinicians, and designated physical spaces.

Bibliography

Abraham T. Patient dumping a symptom of health system woes. Healthcare Dive. Published February 5, 2018. Accessed October 2, 2023. https://www.healthcaredive.com/news/patient-dumping-symptom-of-health-system-woes

Adler L, Ly B, Duffy E, Hannick K, Hall M, Trish E. Ground ambulance billing and prices differ by ownership structure. *Health Aff (Millwood)*. 2023;42(2):227-236.

Agency for Healthcare Research and Quality. Section 3. Measuring emergency department performance. Accessed September 25, 2023. https://www.ahrq.gov/research/findings/final-reports/ptflow/section3.html

Almasi S, Rabiei R, Moghaddasi H, Vahidi-Asl M. Emergency department quality dashboard; a systematic review of performance indicators, functionalities, and challenges. *Arch Acad Emerg Med*. 2021;9(1):1-11.

Alruwaili A, Alanazy ARM. Prehospital time interval for urban and rural emergency medical services: a systematic literature review. *Healthcare (Basel)*. 2022;10(12):2391.

Al-Shaqsi S. Models of International Emergency Medical Service (EMS) systems. *Oman Med J*. 2010;25(4):320.

American College of Emergency Physicians. Emergency care guidelines. *Ann Emerg Med*. 1982;11(4):222-226.

American College of Emergency Physicians. Understanding EMTALA. Accessed September 25, 2023. https://www.acep.org/life-as-a-physician/ethics--legal/emtala/emtala-fact-sheet/

American Medical Association. Teaching medical residents how to make patient handoffs safer. Accessed September 25, 2023. https://www.ama-assn.org/education/improve-gme/teaching-medical-residents-how-make-patient-handoffs-safer

Ansell DA, Schiff RL. Patient dumping. Status, implications, and policy recommendations. *JAMA*. 1987;257(11):1500-1502.

Archibold RC. Dumping of homeless by hospitals stirs debate. *The New York Times*. Published February 23, 2007. Accessed October 2, 2023. https://www.nytimes.com/2007/02/23/us/23dumping.html

Asaro PV, Boxerman SB. Effects of computerized provider order entry and nursing documentation on workflow. *Acad Emerg Med*. 2008;15(10):908-915.

Blazin LJ, Sitthi-Amorn J, Hoffman JM, Burlison JD. Improving patient handoffs and transitions through adaptation and implementation of I-PASS across multiple handoff settings. *Pediatr Qual Saf*. 2020;5(4):e323.

Broida RI, Desai SA, Easter BD, et al. *Emergency Department Crowding: High Impact Solutions*. Emergency Medicine Practice Committee; 2016.

Brown DF, Sullivan AF, Espinola JA, Camargo CA Jr. Continued rise in the use of mid-level providers in US emergency departments, 1993-2009. *Int J Emerg Med*. 2012;5(1):21.

Catalano K. JCAHO'S National Patient Safety Goals 2006. *J Perianesth Nurs*. 2006;21(1):6-11.

Centers for Medicare and Medicaid Services. Clinical quality measures finalized for eligible hospitals and critical access hospitals beginning with FY 2014. https://www.cms.gov/regulations-and-guidance/legislation/ehrincentiveprograms/downloads/2014_cqm_eh_finalrule.pdf

Christie P, Robinson H. Using a communication framework at handover to boost patient outcomes. *Nurs Times*. 2009;105(47):13-15.

Colyer J, Anzaldua A, Blancato R, et al. Access to emergency medical services in rural communities: policy brief and recommendations to the secretary. Health Resources and Services Administration. Published November 2022. Accessed September 27, 2023. https://www.hrsa.gov/sites/default/files/hrsa/advisory-committees/rural/access-to-ems-rural-communities.pdf

Dowell MA. Hill-Burton: the unfulfilled promise. *J Health Polit Policy Law*. 1987;12(1):153-175.

EMS.gov. What is EMS? Accessed September 25, 2023. https://www.ems.gov/what-is-ems/

FAIR Health. Newsroom. Accessed September 25, 2023. https://www.fairhealth.org/press-release/average-estimated-in-network-amount-for-fixed-wing-air-ambulance-transport-rose-76-percent-from-2017-to-2020

Field TS, Tjia J, Mazor KM, et al. Randomized trial of a warfarin communication protocol for nursing homes: an SBAR-based approach. *Am J Med*. 2011;124(2):179.e1-179.e1797.

Friesen MA, White SV, Byers JF. Handoffs: implications for nurses. In: *Patient Safety and Quality: An Evidence-Based Handbook for Nurses*. Published online 2008. Accessed September 25, 2023. https://www.ncbi.nlm.nih.gov/books/NBK2649/

Fryman C, Hamo C, Raghavan S, Goolsarran N. A quality improvement approach to standardization and sustainability of the hand-off process. *BMJ Qual Improv Rep*. 2017;6(1):u222156.w8291.

Füchtbauer L, Nørgaard B, Mogensen C. Emergency department physicians spend only 25% of their working time on direct patient care. *Dan Med J*. 2013;60(1):A4558.

Garmon C, Chartock B. One in five inpatient emergency department cases may lead to surprise bills. *Health Aff (Millwood)*. 2017;36(1):177-181.

Gerard DR. EMS systems of care—JEMS: EMS, Emergency Medical Services—training, paramedic, EMT News. Accessed September 25, 2023. https://www.jems.com/commentary/ems-systems-of-care/

Gopwani PR, Brown KM, Quinn MJ, Dorosz EJ, Chamberlain JM. SOUND: a structured handoff tool improves patient handoffs in a pediatric emergency department. *Pediatr Emerg Care*. 2015;31(2):83-87.

Haig KM, Sutton S, Whittington J. SBAR: a shared mental model for improving communication between clinicians. *Jt Comm J Qual Patient Saf*. 2006;32(3):167-175.

Hollingsworth JC, Chisholm CD, Giles BK, Cordell WH, Nelson DR. How do physicians and nurses spend their time in the emergency department? *Ann Emerg Med*. 1998;31(1):87-91.

Horwitz LI, Moin T, Green ML. Development and implementation of an oral sign-out skills curriculum. *J Gen Intern Med*. 2007;22(10):1470-1474.

Hsia RY, Huang D, Mann NC, et al. A US national study of the association between income and ambulance response time in cardiac arrest. *JAMA Netw Open*. 2018;1(7):e185202.

Institute for Healthcare Improvement. SBAR tool: situation-background-assessment-recommendation. Accessed September 25, 2023. https://www.ihi.org/resources/Pages/Tools/SBARToolkit.aspx

Johnson M, Myers S, Wineholt J, Pollack M, Kusmiesz AL. Patients who leave the emergency department without being seen. *J Emerg Nurs*. 2009;35(2):105-108.

Kachalia A, Gandhi TK, Puopolo AL, et al. Missed and delayed diagnoses in the emergency department: a study of closed malpractice claims from 4 liability insurers. *Ann Emerg Med*. 2007;49(2):196-205.

Kelen GD, Wolfe R, D'Onofrio G, et al. Emergency department crowding: the canary in the health care system. *NEJM Catal Innov Care Deliv*. 2021;2(5).

KFF Health News. The cost of unwarranted ER visits: $32 billion a year. Morning briefing. Published July 25, 2019. Accessed October 2, 2023. https://kffhealthnews.org/morning-breakout/the-cost-of-unwarranted-er-visits-32-billion-a-year/

Klein S, McCarthy D. Sentara Healthcare: making patient safety an enduring organizational value. The Commonwealth Fund; 2011. https://www.commonwealthfund.org/sites/default/files/documents/___media_files_publications_case_study_2011_mar_1476_mccarthy_sentara_case_study_final_march.pdf

Laxmisan A, Hakimzada F, Sayan OR, Green RA, Zhang J, Patel VL. The multitasking clinician: decision-making and cognitive demand during and after team handoffs in emergency care. *Int J Med Inform*. 2007;76(11-12):801-811.

Leap E. Life in Emergistan: 24-hour shifts: an unexpected joy. *Emerg Med News*. 2022; 44(1):23.

Levine RJ, Guisto JA, Meislin HW, Spaite DW. Analysis of federally imposed penalties for violations of the Consolidated Omnibus Reconciliation Act. *Ann Emerg Med*. 1996;28(1):45-50.

Li X, Zhao J, Fu S. SBAR standard and mind map combined communication mode used in emergency department to reduce the value of handover defects and adverse events. *J Healthc Eng*. 2022;2022:8475322.

Loyd JW, Larsen T, Kuhl EA, Swanson D. Aeromedical transport. *StatPearls*. Published online August 14, 2023. Accessed September 25, 2023. https://www.ncbi.nlm.nih.gov/books/NBK518986/

Mahmoodian F, Eqtesadi R, Ghareghani A. Waiting times in emergency department after using the emergency severity index triage tool. *Arch Trauma Res*. 2014;3(4):e19507.

Mariano MT, Brooks V, DiGiacomo M. PSYCH: a mnemonic to help psychiatric residents decrease patient handoff communication errors. *Jt Comm J Qual Patient Saf*. 2016;42(7):316-320.

McKenna RM, Purtle J, Nelson KL, Roby DH, Regenstein M, Ortega AN. Examining EMTALA in the era of the patient protection and Affordable Care Act. *AIMS Public Health*. 2018;5(4):366-377.

Median time from ED arrival to ED departure for admitted ED patients. Accessed September 25, 2023. https://ecqi.healthit.gov/sites/default/files/ecqm/measures/CMS55v6.html

MRSC. Emergency medical services (EMS) levies. Accessed September 25, 2023. https://mrsc. org/explore-topics/finance/revenues/ems-levies

National Academy of Sciences, National Academy of Engineering, National Academy of Medicine. Accidental death and disability. Published online September 1, 1966. https://nap.nationalacademies.org/catalog/9978/accidental-death-and-disability-the-neglected-disease-of-modern-society

National Academy of Sciences, National Academy of Engineering, National Academy of Medicine. Emergency medical services: at the crossroads. Published online June 3, 2007:1-285. https://nasemso.org/wp-content/uploads/EMS-at-Crossroads.pdf

National Emergency Number Association. 9-1-1 statistics. Accessed September 25, 2023. https://www.nena.org/page/911Statistics

NEMSIS. 2021 NEMSIS national EMS data report. Accessed September 25, 2023. https://nemsis.org/2021-nemsis-national-ems-data-report/

Oredsson S, Jonsson H, Rognes J, et al. A systematic review of triage-related interventions to improve patient flow in emergency departments. *Scand J Trauma Resusc Emerg Med*. 2011;19:43.

Peterson-KFF Health System Tracker. Ground ambulance rides and potential for surprise billing. Accessed September 25, 2023. https://www.healthsystemtracker.org/brief/ground-ambulance-rides-and-potential-for-surprise-billing

Pineda RO. Improving patient outcomes and nurse satisfaction through nurse-to-nurse communication (Order No. 3701374). ProQuest Dissertations & Theses Global (1681308941). 2015. https://www.proquest.com/dissertations-theses/improving-patient-outcomes-nurse-satisfaction/docview/1681308941/se-2

PSNet. Handoffs and signouts. Accessed September 25, 2023. https://psnet.ahrq.gov/primer/handoffs-and-signouts

PSNet. Medical errors involving trainees: a study of closed malpractice claims from 5 insurers. Accessed September 25, 2023. https://psnet.ahrq.gov/issue/medical-errors-involving-trainees-study-closed-malpractice-claims-5-insurers

PSNet. Triple handoff. Accessed September 25, 2023. https://psnet.ahrq.gov/web-mm/triple-handoff

Quinones Cardona V, LaBadie A, Cooperberg DB, Zubrow A, Touch SM. Improving the neonatal team handoff process in a level IV NICU: reducing interruptions and handoff duration. *BMJ Open Qual.* 2021;10(1):e001014.

Riebschleger M, Philibert I. New standards for transitions of care: discussion and justification. https://www.acgme.org/globalassets/pdfs/jgme-11-00-57-591.pdf

Rischall ML, Chung AS, Tabatabai R, Doty C, Hart D. Emergency medicine resident shift work preferences: a comparison of resident scheduling preferences and recommended schedule design for shift workers. *AEM Educ Train.* 2018;2(3):229-235.

Rubin DB, Singh SR, Young GJ. Tax-exempt hospitals and community benefit: new directions in policy and practice. *Annu Rev Public Health.* 2015;36:545-557.

Sanghavi P, Jena AB, Newhouse JP, Zaslavsky AM. Outcomes after out-of-hospital cardiac arrest treated by basic vs advanced life support. *JAMA Intern Med.* 2015;175(2):196.

Sax DR, Warton EM, Mark DG, et al. Evaluation of the Emergency Severity Index in US emergency departments for the rate of mistriage. *JAMA Netw Open.* 2023;6(3):e233404.

Schiff RL, Ansell DA, Schlosser JE, Idris AH, Morrison A, Whitman S. Transfers to a public hospital. A prospective study of 467 patients. 1986;314(9):552-557.

Shah MN. The formation of the emergency medical services system. *Am J Public Health.* 2006;96(3):414.

Shahian D. I-PASS handover system: a decade of evidence demands action. *BMJ Qual Saf.* 2021;30(10):769-774.

Shahian DM, McEachern K, Rossi L, Chisari RG, Mort E. Large-scale implementation of the I-PASS handover system at an academic medical centre. *BMJ Qual Saf.* 2017;26(9):760-770.

Shahid S, Thomas S. Situation, background, assessment, recommendation (SBAR) communication tool for handoff in health care—a narrative review. *Saf Health.* 2018;4:7.

Shaikh SB, Jerrard DA, Witting MD, Winters ME, Brodeur MN. How long are patients willing to wait in the emergency department before leaving without being seen? *West J Emerg Med.* 2012;13(6):463-467.

Starmer AJ, Schnock KO, Lyons A, et al. Effects of the I-PASS nursing handoff bundle on communication quality and workflow. *BMJ Qual Saf.* 2017;26(12):949-957.

Starmer AJ, Sectish TC, Simon DW, et al. Rates of medical errors and preventable adverse events among hospitalized children following implementation of a resident handoff bundle. *JAMA.* 2013;310(21):2262-2270.

Starmer AJ, Spector ND, O'Toole JK, et al. Implementation of the I-PASS handoff program in diverse clinical environments: a multicenter prospective effectiveness implementation study. *J Hosp Med.* 2023;18(1):5-14.

Starmer AJ, Spector ND, Srivastava R, et al. Changes in medical errors after implementation of a handoff program. *N Engl J Med.* 2014;371(19):1803-1812.

Starmer AJ, Spector ND, Srivastava R, et al. I-PASS, a mnemonic to standardize verbal handoffs. *Pediatrics.* 2012;129(2):201.

Starmer AJ, Spector ND, West DC, et al. Integrating research, quality improvement, and medical education for better handoffs and safer care: disseminating, adapting, and implementing the I-PASS program. *Jt Comm J Qual Patient Saf.* 2017;43(7):319-329.

Stout J, Pepe PE, Mosesso VN. All-advanced life support vs tiered-response ambulance systems. *Prehosp Emerg Care*. 2000;4(1):1-6.

Terp S, Seabury SA, Arora S, Eads A, Lam CN, Menchine M. Enforcement of the Emergency Medical Treatment and Labor Act, 2005 to 2014. *Ann Emerg Med*. 2017;69(2):155-162.e1.

The Baltimore Sun. 80% of Baltimore 911 calls are non-emergencies. A new plan will make the department more efficient, officials say. Accessed September 25, 2023. https://www.baltimoresun.com/news/crime/bs-md-ci-cr-smart-policing-announcement-20220519-lzdppod7kfdqtopenvdh5tjwu4-story.html

The Joint Commission. Sentinel Event Alert 58: inadequate hand-off communication. Accessed September 25, 2023. https://www.jointcommission.org/resources/sentinel-event/sentinel-event-alert-newsletters/sentinel-event-alert-58-inadequate-hand-off-communication/

Udalova V, Powers D, Robinson S, Notter I. Most vulnerable more likely to depend on emergency rooms for preventable care. United States Census Bureau. Published January 20, 2022. Accessed October 2, 2023. https://www.census.gov/library/stories/2022/01/who-makes-more-preventable-visits-to-emergency-rooms.html

Uscher-Pines L, Pines J, Kellermann A, Gillen E, Mehrotra A. Emergency department visits for nonurgent conditions: systematic literature review. *Am J Manag Care*. 2013;19(1):47-59.

Viccellio P, Zito JA, Sayage V, et al. Patients overwhelmingly prefer inpatient boarding to emergency department boarding. *J Emerg Med*. 2013;45(6):942-946.

Villa-Roel C, Guo X, Holroyd BR, et al. The role of full capacity protocols on mitigating overcrowding in EDs. *Am J Emerg Med*. 2012;30(3):412-420.

Yates GR, Bernd DL, Sayles SM, Stockmeier CA, Burke G, Merti GE. Building and sustaining a systemwide culture of safety. *Jt Comm J Qual Patient Saf*. 2005;31(12):684-689.

Zibulewsky J. The Emergency Medical Treatment and Active Labor Act (EMTALA): what it is and what it means for physicians. *Proc (Bayl Univ Med Cent)*. 2001;14(4):339-346.

Zuabi N, Weiss LD, Langdorf MI. Emergency Medical Treatment and Labor Act (EMTALA) 2002-15: review of Office of Inspector General patient dumping settlements. *West J Emerg Med*. 2016;17(3):245-251.

3

Hospital Care

Clinical Case

The emergency room (ER) clinician mentions to Jessica that she will need to be admitted for further treatment in the hospital. Jessica and her husband, Daniel, check with the clinician to see if there is any possibility that she could be treated from her home instead.

Given Jessica's symptoms, physical examination, and laboratory results, the ER clinician strongly recommends that Jessica receives treatment in the hospital. Furthermore, Jessica is pending consultation from an orthopedic surgeon and may require a possible knee debridement in the hospital operating room. To prepare Jessica for her hospitalization, the ER clinician notifies Jessica that since she is being admitted to a teaching hospital, she will receive care from a team of clinicians that includes students, residents, and the attending physician.

This scenario represents a common occurrence in which a patient meets the criteria to be admitted to the hospital. In modern US health care, the hospital is where patients receive care for many acute illnesses (eg, pneumonia, heart failure). However, until the 19th century, many patients routinely received such care in other settings, such as their homes. Indeed, patients even had surgery performed in their homes. Prior to the 19th century, only lower income individuals were known to be admitted to brick-and-mortar medical facilities such as infirmaries.

Over time, hospitals evolved to play a critical role in providing care for acute illness to all patients. There were many drivers that contributed to the shift of delivering care in hospitals instead of in patients' homes. One key driver was the emergence of third-party payers in the United States, and their influence on the standardization of health care practices in hospitals. In this way, third-party payers represent a crucial systems factor that has contributed to patients receiving care for acute illness in hospitals.

SYSTEMS FACTOR: THIRD-PARTY PAYERS

Third-party payers are public or private entities that pay medical care organizations for medical expenses on behalf of enrolled beneficiaries. In this way, payers play a "third-party" role alongside patients and clinicians or medical care organizations (Figure 3.1). Within this three-party dynamic, beneficiaries pay a premium to payers, who in turn reimburse clinicians and medical care organizations for medical expenses on beneficiaries' behalf.

Third-party payers emerged at a time of significant medical advancements and landmark health policies. During the early 20th century, new medical technology such as x-rays, laboratory tests, and surgical techniques were introduced. The discovery of the first antibiotic, penicillin, changed how clinicians treat patients with acute infections. New medications became available to treat chronic conditions such as rheumatoid arthritis. Vaccines were developed to prevent diseases such as polio. New surgical techniques led to the first successful organ (kidney) transplant.

Landmark policies such as the Hill-Burton Act, enacted in 1946, facilitated extensive public investment in the building of hospitals so that people could conceivably receive the benefits of medical advancements in a centralized location. This combination of medical advancements and public investment in building hospitals began the momentum toward care for acute illness to be delivered centrally in hospitals. However, mechanisms were needed to deliver technologies, techniques, and treatments affordably at scale in hospitals. The emergence of third-party payers was a systems factor that played a key role in shifting care delivery toward hospitals.

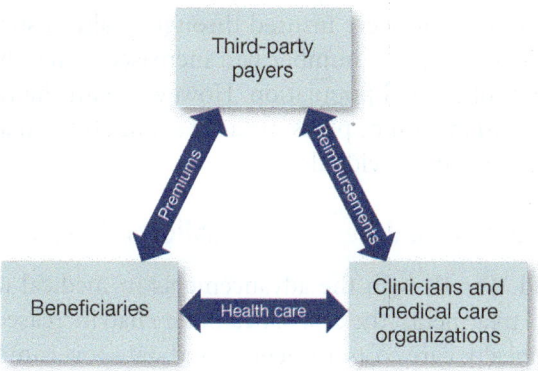

Figure 3.1 Role of Third-Party Payers. (Source: Data from Nowicki M. *The Financial Management of Hospitals and Healthcare Organizations*. Health Administration Press; 2004.)

Emergence and Growth of Private Third-Party Payers

Private organizations were the first third-party entities to pay for hospital care. The first example of a private third-party payer relationship emerged in 1929 when a group of teachers in Dallas, Texas created an employer-sponsored health insurance plan. The Baylor University Hospital in Dallas created an insurance plan, in conjunction with local schools, to provide coverage for hospital care. The plan first enrolled 1250 teachers for a monthly fee of 50 cents. The insurance plan covered 21 days of hospital services annually at Baylor University Hospital.

The precursor to the insurance plans more broadly, the plan created in Dallas later became known as Blue Cross in the 1930s. During the 1930s, other hospitals followed and adapted the Baylor University Hospital concept by offering insurance plans that covered hospital care at more than one hospital. By 1940, there were more than 50 insurance plans with more than 6 million beneficiaries.

During the 1940s, there was a rapid expansion of private employer-sponsored insurance plans. When the Stabilization Act of 1942 limited wage increases amid World War II, US companies needed new ways to recruit and retain employees. Offering an employer-sponsored insurance plan was a way for companies to address wage controls and provide attractive benefits to employees. Employer-sponsored insurance plans were offered as tax-exempt compensation for employees as well as their families.

In 1947, the Taft-Hartley Act defined third-party health insurance as a condition of employment and subject for collective bargaining under organized labor unions. These policy changes contributed to the increase in uptake of employer-sponsored insurance plans. Prior to World War II, approximately 10% of the US population were insured through health insurance plans. By the end of World War II, that number had increased to nearly 23%, then by 1960 close to 70% of the US population. However, with the rapid growth of employer-sponsored insurance plans surfaced a limitation: that they excluded retired and unemployed individuals.

Emergence of Medicare and Medicaid as Public Third-Party Payers

Following World War II, with the advancements in medical technology and discovery of new treatments, the cost of health care had increased. By the 1960s, in light of rising health care costs, the federal and state governments established comprehensive public health insurance programs to make the benefits of health care more affordable to certain populations. In 1965, Congress established Medicare and Medicaid to provide health insurance plans for the older population and low-income individuals, respectively. Upon establishment, Medicare and Medicaid quickly became the largest third-party payers.

Medicare was established to provide health insurance and increase financial security for the older population. Currently, Medicare encompasses health insurance for a number of groups:

- Individuals age 65 or older
- Individuals younger than age 65 with certain disabilities
- Individuals of all ages with end-stage kidney disease or amyotrophic lateral sclerosis

As of 2024, Medicare has four distinct parts:

Medicare Part A (hospital insurance). This part covers facility payments to hospitals, including critical access hospitals, and skilled nursing facilities (SNFs). It also covers hospice care and some home-based care. Most individuals do not pay a premium for Part A because they or their spouses already made their requisite contribution through payroll taxes while employed.

Medicare Part B (medical insurance). This part covers clinicians' services and ambulatory care. It also covers some other medical services that Part A does not, such as physical and occupational therapists, home-based care, and a limited number of prescription drugs. Most individuals pay a monthly premium for Part B.

Individuals enrolled in Medicare Parts A and B are considered insured through "Traditional Medicare."

Medicare Part C (Medicare Advantage). Rather than being incremental to Parts A and B, Part C represents an alternative, Medicare-approved plan offered by a private entity. As an alternative to Traditional Medicare, Part C plans include Parts A and B. In addition, most Medicare Advantage plans include prescription drug benefits. Plans may have lower out-of-pocket costs than Traditional Medicare and offer additional benefits such as vision, hearing, and dental services.

Medicare Part D (prescription drug coverage). This part covers the cost of prescription drugs (including some recommended shots or vaccines). Medicare prescription drug coverage is available to everyone with Medicare and is administered by private entities. Most individuals pay a monthly premium for Part D.

When Medicare was first implemented in 1966, nearly 19 million individuals were enrolled in Medicare Part A (hospital insurance). That number grew to 33.1 million individuals in 1989, and as of 2023, has grown to nearly

66 million individuals enrolled in Medicare Part A through Traditional Medicare and Medicare Advantage plans.

Medicaid was established to insure and cover medical costs for low-income individuals and other groups. In all states, Medicaid in conjunction with the Children's Health Insurance Program provides free or low-cost health coverage to its beneficiaries; some states have expanded their Medicaid program to cover all individuals below a certain income level. While some Medicaid programs pay for patient care directly, others use private payers to provide Medicaid coverage.

Medicaid is jointly financed by the federal and state governments, and therefore coverage for Medicaid beneficiaries varies by state. Medicaid is generally defined as health insurance for the following groups:

- Low-income adults
- Families and children
- Pregnant women
- Older population
- Individuals with disabilities
- Individuals receiving Supplemental Security Income

Of note, the Affordable Care Act in 2010 created the opportunity for states to expand Medicaid coverage to additional low-income individuals younger than 65 years of age. With the support of federal funding, states have been able to expand coverage eligibility for adults with income up to 138% of the federal poverty level. As of 2023, 41 states have expanded Medicaid coverage.

For Medicaid, states establish their own insurance plans that determine the specific type, duration, and scope of services that comply within federal guidelines. Examples of federally mandated benefits include the following:

- Inpatient and outpatient hospital services
- Physician services
- Laboratory and x-ray services
- Home health services

Examples of optional state benefits include the following:

- Prescription drugs
- Case management
- Physical and occupational therapy
- Home- and community-based services

In 1972, Medicaid provided insurance coverage to nearly 18 million beneficiaries, which increased to about 25 million by 1989. By 2023, there were more than 88 million beneficiaries enrolled in Medicaid.

As the agency governing two large national purchasers of health care services, the Centers for Medicare and Medicaid Services (CMS) wields significant influence in how care is delivered in hospitals in two ways: through setting payment policy and establishing care standards for hospitals.

With respect to hospital payment, CMS moved from a cost-based reimbursement system to the Inpatient Prospective Payment System (IPPS). The prospective payment system pays hospitals a predetermined, fixed amount for specific Diagnosis-Related Groups (DRGs). Over time, Medicare's payment system has come to serve as a benchmark or guide for hospital payment rates for private third-party payers.

In its payment to hospitals, CMS also subsidizes facilities for graduate medical education. Medicare is the only third-party payer that explicitly supports graduate medical education in teaching hospitals and does so through two types of payments. First, teaching hospitals receive an adjustment to their IPPS fees to reflect the added indirect patient care costs associated with operating residency training programs. These adjustments to teaching hospitals were reported to be about $4 billion in 1996, which grew to more than $11 billion in 2020. Second, teaching hospitals receive Medicare payments to offset the direct costs of graduate medical education programs. These payments cover salaries of residents and their supervising clinicians, the cost of office space, and other overhead costs. The Medicare payments to offset direct costs of resident training totaled more than $2 billion in 1996, which grew to about $4.5 billion in 2020. In 2023, there are estimated to be more than 1700 teaching hospitals in the United States.

In conjunction with independent accreditation agencies, CMS has established care standards for hospitals. CMS requires accreditation of hospitals as a prerequisite to receive reimbursements for care in hospitals. Independent accreditation agencies such as The Joint Commission accredit more than 20 000 medical care organizations, including hospitals. The mission of The Joint Commission is "to continuously improve health care for the public, in collaboration with other stakeholders, by evaluating medical care organizations and inspiring them to excel in providing safe and effective care of the highest quality and value." While The Joint Commission is the most widely known accreditation agency, there are other agencies such as the Accreditation Commission for Health Care, Det Norske Veritas Health Care Inc, and the Center for Improvement in Healthcare Quality.

Accreditation involves the review of a hospital's compliance with predefined performance standards and safety goals that aim to improve health care quality. For example, the 2009 Joint Commission's National Patient

Safety Goals included regulations targeting the spread of infection due to multidrug-resistant organisms, catheter-related bloodstream infections, and surgical site infections. As a result, hospitals have developed checklists, protocols, and other training methods to decrease infections. In these ways, the CMS, in conjunction with accreditation agencies, guide goals and priorities for the standard of care in hospitals.

Back to the Clinical Case

In this case, because the patient is a Medicare beneficiary, Part A covers her facility payments during her hospitalization. Because she is admitted to a teaching hospital, the patient receives care from clinicians that includes trainees whose costs are funded in part by Medicare.

While in the hospital, the patient would be the recipient of care protocols and interventions, required by independent accreditation agencies, aimed at preventing further infections in the hospital. For instance, upon interacting with the patient, clinicians would take actions to promote patient safety, such as sanitizing their hands when entering her room, wearing appropriate personal protective equipment as relevant, and removing unnecessary catheters.

TAKEAWAYS

- In response to the market need to deliver technologies, techniques, and treatments affordably at scale, third-party payers have played a key role in shifting the delivery of care for acute illnesses toward hospitals.
- Medicare supports graduate medical education in hospitals through dedicated payments.
- In conjunction with independent accreditation agencies, the CMS helps establish hospital care standards.

Clinical Case Continued

Jessica is admitted to the hospital and the ER clinician continues to closely monitor her overnight under "observation status." Jessica continues to have tenderness at her knee with vital signs continuing to show elevated heart and respiratory rates.

Upon finishing the emergent case in the operating room, the orthopedic surgeon, Dr Teres, comes to evaluate Jessica's knee. While the orthopedic surgeon is speaking to Jessica, the ER clinician receives a notification from the lab that Jessica's joint synovial fluid analysis shows an infection with Staphylococcus aureus, a common cause of joint infections in adults. Given the results of the fluid analysis, the ER clinician anticipates that Jessica will require more than monitoring under "observation status" and instead may require more intensive treatments under "inpatient status."

This case represents a common occurrence when a patient receives initial hospital care under a designation called observation status. Patients can be under observation status in the ER or other parts of the hospital, which typically lasts for approximately 24 to 48 hours. If at the end of this time period, patients require further care in the hospital, their status is changed from observation to inpatient status. Conversely, if patients require no further care in the hospital, they can be discharged home from observation status.

In the context of patients receiving care in hospitals, observation status serves to identify patients requiring more time to determine the need for additional treatment. In this way, as one of several designations under which patients can receive care in the hospital, observation status is a systems factor that can affect care for many patients.

SYSTEMS FACTOR: OBSERVATION STATUS

There are more than 2.5 million patients admitted under observation status each year. One common scenario for the use of observation status has been a patient presenting to the ER with acute chest pain or other symptoms potentially worrisome for acute myocardial infarction. In this scenario, a patient can present to the ER with acute chest pain and test negative for an acute myocardial infarction on initial evaluation. However, if clinicians remain concerned on the basis of the clinical presentation and symptoms, the patient can be admitted for further monitoring under observation status.

During this period, the patient is monitored and can receive additional care—in the case of chest pain, potentially repeat tests such as a 12-lead electrocardiogram and serum cardiac biomarkers. If the patient has recurrence of chest pain or subsequently tests positive (eg, changes in 12-electrocardiogram or elevation of serum cardiac biomarkers), the patient can be formally admitted under inpatient status for additional treatment. Conversely, if the symptoms resolve but the patient continues to test negative, the patient can be discharged home from observation status for future follow-up.

There is rationale for the use of observation status to determine whether patients require care under inpatient status or can be discharged home. If they can be diagnosed, treated safely, and then discharged home under observation status, patients are able to avoid potentially high costs and other risks associated with staying longer in the hospital. Thoughtful use of observation versus inpatient status is relevant to payers such as Medicare, which spent nearly 40% of its total expenditures for care under inpatient status in 2021. Since Medicare policy is widely used as a benchmark or starting point for other third-party payers, it is important to understand the history of Medicare observation status.

1983 to 2000: Introduction of Medicare Observation Status

In 1983, Medicare first introduced observation status as a designation for patients who could receive a "set of specific, clinically appropriate services, which include ongoing short-term treatment, assessment, and reassessment that are furnished while a decision is being made regarding whether patients will require further treatment . . . or if they are able to be discharged from the hospital." Services under observation status aimed to treat a group of patients who were too ill to go home but required additional time to determine the need for further treatment. When observation status was first introduced, services were reimbursed on an hourly basis separate from hospital facility payments.

However, observation status was used inconsistently across institutions. There was initial lack of clarity around appropriate clinical conditions and situations to use observation status, which contributed to its initial misuse. A notable example related to scheduled elective procedures. Initially, Medicare only allowed hospitals to use observation status for scheduled elective outpatient procedures in a few instances, one of which was when patients experienced complications and needed extra time for postoperative recovery. In these instances, Medicare allowed hospitals to bill twice: first, for the elective outpatient procedure and, second, for the services under observation status.

However, a number of hospitals were found to be inappropriately billing for both the procedure and observation status. First, hospitals were billing for observation status despite no complications after outpatient procedures. Second, for patients who experienced procedural complications and should have been billed for observation status postoperatively, some hospitals billed erroneously by also counting preoperative and intraoperative time under observation status.

2000 to Early 2010s: Separate Payments for Medicare Observation Status Policy

In 2000, Medicare sought to address misuse of observation status by eliminating separate reimbursements for services under observation status. Instead,

Medicare assigned reimbursements for observation status into payment groups called the Ambulatory Payment Classifications. Instead of hourly reimbursements separate from prospective payments, Medicare added observation services to associated ER or clinic visits and reimbursed those visits at higher amounts. In the years that followed, there was a significant decrease in the use of observation status and a concomitant increase in the number of short hospitalizations under inpatient status. This trend was consistent with new incentives facing hospitals: to avoid delivering care under observation status without significant, additional reimbursement and instead deliver care for patients under inpatient status.

In 2005, however, Medicare reinstituted separate reimbursements for observation status for three specific conditions: chest pain, asthma, and heart failure. Beyond that, Medicare continued to combine costs associated with observation status into payment groups called the Observation Comprehensive Ambulatory Payment Classifications. Under this approach, Medicare made a single payment for "certain costly primary services and all other items and services that are considered adjunctive to the primary service."

By 2008, Medicare further expanded separate reimbursements for observation status to encompass nearly all conditions. Studies found that between 2007 and 2009, there was a 34% increase in the ratio of Medicare patients under observation status relative to inpatient status in the hospital. Similarly, another study showed that between 2006 and 2012, there was an increase in observation status claims from 28 to 53 per 1000 Medicare beneficiaries per year.

2013 to Present: Further Additions to Observation Status

In 2013, Medicare adopted the Two-Midnight Rule to better guide medical care organizations on the use of observation (reimbursed through Medicare Part B) versus inpatient status (reimbursed through Medicare Part A).

The rule helped determine whether a patient meets criteria for inpatient status. The original Two-Midnight Rule stated the following:

- Inpatient status would generally be payable under Part A if the admitting clinician expected the patient to require a hospitalization that crossed two midnights and the medical record supported that reasonable expectation.
- Medicare Part A payment was generally not appropriate for hospitalizations expected to last fewer than two midnights.
- Cases involving a procedure identified on the inpatient-only list or that were identified as "rare and unusual exception" to the Two-Midnight benchmark by CMS were exceptions to this general rule and were deemed to be appropriate for Medicare Part A payment.

- All treatment decisions for patients were based on the medical judgment of clinicians and the Two-Midnight Rule did not prevent the clinician from providing any service at any hospital, regardless of the expected duration of the service.

One of the issues with observation status is patient cost-sharing responsibilities. In particular, because care under observation status is covered under Medicare Part B, patients are subject to Part B cost-sharing rules.

In 2015, to better inform patients regarding the distinction in their care received and cost-sharing responsibilities under observation status, Congress passed a bill called the Notice of Observation Treatment and Implication for Care Eligibility (NOTICE) Act. The NOTICE Act was in response to concerns about a lack of transparency with patients placed under observation status and its consequences with respect to high cost sharing for patients. Although observation status had existed for several decades, patients were not always being notified of their status and unaware of its cost implications. The concerns were mostly 2-fold. First, because services under observation status are covered under Medicare Part B, patients often did not realize they must make co-payments for all clinician fees and hospital services. Secondly, many patients were not aware that being admitted under observation status had implications for their eligibility for a SNF stay.

For patients receiving care under observation status for longer than 24 hours, the bill began to require hospitals to notify them of their status no later than 36 hours after observation status had been initiated. The NOTICE Act required that hospitals provide patients with a standardized notice—the Medicare Outpatient Observation Notice—that can be summarized as follows:

- Explains a patient's observation status as part of Part B (vs Part A) and the reasons as to why their care is under observation status
- Explains the implications of observation status on services rendered, cost-sharing requirements, and subsequent coverage eligibility for services rendered by a SNF
- Provides a verbal explanation alongside the delivery of written notice and must be signed by the patients or persons acting on their behalf to acknowledge receipt

Back to the Clinical Case

In this case, the patient is initially admitted under observation status. So far, she has spent fewer than two midnights at the hospital. If the patient were to remain under observation status for longer than 24 hours, she would receive a written Medicare Outpatient Observation Notice as well as a verbal explanation of the implications of the observation status on services rendered and cost-sharing requirements.

> ### TAKEAWAYS
>
> - Observation status aims to identify patients who are too ill to go home, but require additional time to determine the need for further treatment.
> - Since the 1980s, Medicare observation status policy has been used to address rising hospitalization costs.
> - The Medicare Two-Midnight Rule established the benchmark criteria to determine whether patients meet the criteria for observation versus inpatient status.
> - Hospitals must provide Medicare patients with a standardized notice—the Medicare Outpatient Observation Notice—if under observation status for longer than 24 hours, explaining the reasons for the status and its implications.

Clinical Case Continued

The orthopedic surgeon evaluates Jessica and determines that she requires further treatment in the operating room. The orthopedic surgeon performs a knee debridement and salvages, rather than replaces, her prosthetic joint. The next morning, her first full day of her hospitalization under inpatient status, Jessica is visited by the physical therapist, Dr Singh, who tests Jessica's ability to transfer from a bed to a chair, and observes how she walks to the bathroom and around the room.

Jessica asks the physical therapist why she's being tested so soon after admission, and the physical therapist informs her that the medical and social work teams need to know whether she's able to safely ambulate and can ultimately be discharged home from the hospital, or if she'll need to go to a SNF after her hospital stay. Jessica is confused as to why her teams are already planning for her discharge when she only just had surgery hours ago.

Later that morning, the internal medicine attending physician, Dr Martinez, and her team visit Jessica and her husband on rounds. Jessica's husband mentions that he's been worried that Jessica's memory has gotten worse over the past few years and was wondering if she can get a brain magnetic resonance imaging (MRI) since she's already in the hospital. The attending physician responds that she'll send a note to the primary care clinician to look into Jessica's memory concerns further, but that during this hospital stay they'll have to focus on caring for Jessica's knee. The attending physician suggests that the medical student on the team, Lisa, might return later in the afternoon to perform a memory test. Jessica's husband understands the need to focus on Jessica's knee but is disappointed she will not get an MRI and thought it would be easy to get this test done while Jessica was in the hospital.

These two interactions—between the patient and her physical therapist and between the patient's husband and the attending physician— are commonly observed in US health care. In the first, the patient seeks to understand the focus on coordinating what she'll need upon leaving the hospital so early in her stay; in the second interaction, the patient's husband is disappointed that certain tests may need to be deferred until after hospital discharge.

Broadly speaking, hospitals track and seek to address metrics such as length of stay (the duration that patients are hospitalized) and costs per hospitalization (the costs of evaluation and therapies performed during hospitalization, along with associated indirect costs). This reality is driven in part by the reimbursement system for hospital care in the United States—an important systems factor that can affect patient care.

SYSTEMS FACTOR: REIMBURSEMENT FOR HOSPITAL CARE

While hospitals can be reimbursed for the care for hospitalized patients in several ways, diagnosis-based reimbursement serves as the foundation and most prevalent method in the United States. In particular, instead of being paid via a daily rate or on the basis of reported costs, most hospitals are paid a prospectively determined lump sum based on the diagnosis managed or treatment provided during patients' hospitalizations. This payment approach is used by multiple payers, which vary in how they implement the method to reimburse hospitals.

As the largest payer of hospital care and entity accounting for 26% of national hospital spending, Medicare implements a diagnosis-based reimbursement method that serves as an example or a comparison point for other payers. Therefore, it is important to understand the structure and the history of how Medicare shifted toward this method of reimbursement and how it is implemented.

1965 to 1983: Hospitals Paid Retrospectively Based on "Reasonable Costs"

When Medicare was passed in 1965, Congress was concerned with ensuring that hospitals would voluntarily participate in the new program, as it was the largest government-involved health care financing effort in the nation's history. It therefore decided that Medicare would reimburse for most hospitalizations retrospectively based on "reasonable costs," which meant that hospitals provided services to patients and billed Medicare thereafter; and that so long as services were deemed "reasonable and necessary," Medicare paid hospitals according to the amount hospitals reported that it cost to provide those services. Under this approach, hospitals had considerable leeway to provide services it considered worthwhile with the reassurance that they would be reimbursed at reported values.

One consequence was variation in the resources expended to take care of different patients within a hospital, as well as variation across hospitals and across regions. A cost-based approach also contributed to rapid Medicare hospital expenditure growth, from $3 billion in 1967 to $37 billion in 1983 (Figure 3.2). By 1982, the Medicare trustees predicted that the national hospital fund would be insolvent within 5 years.

Out of concern for this cost growth at hospitals, the Department of Health and Human Services produced a landmark report proposing that Medicare adjust course and implement an IPPS for Medicare hospitalizations at a "reasonable price for a known product."

1983 to Present: Inpatient Prospective Payment Based on Diagnosis-Related Groups

The proposed IPPS, which was passed into law in the Social Security Amendments of 1983, was designed to run off of a DRG method that had been subjected to smaller scale testing. The DRG method was designed in 1967 as a way of identifying hospitalized patients who were similar clinically and in their expected use of hospital resources.

The first step of the method was to group patients based on their principal diagnosis. However, there was recognition that although patients could have the same diagnosis, they could differ with respect to chronic disease burden in ways that might require a different extent and intensity of hospital resources. For example, an otherwise healthy 40-year-old admitted for pneumonia might need fewer hospital resources than an 80-year-old with a history of heart disease and chronic obstructive pulmonary disease also admitted for pneumonia.

Therefore, in addition to accounting for the principal diagnosis for a hospital stay, the DRG method also categorized patients based on their major

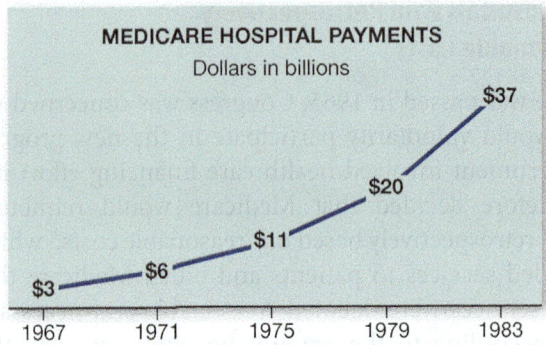

Figure 3.2 Medicare Hospital Expenditures, 1967 to 1983. (Source: Data from U.S. Department of Health and Human Services. Medicare hospital prospective payment system how DRG rates are calculated and updated. Office of Inspector General. August 2001. https://oig.hhs.gov/oei/reports/oei-09-00-00200.pdf)

and minor comorbidities. As of 2023, Medicare groups patients into a total of 767 categories, called Medicare Severity DRGs (MS-DRGs), with each category aiming to include patients with similar hospital resource use based on a shared principal diagnosis, comorbidity burden, or complications related to their principal diagnosis.

Medicare reimburses hospitals a prospectively assigned amount to care for a patient based principally on that patient's MS-DRG category, regardless of the actual resources expended to care for that patient. In order to convert an MS-DRG clinical grouping into a hospital payment in the IPPS, Medicare assigns a weight to each MS-DRG that reflects the national average resources required to care for patients assigned that particular MS-DRG. Each weight assigned to an MS-DRG is relative to the average resources needed to care for all patients in all MS-DRGs nationally.

Each MS-DRG weight is then multiplied by a standard base rate to convert the weight to US dollars. This dollar amount is further adjusted to account for factors that vary across hospitals, such as the cost of labor, disproportionate share of underserved populations, and the presence of trainee physicians completing residency or fellowships in approved training programs (Figure 3.3). Medicare exempts several types of hospitals, such as Children's Hospitals, Long-Term Care Hospitals, Cancer Hospitals, Critical Access Hospitals, Rehabilitation Hospitals, and Psychiatric Hospitals, from the IPPS.

The DRG method poses several implications for hospitals. First, it provides a predictable payment amount based principally on patients' primary diagnosis and morbidities. Second, the DRG method provides payment regardless of the amount of resources or internal costs spent on patient care—that is, reimbursement is the same regardless of the number or nature of tests and treatments performed, or the number of days the patients spend in the

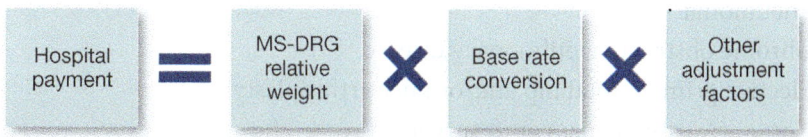

Figure 3.3 Converting an MS-DRG to Hospital Payment. MS-DRG, Medicare Severity Diagnosis-Related Group. (Source: Data from U.S. Department of Health and Human Services. Medicare hospital prospective payment system how DRG rates are calculated and updated. Office of Inspector General. August 2001. https://oig.hhs.gov/oei/reports/oei-09-00-00200.pdf)

hospital. Given these dynamics, the IPPS has the potential to create the following incentives:

Focus resources during hospitalization on patients' main diagnosis or treatment. Since the relative weight assigned to a DRG is intended to reimburse hospitals for the average amount of resources required to care for a patient with a given primary hospital diagnosis, a hospital has the incentive to deploy its resources in a way that focuses on the reason for a patient's hospitalization, as opposed to the array of other secondary or chronic conditions that may exist.

Facilitate expeditious discharge. Since hospital length of stay does not change the reimbursement a hospital receives, duration matters: comparatively shorter stays would contribute to profit (lower internal costs compared to fixed DRG payment) while longer stays would contribute to financial loss (higher internal costs compared to fixed DRG payment). Consequently, diagnosis-based reimbursement can incentivize hospitals to minimize patient length of stay and discharge patients as efficiently as possible.

Collectively, these incentives can create potential unintended consequences. In particular, incentives to discharge patients in a timely manner can inadvertently lead to premature discharges, vulnerability during the immediate postdischarge period, and, in some cases, the need for hospital readmission. In turn, Medicare has employed policies and programs that aim to counterbalance any pressure potentially adverse to patient care.

For instance, to balance the incentive to facilitate expeditious discharge, the Affordable Care Act created the Medicare Hospital Readmission Reduction Problem (HRRP). The program was first implemented in 2012 and held hospitals financially accountable for readmission rates within 30 days of discharge, with the intent of reducing potentially preventable readmissions. As of 2023, the HRRP had evolved to apply to a number of medical conditions or procedures:

- Acute myocardial infarction
- Heart failure

- Pneumonia
- Chronic obstructive pulmonary disease
- Elective primary total hip and/or knee arthroplasty
- Coronary artery bypass graft surgery

Medicare then calculated national average readmissions rates and penalized any hospital whose readmissions rate was above the then national average. Penalties came in the form of reductions in overall hospital payments. Over time, the maximum penalty a hospital could face increased from a 1% reduction in base payments for Medicare inpatient admissions in the program's first year to up to 3% reduction in base payments in HRRP's third year onward.

Ten years after HRRP implementation, 93% of eligible hospitals had faced a penalty at least 1 year, and 41% of hospitals faced a penalty all 10 years. In 2017 alone, Medicare penalties to hospitals amounted to more than $500 million. After HRRP was implemented, readmission rates declined nationally.

Back to the Clinical Case

In this case, the patient is admitted primarily out of concern for an infected knee joint, and the hospital's diagnosis-based reimbursement will reflect the average resources required to care for a patient in that circumstance. However, the reimbursement is not directly connected to evaluation for chronic, nonacutely worsening dementia. Therefore, completing an MRI for cognitive changes would likely be an unreimbursed expenditure from the IPPS perspective, thereby potentially creating incentives for hospitals to defer this evaluation beyond hospital discharge. In addition, since the hospital is reimbursed independent of the number of days the patient stays in the hospital, it has an incentive to work expeditiously toward timely discharge.

TAKEAWAYS

- Since 1983, the most prevalent form of hospital reimbursement has been diagnosis-based reimbursement, in which hospitals are paid prospectively depending on the average amount it costs to care for a hospitalized patient based on a primary diagnosis or treatment, with consideration for major comorbidities and/or complications.
- The diagnosis-based reimbursement system can create incentives for hospitals to focus resource use on needs related to the primary diagnosis and facilitate expeditious discharge.

- Medicare has sought to balance incentives favoring expeditious discharge and potential readmission risks with incentives via programs such as the Hospital Readmissions Reduction Program that penalize hospitals with high readmission rates.

Clinical Case Continued

Jessica's blood cultures return showing that so far, 48 hours after collection, there is no evidence that the infection in her joint spread to her bloodstream. The clinical team shares that Jessica will need to continue with intravenous antibiotics in the hospital for several more days.

Jessica and her husband are worried because she is still in a lot of pain and unable to ambulate independently. The orthopedic surgeon explains that it will take time and physical therapy, much of which will take place after she's left the hospital. The clinical team also explains to Jessica that she'll also need wound care for her surgical site from a trained nurse and a 2-week course of intravenous antibiotics, and that the team social worker, Lynn, will come by and explain Jessica's options for supports to promote recovery after hospital discharge.

It is common for hospitalized patients to require resources and supports beyond hospital discharge to promote continued healing and recovery. While hospitals are a focal point for recovery from acute illness, patients often do not experience the entirety of their recovery in the hospital, and instead need services that are difficult to accommodate in that setting.

For example, as exemplified in this patient's case, some individuals require ongoing medical treatment related to their acute illness (eg, intravenous antibiotics), or physical and/or occupational therapy to safely manage their activities of daily living (eg, transferring in and out of bed, dressing, ambulation). In other circumstances, patients can safely navigate their home but may still have ongoing medical needs related to their acute illness and challenges with instrumental activities of daily living (eg, handling medications, preparing food, housekeeping). One solution for postacute care needs is to transfer patients from hospitals to SNFs.

While the need for posthospitalization supports at SNFs can be common, the ability to access these resources can vary. This dynamic results from the fact that inpatient status serves as a qualifying event for subsequent health care resources for certain insurances, such as Traditional Medicare, but not others, such as Medicaid in many states. Ultimately, the stipulation surrounding qualifying events for SNF care is a systems factor that can affect how health care is delivered and experienced by hospitalized patients.

SYSTEMS FACTOR: HOSPITALIZATION AS A QUALIFYING EVENT FOR SKILLED NURSING FACILITY RESOURCES

Inpatient status can act as a qualifying event that facilitates patient connection with additional health care resources. Since such a significant proportion of Americans who are hospitalized receive insurance through Medicare or Medicaid (in 2019, 60% of all hospital care in the United States was delivered to individuals insured through these programs), it is instructive to understand how these benefits access SNF care following a qualifying hospitalization.

Inpatient Status as a Qualifying Event for Skilled Nursing Facility Care

Medicare includes benefits for care received at nursing home facilities. Typically, these benefits cover "skilled care," which involves services that are delivered at SNFs and provided directly by or under the supervision of licensed medical professionals. Such services can include physical therapy, occupational therapy, and advanced nursing care such as wound care, intravenous injections, or catheter care.

Nursing home facilities also provide "custodial care," which refers to longer term nonmedical care that can be provided by nonlicensed caregivers and involves help with daily activities such as dressing and bathing. When Medicare was first passed, nursing home facilities predominantly provided custodial care and did not frequently provide higher level "skilled care." Under these circumstances, it was important to the safety of patients that they be evaluated at a hospital before admission to a nursing home facility.

As a result, in 1967, Medicare put in place a rule in its SNF benefit design that stipulated that beneficiaries would only qualify for a SNF stay if they first had the following:

- A hospital stay that met criteria for inpatient status
- A hospital stay under inpatient status that lasted at least 3 days

This rule, commonly referred to as the 3-Day Rule, has directly linked inpatient status to Medicare eligibility to receive skilled care at a SNF. In this way, the rule creates a potential disconnect between Medicare beneficiaries who might benefit from such care at a SNF but who do not have a preceding qualifying hospitalization. For instance, SNF services could help Medicare beneficiaries who need physical therapy for mobility-related disability and falls. However, a Medicare beneficiary facing these challenges who has not yet experienced injuries requiring hospitalization could potentially qualify for a dedicated course of physical therapy at home or in the community, but not at a SNF.

Because inpatient status qualifies Medicare beneficiaries for SNF, those admitted under observation status do not qualify regardless of how many days they have been observed in the hospital. This distinction potentially applies to a large number of patients: in 2016, nearly 20% of hospitalized patients completed their hospital stays under observation status. In addition, if a Medicare beneficiary is initially admitted under observation status and later converts to inpatient status (eg, due to worsening of their condition), length of stay is calculated for the purposes of meeting the 3-Day Rule from the time of designation as inpatient status—that is, the days the patient receives care in the hospital under observation do not go toward meeting 3-Day Rule requirements. For example, if a patient was hospitalized for a total of 5 days, where the first and second days were under observation status days and the third through fifth days were under inpatient status, the patient would only be eligible for placement to a SNF after day 5 (Figure 3.4).

When a Medicare beneficiary does qualify for SNF services, Medicare will cover up to 100 days of services in a sliding scale manner, where the beneficiary pays $0 for the first 20 days, $200 a day for the subsequent 80 days (days 21 through 100), and the entirety of costs for all days beyond 100. This means that Medicare will not finance long-term custodial SNF care.

The nature of hospitalization has changed considerably since the 3-Day Rule was implemented. When it was first implemented, the average length of stay for patients age 65 and older was 13.8 days, qualifying many hospital

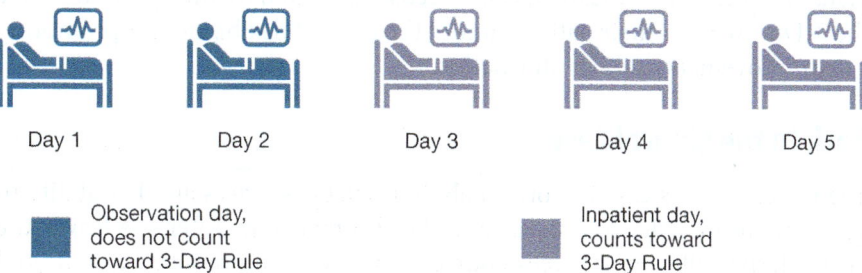

Day 1   Day 2   Day 3   Day 4   Day 5

Observation day, does not count toward 3-Day Rule

Inpatient day, counts toward 3-Day Rule

Figure 3.4 Days in the Hospital and Meeting 3-Day Rule Requirements. (Source: Data from Patel N, Slota JM, Miller BJ. The continued conundrum of discharge to a skilled nursing facility after a Medicare observation stay. *JAMA Health Forum.* 2020;1(5):e200577.)

stays for a subsequent SNF stay. In 2018, the average length of stay for Medicare beneficiaries was 5.5 days.

In contrast to Medicare, there is no national policy requiring state Medicaid beneficiaries to have an inpatient status hospitalization prior to a SNF stay. Although states can differ in approach, a commonly used method is to assess a beneficiary's overall physical functional ability (eg, ability to perform activities of daily living); their combination of health issues and medical needs (eg, whether they need catheter care or intravenous medications); the presence and degree of cognitive impairment; and presence and nature of behavioral problems. Given this approach, many Medicaid beneficiaries can be admitted to a SNF with or without a preceding hospitalization. Unlike Medicare, many Medicaid programs cover both short- and long-term care at nursing facilities, a policy that has made Medicaid the largest payer of nursing facilities in the United States and the insurer covering 6 in 10 nursing home residents.

Efforts to Suspend or Exempt Beneficiaries From the 3-Day Rule

Historically, Medicare has tried suspending the 3-Day Rule a few times. The Medicare Catastrophic Coverage Act, a law passed in 1988 and then repealed in 1989, made a number of changes to Medicare policy, including repealing the 3-Day Rule. This eliminated inpatient status as a qualifying event for SNF care as a systems factor. In the 1 year the law was in effect, Medicare payments to SNFs tripled and there was a 16% increase in covered SNF admissions.

More recently, Medicare waived the 3-Day Rule temporarily during the COVID-19 Public Health Emergency. During that time, 18% of all SNF stays were attributable to patients who sought SNF care without preceding admissions under inpatient status. This was an increase from 3% of SNF stays just prior to the pandemic, in circumstances where the 3-Day Rule was waived only for certain special exceptions. For instance, medical care organizations participating in certain value-based payment models, Medicare Advantage plans, and certain Medicare Special Needs Plans, all have the option to waive the 3-Day Rule for their patients under the aegis of flexibilities for promoting care improvement and transformation.

Back to the Clinical Case

The patient in this case is worried about available services and her ability to access them in order to recover after her hospital stay. After she leaves the hospital, she will need a 2-week course of intravenous antibiotics, a dedicated course of physical therapy, and a wound care nurse. Theoretically, she can receive these services at home, in the community, or in a SNF.

In the Medicare program, she would qualify for a SNF stay if her hospitalization lasts at least 3 days under inpatient status. This circumstance differs from recovery options that were available to her after her initial outpatient knee replacement surgery at the ambulatory surgical center, mentioned in Chapter 1: Ambulatory Care. After that surgery, she only would have qualified for outpatient physical therapy through Medicare because she did not have a 3-day stay under inpatient status associated with her surgery.

Once the patient qualifies for a SNF stay, Medicare would cover the first 20 days of her recovery with no cost sharing, and then up to 100 total days with some cost sharing, after which the patient would have to pay out of pocket if she did not also have Medicaid insurance. However, since this patient also has Medicaid insurance, she could be eligible for a SNF stay even without the 3-day hospital stay under inpatient status, with coverage for SNF for a longer period than would be covered under Medicare.

TAKEAWAYS

- In Medicare, the 3-Day Rule stipulates that beneficiaries would only qualify for a SNF stay if they first had a hospital stay that met criteria for inpatient status that lasted at least 3 days.
- The 3-Day Rule creates a potential disconnect between patients who might benefit from care at a SNF but who do not have a preceding qualifying hospitalization.
- Many Medicaid programs uncouple the requirement for 3-day hospital stay under inpatient status with SNF care eligibility, instead focusing on assessing whether the beneficiary's needs are consistent with requiring "nursing home level of care."
- Periods when the 3-Day Rule was suspended—that is, times in which preceding inpatient status and hospital length of stay requirements were decoupled from subsequent SNF eligibility— were associated with higher SNF use.
- Medical care organizations participating in certain value-based payment models, Medicare Advantage plans, and certain Medicare Special Needs Plans can waive the 3-Day Rule to promote care improvement and transformation.

Implications

The systems factors discussed in this chapter can have implications for access to care. Specifically, since only hospitalization days spent under inpatient status count toward the Medicare 3-Day Rule, providing care to Medicare patients in hospitals under observation status may impact downstream access to postacute care such as SNFs.

This policy is particularly important since approximately 18% of Medicare beneficiaries who are hospitalized are done so under observation status. Indeed, a 2016 report found that patients hospitalized under observation status had less access to postacute care services than patients hospitalized under inpatient status. In 2015, more than 600 000 Medicare beneficiaries had hospitalizations that lasted more than 3 nights, but were hospitalized under observation status, and therefore did not have access to Medicare postacute care benefits.

In addition, the way hospitals are reimbursed has implications for the type of services patients can access during a given hospital stay. A systematic review found that in some instances, DRG reimbursement was associated with lower access to more expensive treatment or diagnostic services for hospitalized patients. In some instances, hospitals preferentially apply inpatient status designations to less clinically complex patients who are expected to have less expensive hospital stays.

The systems factors discussed in this chapter also have implications for quality of care. For instance, among patients hospitalized for heart failure, patients admitted under inpatient status had levels of mortality similar to that of patients admitted under observation status, but had lower readmission rates than patients hospitalized under observation status. Hospital reimbursement mechanisms also pose potential quality implications. Early analyses after the introduction of the IPPS suggested increases in the likelihood that Medicare patients were discharged in unstable conditions without major impact of hospital mortality. Compared to cost-based reimbursement, a systematic review found that DRG-based reimbursement is consistently associated with lower overall hospital length of stay, which can impact quality through dimensions such as risk for hospital acquired infection. However, from a US and international perspective, DRG-based reimbursement can be associated with higher readmission rates than cost-based hospital reimbursement systems.

The systems factors in this chapter also have implications for health care costs. Whether a patient is hospitalized under observation or inpatient status has cost implications. One study found that hospitalizations under inpatient status cost 41% more overall than comparable hospitalizations under observation status among privately insured patients. Out-of-pocket patient costs were also 33% higher for patients hospitalized under inpatient status than those hospitalized for similar reasons under observation status.

However, under the Medicare program, since observation status admissions are reimbursed under Medicare Part B, beneficiaries are responsible to pay 20% coinsurance and there is no maximum for out-of-pocket expenditures. This situation contrasts out-of-pocket costs for beneficiaries hospitalized under inpatient status, which is governed under Medicare Part A, and its policies about patient out-of-pocket maximum contributions. In 10% of observation status hospitalizations, Medicare beneficiaries pay more out of pocket than they would have if admitted under inpatient status.

Tying eligibility for postacute care services to a qualifying preceding hospitalization also has cost implications. One concern is that this Medicare rule leads to unnecessary hospitalizations and longer hospitalizations, each of which could conceivably increase overall health care costs. However, several experiments eliminating the 3-Day Rule yielded mixed cost results. For example, in a 1978 to 1980 study conducted in Oregon and Massachusetts in which the 3-Day Rule was waived, there were negligible changes in Medicare Part A spending on hospital and SNF care. In contrast, when Congress temporarily removed the 3-Day Rule in the Medicare Catastrophic Coverage Act in 1988, Medicare observed decreased hospital days and spending coupled with an increase in patient SNF days. More recently, a 2015 study compared two groups of Medicare Advantage patients who were hospitalized and subsequently admitted to a SNF—one group of patients insured through plans that removed the 3-Day Rule and one group insured through plans that did not—and found that rule removal was associated with overall reduced hospital length of stay.

Lastly, systems factors discussed in this chapter have important equity implications. Studies have found that lower income patients and patients from racial and ethnic minority groups are more likely to be hospitalized under observation status than under inpatient status and face higher costs than higher income patients. In addition, patients living in socially disadvantaged areas are more likely to experience repeat hospitalizations under observation status, compounding the financial burden they face. Within programs such as Medicare that require inpatient status hospitalization prior to SNF care, disproportionate use of observation status in historically marginalized populations also has equity implications for access to SNF care.

Under a DRG-based system, patients from racial and ethnic minority groups have a higher risk of hospital readmission than other groups both before and after implementation of the HRRP. In addition, despite its intention of improving quality of care by reducing readmissions, HRRP was initially designed to evaluate and penalize hospitals using a uniform national readmission rate. One equity consequence was that hospitals that cared for a larger proportion of underserved populations—frequently named "safety net" hospitals—were penalized at higher rates than nonsafety net hospitals. This was addressed in subsequent HRRP adjustments so that hospitals were compared to others caring for communities with similar social complexity.

The role of third-party payers in setting care standards also has important equity implications. For example, after the passage of Title VI of the Civil Rights Act of 1964, which forbade segregation based on race or national origin, many US hospitals still continued to enforce racial segregation. When Medicare was established just 1 year later, the program explicitly tied hospital eligibility for reimbursement to compliance with the Civil Rights Act. Within months of setting this standard, the federal government deployed hundreds of employees and volunteers to ensure that hospitals complied and threatened to withhold federal reimbursements from any hospital that continued to segregate patients based on race. This standard and its implementation represent how a third-party payer can advance health equity.

Multiple-Choice Questions

1. Which of the following entities is a third-party payer that explicitly supports graduate medical education in teaching hospitals?
   A. The Joint Commission
   B. Blue Cross
   C. Medicare
   D. Medicaid

2. An 81-year-old man is evaluated in the ER for acute chest pain. Upon initial evaluation, he tests negative for acute myocardial infarction, but he is admitted under observation status for further monitoring. The patient's observation stay is covered under which part of Medicare?
   A. Part A
   B. Part B
   C. Part C
   D. All the above

3. Medicare reimburses most hospitalizations under inpatient status by which of the following?
   A. Specific costs the hospital incurred to care for the individual patient
   B. Average resources needed to care for a patient with a particular acute illness, comorbidities, and complications
   C. Fee-for-service basis, where each individual service the hospital provides is assigned a relative value unit and then converted to US dollars
   D. Flat daily fee for each day a patient is hospitalized

4. An 80-year-old man insured through Medicare is admitted to the hospital for pneumonia 2 weeks after hip replacement surgery. Under what circumstances would this patient qualify for a SNF stay?
   A. Two-day hospitalization under observation status
   B. Six-day hospitalization under inpatient status with ongoing nursing and therapy needs at the time of discharge
   C. Six-day hospitalization under inpatient status without ongoing nursing or therapy needs at the time of discharge
   D. Four-day hospitalization, inclusive of 2 days under observation status and 2 days under inpatient status

Answers

1. The correct answer is C. Medicare is the only third-party payer that explicitly supports graduate medical education in teaching hospitals through two types of payments (direct and indirect).

2. The correct answer is B. Care under observation status is reimbursed through Medicare Part B, while care under inpatient status is reimbursed through Medicare Part A.

3. The correct answer is B. Hospitals are paid via diagnosis-based reimbursement, which is based on the average resources needed to care for a patient with a particular acute illness, comorbidities, and complications.

4. The correct answer is B. This is the only patient whose hospitalization under inpatient status would satisfy Medicare's 3-Day Rule to qualify for a SNF stay.

Bibliography

Accreditation Commission for Health Care. About ACHC accreditation. https://www.achc.org/about-accreditation/

Alliance for Health Policy. Third party payer. https://www.allhealthpolicy.org/glossary/third-party-payer

American College of Emergency Physicians. APC (Ambulatory Payment Classifications) FAQ. https://www.acep.org/administration/reimbursement/reimbursement-faqs/apc-ambulatory-payment-classifications-faq

American Council on Aging. What is nursing home level of care & its importance to Medicaid eligibility. https://www.medicaidplanningassistance.org/nursing-home-level-of-care/

American Hospital Association. Underpayment by Medicare and Medicaid fact sheet. Published January 2019. https://www.aha.org/system/files/2019-01/underpayment-by-medicare-medicaid-fact-sheet-jan-2019.pdf

American Medical Student Association. The health equity legacy of Medicare and Medicaid. Published July 30, 2021. https://www.amsa.org/the-health-equity-legacy-of-medicare-and-medicaid/

American Society for Health Care Engineering. Academic medical centers. https://www.ashe.org/advocacy/orgs/amc

Aminov RI. A brief history of the antibiotic era: lessons learned and challenges for the future. *Front Microbiol*. 2010;1:134.

Anderson A, Mills CW, Willits J, et al. Follow-up post-discharge and readmission disparities among Medicare fee-for-service beneficiaries, 2018. *J Gen Intern Med*. 2022;37(12):3020-3028.

Association of American Medical Colleges. Graduate medical education (GME): payments to teaching hospitals. https://www.aamc.org/about-us/mission-areas/health-care/graduate-medical-education-gme-payments-teaching-hospitals

Audit of Observation Service Billing by PPS Hospitals. Office of the Inspector General OoAS, H.H.S. Common Identification Number: A-06-01-00028. https://oig.hhs.gov/documents/audit/4786/A-06-01-00028-Complete%20Report.pdf

Banerjee S, Paasche-Orlow MK, McCormick D, Lin MY, Hanchate AD. Readmissions performance and penalty experience of safety-net hospitals under Medicare's hospital readmissions reduction program. *BMC Health Serv Res.* 2022;22(1).

Barouni M, Ahmadian L, Anari HS, Mohsenbeigi E. Challenges and adverse outcomes of implementing reimbursement mechanisms based on the diagnosis-related group classification system: a systematic review. *Sultan Qaboos Univ Med J.* 2020;20(3):260-270.

Beazley S. *Eight Decades of Health Care.* Hospital and Health Networks; 2007.

Berwanger O, Polanczyk CA, Rosito G. Chest pain observation units for patients with symptoms suggestive of acute cardiac ischaemia. *Cochrane Database Syst Rev.* 2017;2017(11).

Boccuti C, Casillas G. Aiming for fewer hospital U-turns: the Medicare hospital readmission reduction program. Kaiser Family Foundation. Published March 10, 2017. https://www.kff.org/medicare/issue-brief/aiming-for-fewer-hospital-u-turns-the-medicare-hospital-readmission-reduction-program/

Carter GM, Jacobson PD, Kominski GF, Perry MJ. Use of diagnosis-related groups by non-Medicare payers. *Health Care Financ Rev.* 1994;16(2):127.

Catlin A, Cowan C. National health spending 1960-2013. *Health Aff.* 2015. https://www.healthaffairs.org/content/forefront/national-health-spending-1960-2013

Center for Improvement in Healthcare Quality. Welcome: hospitals. https://cihq.org/acc-default-hospitals.asp

Centers for Medicare and Medicaid Services. Benefits. https://www.medicaid.gov/medicaid/benefits/index.html

Centers for Medicare and Medicaid Services. CMS Manual System. Department of Health & Human Services (DHHS). Pub 100-02 Medicare Benefit Policy. Transmittal 215. January 2016 Update of the Hospital Outpatient Prospective Payment System (OPPS). https://www.cms.gov/regulations-and-guidance/guidance/transmittals/downloads/r215bp.pdf

Centers for Medicare and Medicaid Services. Custodial care vs. skilled care. https://www.cms.gov/Medicare-Medicaid-Coordination/Fraud-Prevention/Medicaid-Integrity-Education/Downloads/infograph-CustodialCarevsSkilledCare-%5BMarch-2016%5D.pdf

Centers for Medicare and Medicaid Services. Fact sheet: two-midnight rule. https://www.cms.gov/newsroom/fact-sheets/fact-sheet-two-midnight-rule

Centers for Medicare and Medicaid Services. February 2024 Medicaid & CHIP enrollment data highlights. https://www.medicaid.gov/medicaid/program-information/medicaid-and-chip-enrollment-data/report-highlights/index.html

Centers for Medicare and Medicaid Services. Hospital outpatient prospective payment system (OPPS). https://www.cms.gov/cms-guide-medical-technology-companies-and-other-interested-parties/payment/opps

Centers for Medicare and Medicaid Services. Hospital Readmissions Reduction Program (HRRP). https://www.cms.gov/medicare/payment/prospective-payment-systems/acute-inpatient-pps/hospital-readmissions-reduction-program-hrrp

Centers for Medicare and Medicaid Services. Medicaid eligibility. https://www.medicaid.gov/medicaid/eligibility/index.html

Centers for Medicare and Medicaid Services. Medicare CY 2016 outpatient prospective payment system (OPPS) proposed rule claims accounting. http://www.cms.gov/medicare/medicare-fee-for-service-payment/hospitaloutpatientpps/downloads/cms-1633-p-opps-claims-accounting.pdf

Centers for Medicare and Medicaid Services. Medicare monthly enrollment. https://data.cms.gov/summary-statistics-on-beneficiary-enrollment/medicare-and-medicaid-reports/medicare-monthly-enrollment/data

Centers for Medicare and Medicaid Services. Medicare Outpatient Observation Notice (MOON). https://www.cms.gov/newsroom/fact-sheets/medicare-outpatient-observation-notice-moon

Centers for Medicaid and Medicaid Services. Medicare program—general information. https://www.cms.gov/about-cms/what-we-do/medicare

Centers for Medicare and Medicaid Services. MS-DRG classifications and software. https://www.cms.gov/medicare/payment/prospective-payment-systems/acute-inpatient-pps/ms-drg-classifications-and-software

Centers for Medicare and Medicaid Services. New steps to encourage efficiency and quality for Medicare hospital outpatient services in 2008. Published November 1, 2007. https://www.cms.gov/newsroom/press-releases/new-steps-encourage-efficiency-and-quality-medicare-hospital-outpatient-services-2008

Centers for Medicare and Medicaid Services. NHE fact sheet. https://www.cms.gov/data-research/statistics-trends-and-reports/national-health-expenditure-data/nhe-fact-sheet

Centers for Medicare and Medicaid Services. Parts of Medicare. https://www.medicare.gov/basics/get-started-with-medicare/medicare-basics/parts-of-medicare

Centers for Medicare and Medicaid Services. PPS-exempt cancer hospitals (PCHs). https://www.cms.gov/medicare/payment/prospective-payment-systems/acute-inpatient-pps/pps-exempt-cancer-hospitals-pchs

Centers for Medicare and Medicaid Services. Recovery auditing in Medicare for fiscal year 2014—FY 2014 report to Congress as required by Section 1893(h) of the Social Security Act. https://www.cms.gov/Research-Statistics-Data-and-Systems/Monitoring-Programs/Medicare-FFS-Compliance-Programs/Recovery-Audit-Program/Downloads/FY-2014-Medicare-FFS-RAC-Report-to-Congress---.pdf

Centers for Medicare and Medicaid Services. Rules and regulations. *Fed Regist.* 2007;72(227): 66580-67225. https://www.govinfo.gov/content/pkg/FR-2007-11-27/html/07-5507.htm

Centers for Medicare and Medicaid Services. Skilled nursing facility (SNF) care. https://www.medicare.gov/coverage/skilled-nursing-facility-snf-care

Centers for Medicare and Medicaid Services. Skilled nursing facility (SNF) situations. https://www.medicare.gov/what-medicare-covers/skilled-nursing-facility-snf-situations

Centers for Medicare and Medicaid Services, HHS, ed. Medicare program: changes to the hospital outpatient prospective payment system for calendar year 2008; final rule. *Fed Regist.* 2007;72(227): 66646-66652.

Chaiyachati KH, Qi M, Werner RM. Changes to racial disparities in readmission rates after Medicare's hospital readmissions reduction program within safety-net and non–safety-net hospitals. *JAMA Netw Open.* 2018;1(7):e184154.

Chen YJ, Zhang XY, Yan JQ, Xue-Tang, Qian MC, Ying XH. Impact of diagnosis-related groups on inpatient quality of health care: a systematic review and meta-analysis. *Inquiry.* 2023;60:1-16.

Chidambaram P, Burns A. A look at nursing facility characteristics between 2015 and 2023. Kaiser Family Foundation. Published January 5, 2024. https://www.kff.org/medicaid/issue-brief/a-look-at-nursing-facility-characteristics/

Clark LJ, Field MJ, Koontz TL, Koontz VL. The impact of Hill-Burton: an analysis of hospital bed and physician distribution in the United States, 1950-1970. *Med Care*. 1980;18(5):532-550.

Coffey RM, Barrett ML, Steiner S. Final report observation status related to hospital records. HCUP Methods Series Report #2002-3. Agency for Healthcare Research and Quality. Published online September 27, 2002. https://hcup-us.ahrq.gov/reports/methods/FinalReportonObservationStatus_v2Final.pdf

Collins AS. Preventing health care–associated infections. In: Hughes RG, ed. *Patient Safety and Quality: An Evidence-Based Handbook for Nurses*. Agency for Healthcare Research and Quality (US). Published online 2008. https://www.ncbi.nlm.nih.gov/books/NBK2683/

Congressional Research Service. Medicare graduate medical education payments: an overview. https://crsreports.congress.gov/product/pdf/IF/IF10960

Cubanski J, Neuman T. What to know about Medicare spending and financing. Kaiser Family Foundation. Published January 19, 2023. https://www.kff.org/medicare/issue-brief/what-to-know-about-medicare-spending-and-financing/

Department of Health & Human Services, Centers for Medicare and Medicaid Services. CMS Manual System. Department of Health & Human Services (DHHS). Pub. 100-07 State Operations. Provider certification II. Centers for Medicare and Medicaid Services; 2020.

DNV Healthcare USA Hospital Accreditation for Acute Care, Critical Access, and Psychiatric. https://www.dnv.us/services/hospital-accreditation-218999/

Goldstein JN, Zhang Z, Schwartz JS, Hicks LRS. Observation status, poverty and high financial liability among Medicare beneficiaries. *Am J Med*. 2018;131(1):101.e9.

Gonçalves-Bradley DC, Lannin NA, Clemson L, Cameron ID, Shepperd S. Discharge planning from hospital. *Cochrane Database Syst Rev*. 2022;2(2).

Grebla RC, Keohane L, Lee Y, Lipsitz LA, Rahman M, Trivedi AN. Waiving the three-day rule: admissions and length-of-stay at hospitals and skilled nursing facilities did not increase. *Health Aff (Millwood)*. 2015;34(8):1324-1330.

Health Care Financing Administration, HHS, ed. Medicare program: prospective payment system for hospital outpatient services proposed rule. *Fed Regist*. 1998;63(173):47570.

Health Care Financing Administration, HHS, ed. Medicare program: prospective payment system for hospital outpatient services; final rule. *Fed Regist*. 2000;65(68):18443, 18448, 18450.

Hyndman IJ. Rheumatoid arthritis: past, present and future approaches to treating the disease. *Int J Rheum Dis*. 2017;20(4):417-419.

Institute of Medicine (US) Committee on Employment-Based Health Benefits, Field MJ, Shapiro HT, eds. *Origins and Evolution of Employment-Based Health Benefits*. National Academies Press. Published online 1993. https://www.ncbi.nlm.nih.gov/books/NBK235989/

Institute of Medicine (US) Committee on Implementing a National Graduate Medical Education Trust Fund. *Appendix B: History and Current Status of Medicare Graduate Medical Education Funding*. National Academies Press. Published online 1997. https://www.ncbi.nlm.nih.gov/books/NBK233563/

Jeon CY, Neidell M, Jia H, Sinisi M, Larson E. On the role of length of stay in healthcare-associated bloodstream infection. *Infect Control Hosp Epidemiol*. 2012;33(12):1213-1218.

Joynt KE, Orav EJ, Jha AK. Thirty-day readmission rates for Medicare beneficiaries by race and site of care. *JAMA*. 2011;305(7):675-681.

Kaiser Family Foundation. Medicaid's role in nursing home care. Published June 20, 2017. https://www.kff.org/infographic/medicaids-role-in-nursing-home-care/

Kaiser Family Foundation. Status of state Medicaid expansion decisions: interactive map. Published December 1, 2023. https://www.kff.org/medicaid/issue-brief/status-of-state-medicaid-expansion-decisions-interactive-map/

Legal Information Institute. Electronic Code of Federal Regulations (e-CFR): 42 CFR § 409.30—basic requirements. *US Law*. https://www.law.cornell.edu/cfr/text/42/409.30

Levinson DR. Vulnerabilities remain under Medicare's 2-midnight hospital policy. Department of Health and Human Services, Office of the Inspector General; 2016. https://oig.hhs.gov/oei/reports/oei-02-15-00020.asp

Lopez E, Neuman T, Jacobson G, Levitt L. How much more than Medicare do private insurers pay? A review of the literature. Kaiser Family Foundation. Published April 15, 2020. https://www.kff.org/medicare/issue-brief/how-much-more-than-medicare-do-private-insurers-pay-a-review-of-the-literature/

Mann C, Striar A. How differences in Medicaid, Medicare, and commercial health insurance payment rates impact access, health equity, and cost. Commonwealth Fund. Published August 17, 2022. https://www.commonwealthfund.org/blog/2022/how-differences-medicaid-medicare-and-commercial-health-insurance-payment-rates-impact

Masri A, Althouse AD, McKibben J, et al. Outcomes of heart failure admissions under observation versus short inpatient stay. *J Am Heart Assoc*. 2018;7(3):e007944.

Medicare.gov. Frequently asked questions: Medicare Outpatient Observation Notice. Centers for Medicare and Medicaid Services; 2016. https://www.cms.gov/Medicare/Medicare-General-Information/BNI/Downloads/MOON-FAQs.docx

Medicare Learning Network. Information for critical access hospital. Centers for Medicare and Medicaid Services; 2018. https://www.cms.gov/files/document/mln006400-information-critical-access-hospitals.pdf

Medicare Payment Advisory Commission. Report to the Congress: Medicare payment policy. Hospital inpatient and outpatient services. Published March 2014. https://www.medpac.gov/wp-content/uploads/import_data/scrape_files/docs/default-source/reports/mar14_entirereport.pdf

Meng Z, Hui W, Cai Y, Liu J, Wu H. The effects of DRGs-based payment compared with cost-based payment on inpatient healthcare utilization: a systematic review and meta-analysis. *Health Policy*. 2020;124(4):359-367.

Mor V. A brief history of the 3-day hospital stay rule. *JAMA Intern Med*. 2023;183(7):645-646.

Morrisey MA. *Health Insurance*. Health Administration Press; 2014.

Nordham KD, Ninokawa S. The history of organ transplantation. *Proc (Bayl Univ Med Cent)*. 2022;35(1):124.

Nowicki M. *The Financial Management of Hospitals and Healthcare Organizations*. Health Administration Press; 2004.

Patel N, Slota JM, Miller BJ. The continued conundrum of discharge to a skilled nursing facility after a Medicare observation stay. *JAMA Health Forum*. 2020;1(5):e200577.

Quinn K. After the revolution: DRGs at age 30. *Ann Intern Med*. 2014;160(6):426-429.

Rahman M, Meyers DJ, Wright B. Unintended consequences of observation stay use may disproportionately burden Medicare beneficiaries in disadvantaged neighborhoods. *Mayo Clin Proc*. 2020;95(12):2589-2591.

Rambachan A, Abe-Jones Y, Fernandez A, Shahram Y. Racial disparities in 7-day readmissions from an adult hospital medicine service. *J Racial Ethn Health Disparities*. 2022;9(4):1500-1505.

Rau J. 10 years of hospital readmissions penalties. Kaiser Family Foundation. Published November 4, 2021. https://www.kff.org/affordable-care-act/slide/10-years-of-hospital-readmissions-penalties/

Rep. Stark FP [D C 9]. H.R.2470—100th Congress (1987-1988): Medicare Catastrophic Coverage Act of 1988. Published online 1988. https://www.congress.gov/bill/100th-congress/house-bill/2470

Rice T, Desmond K, Gabel J. The Medicare Catastrophic Coverage Act: a post-mortem. *Health Aff (Millwood)*. 1990;9(3):75-87.

Rogers WH, Draper D, Kahn KL, et al. Quality of care before and after implementation of the DRG-based prospective payment system: a summary of effects. *JAMA*. 1990;264(15):1989-1994.

Rogstad TL, Gupta S, Connolly J, Shrank WH, Roberts ET. Social risk adjustment in the hospital readmissions reduction program: a systematic review and implications for policy. *Health Aff (Millwood)*. 2022;41(9):1307-1315.

Rosenberg CE. *The Care of Strangers: The Rise of America's Hospital System*. Johns Hopkins University Press; 1987.

Ross MA, Granovsky M. History, principles, and policies of observation medicine. *Emerg Med Clin North Am*. 2017;35(3):503-518.

Sabbatini AK, Joynt-Maddox KE, Liao J, et al. Accounting for the growth of observation stays in the assessment of Medicare's hospital readmissions reduction program. *JAMA Netw Open*. 2022;5(11):e2242587.

Sabbatini AK, Wright B, Hall MK, Basu A. The cost of observation care for commercially insured patients visiting the emergency department. *Am J Emerg Med*. 2018;36(9):1591-1596.

Schotland S, Werner RM, Weiner J. Medicare payment policy for post-acute care in nursing homes. Penn Leonard Davis Institute of Health Economics. Published September 14, 2023. https://ldi.upenn.edu/our-work/research-updates/medicare-payment-policy-for-post-acute-care-in-nursing-homes/

Social Security Administration. How social security helped desegregate America's hospitals. Published February 19, 2021. https://blog.ssa.gov/how-social-security-helped-desegregate-americas-hospitals/

Society of Hospital Medicine. Policy & advocacy: current issues: observation care. https://www.hospitalmedicine.org/policy--advocacy/current-issues/observation-status/

Tan SY, Ponstein N. Jonas Salk (1914–1995): a vaccine against polio. *Singapore Med J*. 2019;60(1):9.

The Joint Commission announces the 2009 National Patient Safety Goals and requirements. *Jt Comm Perspect*. 2008;28(7):1-15.

The Joint Commission. Hospital accreditation. https://www.jointcommission.org/what-we-offer/accreditation/health-care-settings/hospital/

The Joint Commission. Hospital: 2024 National Patient Safety Goals. https://www.jointcommission.org/standards/national-patient-safety-goals/hospital-national-patient-safety-goals/

Ulyte A, Waken RJ, Epstein AM, et al. Medicare skilled nursing facility use and spending before and after introduction of the public health emergency waiver during the COVID-19 pandemic. *JAMA Intern Med*. 2023;183(7):637-645.

Villagrana MA, Heisler EJ, Romero PD. Closed, converted, merged, and new hospitals with Medicare rural designations: January 2018-November 2022. Assistant Secretary for Planning and Evaluation; 2023. https://crsreports.congress.gov/product/pdf/R/R47526

Wall BM. Healthcare as product: Catholic sisters confront charity and the hospital marketplace, 1865-1925. In: Strasser S, ed. *Commodifying Everything: Relationships of the Market*. Routledge; 2003:143-168.

Washington State Health Care Authority. Hospital reimbursement. https://www.hca.wa.gov/billers-providers-partners/prior-authorization-claims-and-billing/hospital-reimbursement

Weiner SM. "Reasonable Cost" Reimbursement for inpatient hospital services under Medicare and Medicaid: the emergence of public control. *Am J Law Med*. 1977;3(1):1-47.

Wiler JL, Ross MA, Ginde AA. National study of emergency department observation services. *Acad Emerg Med*. 2011;18(9):959-965.

Wright B, Dusetzina SB, Upchurch G. Medicare's variation in out-of-pocket costs for prescriptions: the irrational examples of in-hospital observation and home infusion. *J Am Geriatr Soc*. 2018;66(12):2249-2253.

Zuckerman S, Skopec L, Aarons J. Medicaid physician fees remained substantially below fees paid by Medicare in 2019. *Health Aff*. 2021;40(2):343-348.

4

Transitions After Hospital Care

Clinical Case

The team social worker (Lynn) and the team discharge planner (Joseph) come to Jessica's room to explain the care supports that she may need to continue her recovery after hospital discharge. Jessica explains that she has never been hospitalized before and does not know much about the resources she will need. Jessica asks how the hospital will work to ensure that she continues to recover upon leaving and that her condition does not worsen resulting in a repeat hospitalization.

While multiple factors affect patient care within specific care settings (eg, ambulatory, emergency room [ER], hospital), systems factors also drive how patients transition between settings. Broadly, transitions of care are defined by the Centers for Medicare and Medicaid Services as "movement of a patient from one setting of care to another, which may include hospitals, ambulatory primary care practices, ambulatory specialty care practices, long-term care facilities, home health, and rehabilitation facilities." Among different types of transitions, the one between hospital and postdischarge care settings can be particularly salient given the need for care coordination of treatment plans, medications, and other changes made during hospitalization that require subsequent follow-up management. In this way, the elements of high-quality transitions after hospital care are an important systems factor for patients.

SYSTEMS FACTOR: ELEMENTS OF HIGH-QUALITY TRANSITIONS AFTER HOSPITAL CARE

High-quality transitions after hospital care tend to have two elements. First, patients must have timely access to follow-up visits with their ambulatory care clinicians and care teams. Secondly, ambulatory clinicians and teams must

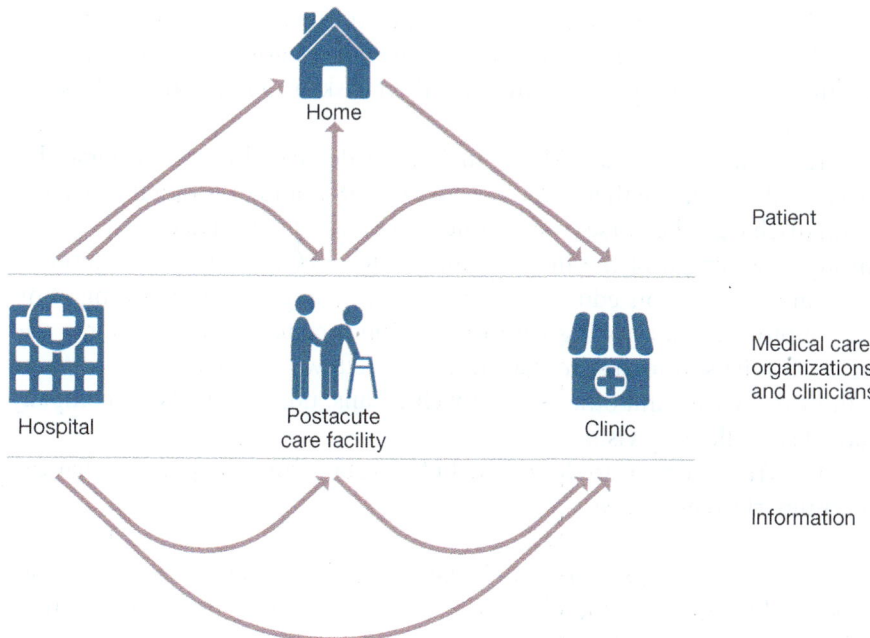

Figure 4.1 High-Quality Transitions After Hospital Care. (Source: Data from Workshop images from Design Institute for Health at the University of Texas at Austin.)

have comprehensive and actionable information regarding patients' hospitalization. Without this information, ambulatory care clinicians may not be aware of critical test results, medication changes, or new treatment plans enacted during patients' hospitalizations. Information regarding patients' hospitalization must be communicated from the clinicians in the hospital to those in the ambulatory setting (Figure 4.1). ·

Approaches to Transitions to Home After Hospital Care

A number of approaches have emerged for achieving high-quality transitions to home after hospital care. Three notable examples targeting transitions from hospital to home settings include the Transitional Care Model, the Care Transitions Intervention, and Project Better Outcomes for Older adults through Safe Transitions (BOOST).

Transitional Care Model

Developed in 1981, the Transitional Care Model is a nurse-led intervention originally designed to improve transitions for chronically ill, older patients transitioning from hospital to home. First, the model identifies patients with higher risk of readmissions based on the following factors: one or more chronic illnesses, more than one hospitalization within the past 6 months, polypharmacy, and living alone. Once identified, patients are enrolled into the model with the goal of reducing their risk of 30- to 60-day hospital readmissions.

The Transitional Care Model includes a dedicated program nurse that meets with patients either prior to or within 48 hours of hospital discharge. Upon discharge, the nurse conducts home visits and is available 7 days a week through the length of the intervention, which can extend up to 2 months. The nurse focuses on educating patients and caregivers, monitoring clinical symptoms, and assisting with medication reconciliation. The nurse also serves as a liaison to ensure that necessary follow-up visits are coordinated with primary care and other specialty clinicians; nurses can also accompany patients to follow-up visits.

The Transitional Care Model includes certain core components that can be summarized as follows:

Delivering services from hospital to home. In the model, patient visits by nurses begin during a hospital admission and continue after the patient returns home following discharge.

Screening at-risk older adults. The model involves the use of a standardized protocol to identify and enroll hospitalized older adults who are at risk for poor outcomes.

Relying on nurses. The model relies on nurses to assume primary responsibility for services focused on managing patients throughout episodes of acute illness.

Promoting continuity. The model is designed to prevent breakdowns in care from hospital to home by having a nurse involved across these care settings. During visits with patients, the nurse uses evidence-based strategies to communicate patients' highest priority needs, goals, and plans of care.

Coordinating care. The model seeks to promote communication and connections between clinicians in hospital and ambulatory settings.

Collaborating with patients, caregivers, and the care team. The model promotes collaboration and consensus on a plan of care between older adults, family caregivers, and members of the care team.

Maintaining relationships with patients and caregivers. The model seeks to enable the nurse to establish and maintain a trusting relationship with patients and their caregivers.

Engaging patients and caregivers. The model engages older adults in design and implementation of the plan of care aligned with their goals, preferences, and values.

Managing symptoms and other risks. The model identifies and addresses patients' priority risk factors and symptoms.

Educating and promoting self-management. The model prepares patients and caregivers to identify and respond quickly to worsening symptoms.

The Transitional Care Model has been associated with lower readmission risk and related costs for medical care organizations. In particular, studies have demonstrated that patients enrolled in the model experienced reductions in preventable hospital readmissions at 6 weeks, 6 months, and 1 year after hospital discharge. These patients also had improvements in health outcomes, such as overall quality of life and patient satisfaction. Furthermore, a study among Medicare Advantage patients found that those receiving care under the Transitional Care Model exhibited a per-patient cost savings of $2170 over the 1-year period compared to patients in a control group.

Care Transitions Intervention

Developed in 2003, the Care Transitions Intervention is another approach that seeks to improve the quality of care during transitions from hospital to home. Designed on the basis of inputs from patients and their caregivers, the intervention aims to engage and activate patients in managing their health conditions. The intervention is designed to last 30 days and targets patients 65 years and older who often have chronic illnesses such as congestive heart failure, chronic obstructive pulmonary disease, and diabetes.

The Care Transitions Intervention comprises five visits and a "transitions coach." The model begins with a visit while the patient is in the hospital. A transitions coach—a nurse, social worker, community worker, or trained volunteer—meets with the patient and caregivers to discuss any concerns. Upon discharge, the coach conducts a follow-up home visit and three follow-up phone calls, with interactions focused on increasing the patient's and/or their caregivers' confidence in the following Four Pillars of the Care Transitions Intervention, which can be summarized as follows:

Medication self-management. Comprehending and managing their medications

Dynamic patient-centered health record. Using the electronic health record to facilitate communication and continuity of care across clinicians and settings

Primary care and specialist follow-up. Scheduling and completing follow-up visits with clinicians as an active participant in their care

Knowledge of red flags. Understanding about when their condition is worsening and an action plan for how to respond

The Care Transitions Intervention has been associated with reductions in hospital readmissions and related costs. Studies show that patients who are enrolled in the intervention experience fewer hospital readmissions at 30, 60, and 180 days after hospital discharge. In addition, studies show that Medicare patients receiving care through the intervention can have lower health care costs and utilization during the 180 days after hospital discharge, leading to an average cost savings of $3762 compared to those not enrolled in the intervention.

Project Better Outcomes for Older adults through Safe Transitions (Project BOOST)

Developed in 2008, BOOST is a project that aims to reduce medication-related errors, reduce 30-day readmission rates, and improve clinician workflow. The project is intended for use by clinicians and nonclinicians (case managers, social workers, etc) in the care team and is designed to span several months. Desired outcomes are anticipated after 12 months of implementation.

Medical care organizations implementing BOOST join a learning network of participating peer organizations around the country to share challenges and lessons learned. Although there are some differences across participating organizations, they share key characteristics, which can be summarized as follows:

Assessing the patient's risk for adverse events after hospital discharge. Participants use the 8Ps Risk Assessment tool—which assesses problems with medications, psychological needs, principal diagnosis, physical limitations, poor health literacy, poor social support, prior hospitalizations, and palliative care—as a checklist of risks that should be identified and addressed.

Assessing the patient's preparedness for transitioning out of the hospital. Participants use the General Assessment of Preparedness checklist to identify the patient's logistic and psychological preparedness to transition out of the hospital.

Patient-centered written discharge instructions. Participants use two tools—the Patient Preparation to Address Situations Successfully tool and the Discharge Patient Education tool—to compile and convey essential information at hospital discharge at an appropriate literacy level.

Teach-back method. Participants use the teach-back method, a patient-centered communication style, designed to ensure that the patient comprehends information from clinicians and can explain in their own words what they have learned.

Follow-up telephone calls. Participants make follow-up phone calls to the patient in order to address common difficulties, such as medication reconciliation.

Follow-up visits. Participants assist the patient and their caregivers with scheduling follow-up visits and identifying potential barriers such as transportation.

Interprofessional rounds. Participants conduct interprofessional or interdisciplinary rounds to improve communication and coordination among care team members.

Postacute care transitions. Participants leverage existing partnerships between hospitals and skilled nursing facilities to improve care transitions.

Medication reconciliation. Participants use best practices to reduce medication discrepancies and identify if a patient is at high risk for developing medication-related complications.

Project BOOST has been associated with reductions in 30-day readmissions after 12 months of implementation, but, historically, data about cost implications have been scant. The 8Ps Risk Assessment tool has also been shown to predict approximately 90% of readmissions for patients 65 years and older.

Back to the Clinical Case

If offered at the patient's hospital, approaches such as the Transitional Care Model, the Care Transitions Intervention, and Project BOOST could benefit the patient by promoting high-quality transitions from hospital after discharge. Although specific processes and methods vary across different approaches, the patient could benefit from the shared emphasis on early planning (eg, beginning during hospitalization and before discharge) and coordinated services across the transition period (eg, visits or interactions with clinical team members).

TAKEAWAYS

- High-quality transitions involve patients having timely access to follow-up visits with their ambulatory clinicians who have comprehensive and actionable information regarding patients' hospitalization.
- Approaches such as the Transitional Care Model, the Care Transitions Intervention, and Project BOOST have been widely adopted to improve patient transitions from hospital to home.
- Implementation of these approaches has been associated with benefits including fewer readmissions and lower health care costs.

Clinical Case Continued

The discharge planner explains that the first step of planning for Jessica's transition after hospitalization is to identify medical or nonmedical barriers that could impede a timely discharge. With respect to medical barriers, the discharge planner convenes with Jessica's clinicians about her postacute care rehabilitation needs, as well as any cognitive impairment that could hinder decision-making. The discharge planner also assesses for nonmedical barriers and confirms that Jessica is safely housed and lives with her husband.

Timely treatment and discharge from the hospital can decrease patients' risk of hospital-acquired infections, falls, and functional decline. Delayed discharges can also negatively impact cognitive and mental health for older patients. For medical care organizations, delayed discharges contribute to higher patient censuses, greater clinician workload, and greater costs. Higher patient censuses can affect hospital operations by increasing the number of patients waiting in the ER for hospital beds, delaying transfers within and between hospitals, and contributing to cancellation of elective procedures. Simply put, delayed discharges can be detrimental to both patients and medical care organizations.

To prevent delays in patient discharges, clinicians and care teams must address medical and nonmedical barriers to discharge. Medical barriers refer to obstacles that prevent patients who are otherwise sufficiently recovered from their acute conditions to safely leave the hospital. Nonmedical barriers refer to possible financial, health system, decision-making capacity, or other obstacles that hinder patients from being discharged. Unfortunately, there are an increasing number of patients who have recovered from their acute illness or reason for hospitalization who nonetheless remain hospitalized due to nonmedical barriers to discharge. Such barriers to discharge represent a systems factor that can meaningfully affect patient care.

SYSTEMS FACTOR: NONMEDICAL BARRIERS TO PATIENT DISCHARGE

Nonmedical barriers can be categorized into six groups: postacute care facility needs, financial needs, decision-making capacity, disruptive or dangerous patient behaviors, disagreement with discharge plans, and unstable housing (Figure 4.2). The most common barriers are postacute care facility needs and financial needs.

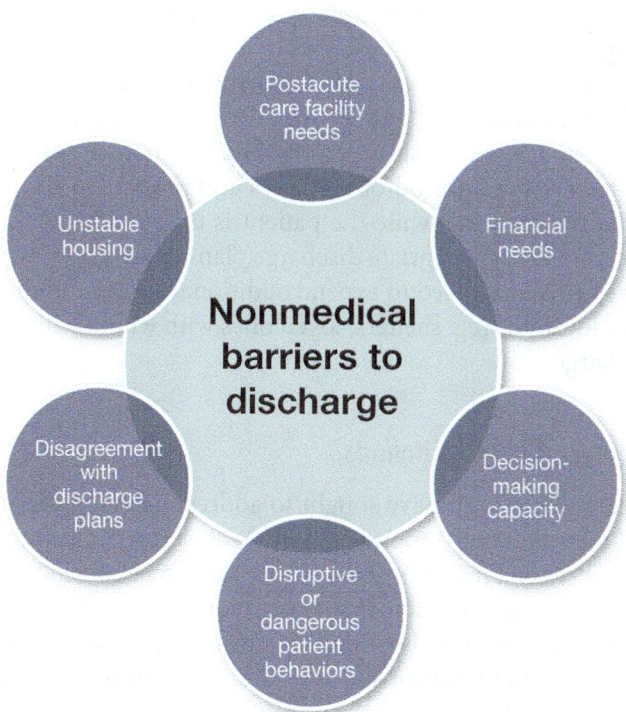

Figure 4.2 Nonmedical Barriers to Discharge. (Source: Data from Meo N, Liao JM, Reddy A. Hospitalized after medical readiness for discharge: a multidisciplinary quality improvement initiative to identify discharge barriers in general medicine patients. *Am J Med Qual.* 2020;35(1):23-28.)

In the case of postacute care facility needs, barriers can include inability to accommodate certain patient care needs, such as dialysis coordination or isolation rooming due to multidrug-resistant organisms. In the case of financial needs, barriers can consist of issues such as lack of insurance; the need for obtaining insurance authorization for postdischarge services; or facility refusal because of patients' unpaid bills from prior stays. In particular, the need to obtain Medicaid coverage—that is, situations in which individuals with low income and no insurance coverage must remain in the hospital until they can obtain Medicaid and become eligible for subsequent care—has been identified to account for more than 40% of delays in patients with delayed discharges.

In the case of decision-making capacity, barriers can include the need to identify surrogate decision-makers or pursue court-appointed guardianship for hospitalized patients, which can take weeks if not longer. Documentation of disruptive patient behaviors, such as physical or verbal aggression, can become barriers that delay or narrow discharge options.

Disagreements with discharge plans between the patient and their caregiver or hospital care team can also create barriers to discharge. An example would be disagreement about the posthospital discharge care setting and plan, with the patient desiring one approach (eg, discharge home to self-care) and caregivers and/or care teams recommending another (eg, discharge to a postacute facility for a period of therapies and monitored recovery). Such situations can require time while the patient is hospitalized to achieve consensus and create safe, appropriate discharge plans. For patients with unstable housing, care teams may need to expend additional efforts and time identifying discharge locations (eg, shelters, loved ones with whom patients can stay) prior to discharge.

Multidisciplinary Discharge Rounds

Medical care organizations have sought to address delays in discharge using multidisciplinary discharge rounds (MDRs), structured meetings in which different members of a patient's hospital care team meet during the course of their hospitalization and collaboratively plan for their discharge.

MDRs typically involve an attending physician, nurses, discharge planners (typically, case managers or social workers), pharmacists, and therapists. MDRs can also include nutritionists, utilization management specialists, and others as available or necessary. All these members can help identify potential nonmedical discharge barriers, such as placement to postacute care facilities or the need for further education regarding medication management.

Typically, MDRs are held at regular times on a recurring basis and organized by either hospital unit (eg, second floor, southeast wing) or service line (eg, internal medicine, emergency general surgery). MDRs can be held in person, virtually, or as a hybrid of both, based on team members' availability and location. Some units or service lines may need to meet more frequently than others.

Organizations can create scripts to ensure that desired topics and questions are being addressed during MDRs in a standardized format. The team starts with demographic information (eg, patient name, age, room number, admission date) and then discusses topics such as anticipated discharge date, discharge location, and care needs (Table 4.1).

In addition to the script, medical care organizations can incorporate a whiteboard (physical or electronic) into MDRs (Figure 4.3). When electronic, the whiteboard is typically a spreadsheet at the nurses' station with a stoplight-based color system to indicate patients' anticipated discharge timeline (red, >2 days to anticipated discharge; yellow, 1-2 days to anticipated discharge; green, day of anticipated discharge). Whiteboards are updated regularly to track patient progress in ways that are visible to all participants in MDRs.

Table 4.1 Example Multidisciplinary Discharge Rounds Script

Discharge Planner	■ Patient name, room number, and admission date ■ When will the patient be discharged (eg, today, within 2 d, >2 d)? ■ What will the patient need for discharge (eg, durable medical equipment, home intravenous antibiotics)? ■ Does the patient have any potential insurance challenges or social work needs? ■ Is this a patient who has complex discharge needs?
Pharmacist	■ What will the patient need for discharge (eg, prior authorizations, medication reconciliation, medication education)? ■ Does the patient have any new medications on discharge? ■ Does the patient have any "high-risk" or "high-cost" medications for discharge? ■ Does the patient have any challenges with medication adherence?
Nurse	■ Does the patient require any lines, tubes, or drains upon discharge? ■ Does the patient have any wound care needs? ■ Does the patient have all of the discharge instructions?

Source: Data from Patel H, Yirdaw E, Yu A, et al. Improving early discharge using a team-based structure for discharge multidisciplinary rounds. *Prof Case Manag*. 2019;24(2):83-89.

MDRs have been associated with a number of benefits. These meetings can reduce the number of delayed discharge days due to nonmedical barriers by nearly 25% and lower the average length of stay by 16%. MDRs have been associated with lower 30-day readmission rates (12.6% in pilot vs 18.9% in control) and greater patient satisfaction percentages on survey results (54.2% in pilot vs 35.1% in control).

Patient	Diagnosis	Discharge Planner	Pharmacist	Nurse	Attending	Notes	Anticipated DC
Patient A	Pneumonia	✓	✓			Wean off O$_2$	
Patient B	CHF					Still sick	
Patient C	UTI, nausea/vomiting		✓	✓	✓	Awaiting placement	
Patient D	Persistent atrial fibrillation	✓	✓	✓	✓	Ready for DC	
Patient E	Constipation	✓	✓	✓	✓	Ready for DC	

Figure 4.3 Multidisciplinary DC Rounds Electronic Whiteboard. CHF, congestive heart failure; DC, discharge; UTI, urinary tract infection. (Source: Data from Bumpas J, Copeland DJ. Standardizing multidisciplinary discharge planning rounds to improve patient perceptions of care transitions. *J Nurs Adm*. 2021;51(2):101-105.)

Back to the Clinical Case

In this patient's case, the care team can address potential nonmedical barriers early on during the patient's hospitalization via MDRs. Using an MDR script, they can identify her care needs (eg, physical therapy for her knee) as well as key considerations and potential obstacles, including nonmedical barriers, to discharge. The care team can anticipate that the patient will likely be discharged during the next 1 to 2 days and can mark her as yellow on the electronic whiteboard.

TAKEAWAYS

- Delayed discharges due to nonmedical barriers—obstacles that result in patients remaining hospitalized despite medical readiness for discharge—can be detrimental to patients and medical care organizations.
- Common nonmedical barriers to patient discharge are postacute facility needs, financial needs, decision-making capacity, disruptive or dangerous patient behaviors, disagreement with discharge plans, and unstable housing.
- Medical care organizations have utilized MDRs to minimize delays in discharge.

Clinical Case Continued

The internal medicine clinician begins to prepare a note summarizing Jessica's hospitalization. The clinician's note provides a brief overview of Jessica's hospitalization, highlighting her tests, diagnoses, and treatments received so far.

The clinician then begins to outline the discharge care plan. Jessica will continue intravenous antibiotics, will need more intensive physical therapy, and will require a close follow-up visit with her orthopedic surgeon upon discharge. The clinician makes note of these key items that Jessica and her primary care clinician will need to know for Jessica's post hospital recovery.

Prior to the 1990s, many primary care clinicians cared for their patients in both the ambulatory and hospital setting. These clinicians generally rounded on patients at the hospital in the mornings, evaluated patients at the clinic in the afternoons, and ended their day with a return to the hospital to follow-up on or admit new patients. Although a number of clinicians still practice in this way, most primary care clinicians now practice exclusively in the ambulatory setting. As a result, patients frequently receive care from different clinicians in the hospital and ambulatory settings.

This dynamic has increased the importance of clear communication during transitions after hospital care. As written summaries of patients' hospital courses and necessary follow-up items, discharge summaries serve as the predominant and, often, the only mode of communication between hospital- and ambulatory-based clinicians. In these ways, thorough and well-written hospital discharge summaries are a key systems factor for promoting safe, high-quality care for individuals discharging from the hospital.

SYSTEMS FACTOR: HOSPITAL DISCHARGE SUMMARIES

Studies show that communication—in the form of hospital discharge summaries—between hospital and ambulatory clinicians only occurs in about 23% to 38% of hospital discharges. Discharge summaries not completed within 3 days of patient discharge have been associated with higher odds of readmissions.

Even for those that are completed on time, discharge summaries have been found to be frequently missing key elements such as a summary of hospital course, test results, and discharge medications. Comprehensive, accurate discharge summaries are crucial for promoting continuity of patient care across hospital and ambulatory settings to decrease the risk of readmissions and decrease overuse of health care (eg, redundant tests, unnecessary medications).

To improve the completeness and accuracy of discharge summaries, The Joint Commission has standardized six mandatory components for accreditation that it believes should be included in all hospital discharge summaries:

- Reason for hospitalization
- Significant findings
- Procedures and treatment provided
- Patient's discharge condition
- Patient and family instructions (as appropriate)
- Attending physician's signature

How these components are organized and composed in discharge summaries vary by clinicians and their medical care organizations.

Over time, primary care clinicians—a major end user group of hospital discharge summaries—have identified more specific content that should be included and content that should be excluded. In particular, primary care clinicians have advocated for inclusion of an actionable to-do list, identification of incidental findings, justification of medication changes, and duration of medication therapy in all discharge summaries. Furthermore, clinicians have reported frustrations with information that they perceive as not pertinent to the ambulatory setting (Table 4.2).

Table 4.2 Primary Care Clinicians' Recommendations on Discharge Summaries

Recommendations	Description	Examples
Inclusion of an actionable to-do list	Include actionable items that the primary care clinician needs to complete in follow-up.	■ Laboratory tests needed within a few days of discharge ■ Pending pathology or cultures ■ Referrals to be placed by the primary care clinician
Identification of incidental findings	List incidental findings.	■ Thyroid or lung nodules
Justification of medication changes	Explain changes in the medication regimen (ie, medications added, discontinued, or modified).	■ Lisinopril was held in a patient with acute kidney injury. ■ Metoprolol was modified to carvedilol (different β-blocker class).
Duration of medication therapy	Provide detailed timing of antibiotics and other high-risk medications.	■ Antibiotics: Start and stop dates, include specific duration for outpatient completion. ■ Anticoagulation: Number of weeks/months expected to be on therapy ■ Opioids: Plan for taper and refills by primary care clinician.
Removal of hospital care–specific information	Avoid including care plans not relevant to ambulatory care.	■ Intravenous potassium repletion ■ Transfusion for hemoglobin levels <7%
Exclusion of irrelevant day-to-day details	Provide a summary rather than day-to-day details during the hospitalization.	■ Instead of listing the variable levels of oxygen needed each day during hospitalization, write a summary such as: "Patient required as much as 3 L of supplemental oxygen due to pneumonia, but at the time of discharge the patient was stable on room air."

Source: Data from Chatterton B, Chen J, Schwarz EB, Karlin J. Primary care physicians' perspectives on high-quality discharge summaries. *J Gen Intern Med*. 2024;39(8):1438-1443.

Discharge Summary Curricula and Tools

Given the importance of hospital discharge summaries, a number of medical centers have designed curricula to improve how clinicians write and prepare these documents. Curricula can include didactic sessions to improve hospital clinicians' understanding of how the summaries are used by their ambulatory-based colleagues, as well as workshops where deidentified example discharge summaries are reviewed for deficiencies and improvement areas. Clinicians can also participate in longitudinal workshops through which they receive serial feedback on their discharge summaries over time.

Medical care organizations have also sought to systematize discharge summary content by developing checklists and templates. For instance, some organizations use pocket-sized laminated checklists to guide clinicians on what should be and should not be written into discharge summaries (Figure 4.4).

Other organizations incorporate discharge summary guidance into electronic health records. Clinicians can access standardized templates (Figure 4.5) meant to promote consistent (eg, via autopopulated fields or prepopulated drop-down menu options), high-quality, and readable documents that provide guidance while permitting flexibility (eg, via open-ended free text fields).

Curricula and tools can be effective in improving the quality of discharge summaries. Some programs have been associated with up to 70% reductions in the average time to discharge summary completion. Some educational

Writing Prototype: Checklist

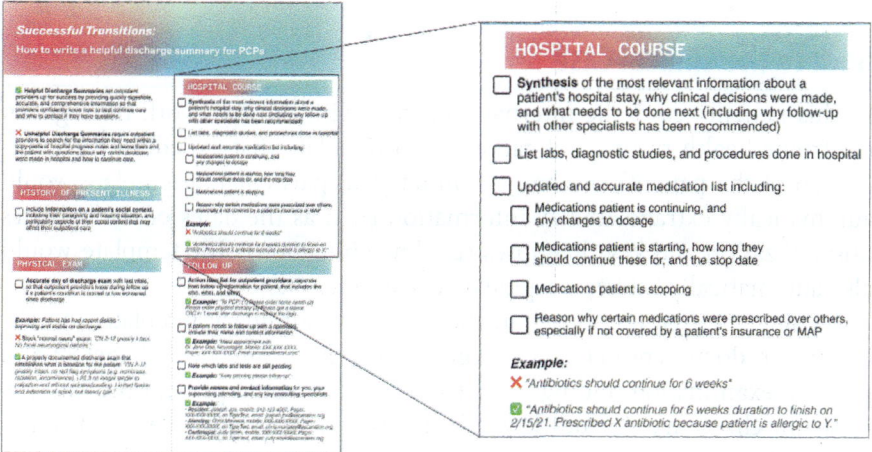

Figure 4.4 Example of a Discharge Summary Checklist. (Source: Reproduced with permission from the University of Texas at Austin.)

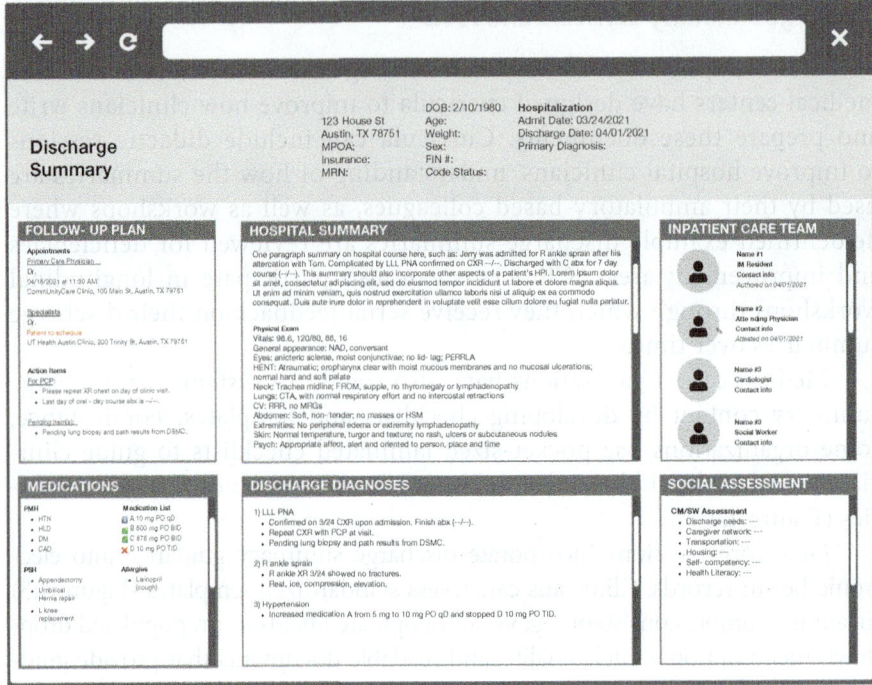

Figure 4.5 Example of a Discharge Summary Template. (Source: Reproduced with permission from the University of Texas at Austin.)

programs have also been associated with 44% reduction in the proportion of discharge summaries that have deficiencies or have been defined as inaccurate or missing key information.

Back to the Clinical Case

In this patient's case, the internal medicine clinician can work through an electronic health record and can access a template that expedites the completion of the patient's discharge summary. In particular, a template would automatically extrapolate key information such as the dates of the patient's hospitalization and key diagnoses (eg, knee infection). The template would also automatically list key hospital care team members.

Using the free text boxes in the discharge summary template, the clinician can document pertinent diagnoses (eg, knee infection, diabetes) and physical examination findings. The template also would prompt the internal medicine clinician to include key information, such as the start and stop dates of the patient's antibiotic treatment, including duration of required outpatient treatment, and needed postdischarge follow-up visit information.

> ## TAKEAWAYS
>
> - As written summaries of patients' hospital courses and necessary follow-up items, discharge summaries serve as the predominant and, often, the only mode of communication between hospital- and ambulatory-based clinicians.
> - Comprehensive, accurate discharge summaries are crucial for promoting continuity of patient care across hospital and ambulatory settings to decrease the risk of readmissions and decrease overuse of health care.
> - While The Joint Commission has standardized mandatory discharge summary components for accreditation, how these components are written vary by clinicians and their medical care organizations.
> - Curricula and tools have been developed to improve the timeliness and quality of discharge summaries.

Clinical Case Continued

Given Jessica's age, past medical history, and hospital course, her hospital care team asks the discharge planner to schedule postdischarge follow-up visits with her primary care clinician and orthopedic surgeon. These are scheduled at the next available date 3 weeks away.

Jessica is discharged home. Five days later, Jessica develops fever and severe pain in her knee in the middle of the night. Unable to arrange an urgent appointment with her ambulatory care clinicians and worried about her worsening condition, the patient returns to the hospital and is readmitted.

Timely follow-up in the ambulatory care setting is vital to high-quality transitions after hospital care. However, the average wait time for patients requiring post-discharge follow-up—the time from scheduling a visit to being seen—has continued to increase in the United States. In 2022, the average wait time was 26 days compared to 21 days in 2004. The average wait time in 2022 for patients to be seen by clinicians in family medicine was about 21 days, compared with 31 days to be seen by clinicians in obstetrics and gynecology, 27 days to be seen by clinicians in cardiology, 17 days to be seen by clinicians in orthopedic surgery, and 35 days to be seen by clinicians in dermatology.

Long wait times can leave patients vulnerable to complications. Patients may need urgent clarification regarding their medication regimen, further instructions on how to dress their wounds, or a better understanding of which clinical symptoms should or should not be cause for concern. If such questions or concerns are not able to be addressed in a timely manner, patients may be left without a choice but to go to the hospital for care. These concerns can be particularly salient for individuals with multiple chronic conditions or complex care needs. In these ways, long visit wait times can be a systems factor that impact transitions after hospital care.

SYSTEMS FACTOR: LONG VISIT WAIT TIMES

Long visit wait times can cause delays in medical care and in turn increase morbidity and mortality risk among patients. Although timely visits with ambulatory clinicians have been shown to improve long-term health outcomes, ambulatory access issues can drive patients to instead seek care in ERs. Among patients who do have an established relationship with a primary care clinician, approximately 70% of patients express that it's easier for them to go to the ER for urgent medical issues than to schedule a clinic visit. Delays in ambulatory care can have significant consequences and lead to hospital readmissions; studies have shown that hospital readmission within 30 days of discharge is responsible for a large proportion of national health care expenditures.

Transitional Care Management Services and Codes

In 2013, the Centers for Medicare and Medicaid Services created billing codes for Transitional Care Management (TCM) services as one way to improve transitions after hospital care while providing clinician incentives to see patients in a timely manner following hospital discharge. TCM services are intended for patients that require moderate- or high-complexity medical decision-making, with the goal to "oversee management and coordination of services, as needed, for all medical conditions, psychosocial needs, and activity of daily living support." Of note, TCM services and their associated billing codes are independent of the nurse-led Transitional Care Model from earlier in this chapter.

Medicare covers TCM services during the 30-day period that begins after a patient is discharged after one of the following circumstances/settings:

- Inpatient status hospitalization
- Observation status hospitalization
- Long-term care hospitalization
- Inpatient rehabilitation facility stay
- Skilled nursing facility stay

- Psychiatric hospitalization
- Partial hospitalization at a community mental health center

For TCM services to be reimbursed, the patient must be discharged to home, domiciliary (eg, group home or boarding house), nursing home, or assisted living facility. TCM services must include both virtual (telephone, video, email) and in-person visits and can be provided by the following clinicians:

- Physicians (any specialty)
- Physician assistants
- Nurse practitioners
- Clinical nurse specialists
- Certified nurse-midwives

Clinicians must have interactive contact (ie, usually a virtual visit) within 2 business days after the patient's discharge. During such a visit, clinicians can review the patient's need for diagnostic tests and treatments, educate the patient and caregivers, and help establish referrals and arrange community-based resources.

In addition, clinicians must also provide an in-person visit within either 1 or 2 weeks of a patient's hospital discharge. For a patient that requires at least moderate-level complexity of medical decision-making, clinicians must see the patient within 14 days of discharge; clinicians must see a patient that requires high-level complexity of medical decision-making within 7 days of discharge.

Postdischarge Clinics

One method of addressing long visit wait times is the use of postdischarge clinics. Postdischarge clinics are intended to bridge care between the hospital and ambulatory clinicians, offering up to several visits to promote continuity of care and complement patients' follow-up with their established ambulatory clinicians.

Postdischarge clinics can be a particularly helpful solution for safety net organizations to secure follow-up visits for patients. For instance, Harborview Medical Center established a postdischarge clinic in Seattle, Washington in 2007 for patients with limited or poor access to other forms of primary care, with the goal of linking patients with long-term primary care at other care sites.

As another example, CareMore Health System—an integrated health plan and medical care organization for Medicare and Medicaid patients—has established postdischarge clinics staffed by clinicians called extensivists. Extensivists help bridge care needs for a panel of patients, including those with complex care needs and multiple chronic conditions. In particular, extensivists follow up their panel of patients for several months across care settings, extending their scope beyond clinics into hospitals and postacute care and providing a range of services including intensive ambulatory management (eg, intravenous antibiotics and fluids) until patients connect to longer term primary care clinicians. The intent of the extensivist is to provide patients with improved access to care, including in the period following hospital discharge. Implementation of extensivists has been associated with nearly a 40% reduction in 30-day hospital readmission rates for Medicare beneficiaries compared to the national average.

Patients with certain diagnoses may derive particular benefit from postdischarge clinics. For instance, nearly a quarter of patients diagnosed with congestive heart failure can be readmitted within 30 days of hospital discharge. In patients with frequent congestive heart failure exacerbations, a postdischarge visit to monitor volume status, weight, and medication adherence can reduce the frequency of readmissions. Other examples of populations that can benefit from close follow-up and services provided through postdischarge clinics include patients diagnosed with end-stage renal disease and chronic obstructive pulmonary disease.

Back to the Clinical Case

Due to long visit wait times, the patient could have benefited from receiving TCM services from a clinician or a postdischarge clinic visit, if such options were available. In the absence of these options, the patient in this case returned to the hospital for evaluation and care.

TAKEAWAYS

- Long visit wait times can cause delays in medical care and in turn increase morbidity and mortality risk among patients.
- TCM services are a combination of initial virtual contact and a subsequent in-person visit to support transitions after hospital discharge among patients whose care requires moderate- or high-complexity medical decision-making.
- Postdischarge clinics are intended to bridge care between the hospital and ambulatory clinicians.
- Patients with certain diagnoses such as congestive heart failure, end-stage renal disease, and chronic obstructive pulmonary disease may benefit more than others from postdischarge clinics.

Implications

The systems factors discussed in this chapter can pose implications for access to care. For patients transitioning after hospital care, long visit wait times can lead to significant consequences. Studies show that some patients consider ER clinicians as their primary care clinicians and utilize the ER even for nonurgent medical issues. Such patient perspectives are hypothesized to be contributing to the concomitant rise in ER wait times across the United States.

In turn, postdischarge clinics can be a way to improve the access to care for patients with certain medical conditions and insurance status. Postdischarge clinics have been associated with improved outcomes in patients with congestive heart failure, end-stage renal disease, and chronic obstructive pulmonary disease; medical care organizations can stratify patients who benefit more from access to intensive follow-up visits. Socioeconomic factors are increasingly being recognized as a factor that drives hospital readmissions. Postdischarge clinics can also help connect patients with longer term ambulatory care at federally qualified health centers or other surrounding clinics.

The systems factors also pose implications for quality of care. The approaches reviewed—the Transitional Care Model, Care Transitions Intervention, and Project BOOST—can be effective in decreasing patient risk of readmissions. Minimizing the delays in patient discharge due to nonmedical barriers can also promote quality by decreasing the patient risk of in-hospital complications such as falls, infections, and deep vein thromboses.

Delays and inaccurate discharge summaries have been associated with poor quality of care. More than 20% of patients experience a preventable adverse event within 3 weeks of hospital discharge, nearly one-third of which are thought to be related to medication errors. Templates, curricula, and tools that improve accuracy and comprehensiveness of hospital discharge summaries can improve the quality of care, in part, through decreasing the likelihood of medication errors or other safety concerns.

The systems factors also have significant cost ramifications. Delayed discharges due to nonmedical barriers can increase patients' length of stay. According to a 2021 study, the average cost of US hospital expenses per day was $2883. Incomplete and inaccurate discharge summaries can put patients at higher risk for hospital readmission, which occurs for nearly 20% of Medicare patients within 30 days of discharge, costing more than $26 billion annually. Furthermore, low-quality transitions of care can lead to patients receiving redundant or unnecessary care, which is estimated to exceed $200 billion annually. Lastly, increases in patient visit wait times after hospital discharge can lead to overutilization of ER care; ER treatments can be up to 12 times more expensive than if the same treatments are delivered in an ambulatory setting.

Finally, the systems factors discussed in this chapter have important equity implications. Medicaid beneficiaries tend to experience more delays in discharge due to nonmedical barriers than individuals insured through other public or private insurance sources. There are also disparities with respect to discharge communication; studies from 2009 to 2014 reported that Black and Asian patients were less likely than White patients to receive high-quality discharge communication.

Race and ethnicity, income, nonmedical drivers of health (as reflected in dual eligibility for Medicare and Medicaid), and potentially disabling conditions (ie, mobility, cognitive, hearing, and vision) can also be associated with disparities in 30-day readmission rates. In 2020, the readmission rates for non-Hispanic White patients were 13.8% compared to 19.4% among non-Hispanic Black patients. Readmission rates were 16.8% among Hispanic patients, 15.9% among American Indian/Alaska Native patients, and 14.3% among Asian patients. Nearly 20% of patients with dual eligibility experienced 30-day readmissions compared with 12.3% of those without dual eligibility. Readmission rates among patients with potentially disabling conditions were 18.3% compared with 11.9% for patients without potentially disabling conditions.

Multiple-Choice Questions

1. Which of the following approaches were designed to improve transitions after hospital care using five visits and a transitions coach?
   A. Project BOOST
   B. Care Transitions Intervention
   C. Transitional Care Model
   D. All the above

2. Which of the following is not a common nonmedical barrier that can delay patient discharges?
   A. Postacute care facility needs
   B. Disruptive or dangerous patient behaviors
   C. Financial needs
   D. Transportation needs

3. Which of the following is not a primary care clinician recommendation for what should be included in discharge summaries?
   A. Identification of incidental findings
   B. Justification of medication changes
   C. Inclusion of all hospital day-to-day details
   D. Duration of medication therapy

4. To be reimbursed by the Centers for Medicare and Medicaid Services for TCM services, clinicians must see patients requiring high-complexity decision-making within how many days of hospital discharge?

A. 2 days

B. 7 days

C. 14 days

D. 30 days

Answers

1. The correct answer is B. Designed to last 30 days, the Care Transitions Intervention comprises five visits, the first of which occurs while the patient is in the hospital. A transitions coach—a nurse, social worker, community worker, or trained volunteer—meets with the patient and caregivers to discuss any concerns.

2. The correct answer is D. Transportation needs are not among the six common nonmedical barriers that can delay patient discharges.

3. The correct answer is C. Primary care clinicians have recommended the exclusion of hospital day-to-day details that may be irrelevant to the ambulatory setting.

4. The correct answer is B. To be reimbursed by the Centers for Medicare and Medicaid Services for TCM services, clinicians must see patients that require a high level of medical decision-making within 7 days of hospital discharge.

Bibliography

Agency for Healthcare Research and Quality. Overview of clinical conditions with frequent and costly hospital readmissions by payer, 2018 #278. https://hcup-us.ahrq.gov/reports/statbriefs/sb278-Conditions-Frequent-Readmissions-By-Payer-2018.jsp

Agency for Healthcare Research and Quality. Project BOOST increases patient understanding of treatment and follow-up care. PSNet. https://psnet.ahrq.gov/innovation/project-boost-increases-patient-understanding-treatment-and-follow-care

Agency for Healthcare Research and Quality. Readmissions and adverse events after discharge. PSNet. https://psnet.ahrq.gov/primer/readmissions-and-adverse-events-after-discharge

Agency for Healthcare Research and Quality. Transitions of care. Chartbook on care coordination. 2018. https://www.ahrq.gov/research/findings/nhqrdr/chartbooks/carecoordination/measure1.html

Andrew Josephson S. Focusing on transitions of care: a change is here. *Neurol Clin Pract.* 2016;6(2):183-189.

Auerbach AD, Davis RB, Phillips RS. Physician views on caring for hospitalized patients and the hospitalist model of inpatient care. *J Gen Intern Med*. 2001;16(2):116-119.

Axon RN, Penney FT, Kyle TR, et al. A hospital discharge summary quality improvement program featuring individual and team-based feedback and academic detailing. *Am J Med Sci*. 2014;347(6):472-477.

Banker SL, Lakhaney D, Hooe BS, McCann TA, Kostacos C, Lane M. A quality improvement approach to improving discharge documentation. *Pediatr Qual Saf*. 2022;7(1):e428.

Bann M, Meo N, Lopez JP, et al. Medically ready for discharge: a multisite "point-in-time" assessment of hospitalized patients. *J Hosp Med*. 2023;18(9):795-802.

Bann M, Rosenthal MA, Meo N. Optimizing hospital capacity requires a comprehensive approach to length of stay: opportunities for integration of "medically ready for discharge" designation. *J Hosp Med*. 2022;17(12):1021-1024.

Beauvais B, Whitaker Z, Kim F, Anderson B. Is the hospital value-based purchasing program associated with reduced hospital readmissions? *J Multidiscip Healthc*. 2022;15:1089.

Bell CM, Schnipper JL, Auerbach AD, et al. Association of communication between hospital-based physicians and primary care providers with patient outcomes. *J Gen Intern Med*. 2009;24(3):381-386.

Beresford L. Is a post-discharge clinic in your hospital's future?—The Hospitalist. Accessed February 27, 2024. https://www.the-hospitalist.org/hospitalist/article/124553/qi-initiatives/post-discharge-clinic-your-hospitals-future

Bumpas J, Copeland DJ. Standardizing multidisciplinary discharge planning rounds to improve patient perceptions of care transitions. *J Nurs Adm*. 2021;51(2):101-105.

Cai C, Lindquist K, Bongiovanni T. Factors associated with delays in discharge for trauma patients at an urban county hospital. *Trauma Surg Acute Care Open*. 2020;5(1):e000535.

Capp R, Camp-Binford M, Sobolewski S, Bulmer S, Kelley L. Do adult Medicaid enrollees prefer going to their primary care provider's clinic rather than emergency department (ED) for low acuity conditions? *Med Care*. 2015;53(6):530-533.

Centers for Medicare and Medicaid Services. Community-based Care Transitions Program. https://www.cms.gov/priorities/innovation/innovation-models/cctp

Centers for Medicare and Medicaid Services. Definition of terms. Eligible professional meaningful use menu set measures measure 7 of 9. https://www.cms.gov/regulations-and-guidance/legislation/ehrincentiveprograms/downloads/8_transition_of_care_summary.pdf

Centers for Medicare and Medicaid Services Learning Network. Transitional Care Management Services. 2023. https://www.cms.gov/files/document/mln908628-transitional-care-management-services.pdf

Chatterton B, Chen J, Schwarz EB, Karlin J. Primary care physicians' perspectives on high-quality discharge summaries. *J Gen Intern Med*. 2024;39(8):1438-1443.

Chi JT, Handcock MS. Identifying sources of health care underutilization among California's immigrants. *J Racial Ethn Health Disparities*. 2014;1(3):207-218.

Coffey C, Greenwald J, Budnitz T, Williams MV. *Project Boost ® Implementation Guide 2nd ed.* www.hospitalmedicine.org/Boost

Coleman EA, Parry C, Chalmers S, Min SJ. The care transitions intervention: results of a randomized controlled trial. *Arch Intern Med*. 2006;166(17):1822-1828.

Coleman EA, Smith JD, Frank JC, Min SJ, Parry C, Kramer AM. Preparing patients and caregivers to participate in care delivered across settings: the care transitions intervention. *J Am Geriatr Soc*. 2004;52(11):1817-1825.

Dharmarajan K, Hsieh AF, Lin Z, et al. Diagnoses and timing of 30-day readmissions after hospitalization for heart failure, acute myocardial infarction, or pneumonia. *JAMA*. 2013;309(4):355-363.

Doctoroff L. Postdischarge clinics and hospitalists: a review of the evidence and existing models. *J Hosp Med*. 2017;12(6):467-471.

Earl T, Katapodis N, Schneiderman S. Care transitions. *Making Healthcare Safer III: A Critical Analysis of Existing and Emerging Patient Safety Practices*. NCBI Bookshelf. https://www.ncbi.nlm.nih.gov/books/NBK555516/

Elliott K, Klein JW, Basu A, Sabbatini AK. Transitional care clinics for follow-up and primary care linkage for patients discharged from the ED. *Am J Emerg Med*. 2016;34(7):1230-1235.

Erickson KF, Winkelmayer WC, Chertow GM, Bhattacharya J. Physician visits and 30-day hospital readmissions in patients receiving hemodialysis. *J Am Soc Nephrol*. 2014;25(9):2079-2087.

Feigal J, Park B, Bramante C, Nordgaard C, Menk J, Song J. Homelessness and discharge delays from an urban safety net hospital. *Public Health*. 2014;128(11):1033.

Foer D, Ornstein K, Soriano TA, Kathuria N, Dunn A. Nonmedical factors associated with prolonged hospital length of stay in an urban homebound population. *J Hosp Med*. 2012;7(2):73-78.

FPM Blogs. Appointment wait times increase across specialties, but not in family medicine. AAFP. https://www.aafp.org/pubs/fpm/blogs/inpractice/entry/wait-times.html

Garg V, Molosky A, Palakodeti S, Jain SH. Rethinking how Medicaid patients receive care. Harvard Business Review. https://hbr.org/2018/10/rethinking-how-medicaid-patients-receive-care

Gertz AH, Pollack CC, Schultheiss MD, Brownstein JS. Delayed medical care and underlying health in the United States during the COVID-19 pandemic: a cross-sectional study. *Prev Med Rep*. 2022;28:101882.

Gurses AP, Xiao Y. A systematic review of the literature on multidisciplinary rounds to design information technology. *J Am Med Inform Assoc*. 2006;13(3):267.

Hansen LO, Greenwald JL, Budnitz T, et al. Project BOOST: effectiveness of a multihospital effort to reduce rehospitalization. *J Hosp Med*. 2013;8(8):421-427.

HealthLeaders Media. The extensivist model. https://www.healthleadersmedia.com/strategy/extensivist-model

Hernandez AF, Greiner MA, Fonarow GC, et al. Relationship between early physician follow-up and 30-day readmission among Medicare beneficiaries hospitalized for heart failure. *JAMA*. 2010;303(17):1716-1722.

Hostetter M, Klein S, McCarthy D. CareMore: Improving outcomes and controlling health care spending for high-needs patients. The Commonwealth Fund; 2017.

Hoyer EH, Odonkor CA, Bhatia SN, Leung C, Deutschendorf A, Brotman DJ. Association between days to complete inpatient discharge summaries with all-payer hospital readmissions in Maryland. *J Hosp Med*. 2016;11(6):393-400.

Ibrahim H, Harhara T, Athar S, Nair SC, Kamour AM. Multi-disciplinary discharge coordination team to overcome discharge barriers and address the risk of delayed discharges. *Risk Manag Healthc Policy*. 2022;15:141.

Jackson C, Shahsahebi M, Wedlake T, Dubard CA. Timeliness of outpatient follow-up: an evidence-based approach for planning after hospital discharge. *Ann Fam Med*. 2015;13(2):115-122.

Kaiser Family Foundation. Hospital adjusted expenses per inpatient day. https://www.kff.org/health-costs/state-indicator/expenses-per-inpatient-day

Khau M, Maksut J, Mills C, Gaiser M, Saunders R, Scholle SH. Impact of hospital readmissions reduction initiatives on vulnerable populations. 2020.

Kind AJH, Smith MA. Documentation of mandated discharge summary components in transitions from acute to subacute care. *Advances in Patient Safety: New Directions and Alternative Approaches (Vol 2: Culture and Redesign)*. Published online 2008. https://www.ncbi.nlm.nih.gov/books/NBK43715/

Larrow A, Chong A, Robison T, et al. A quality improvement initiative to improve discharge timeliness and documentation. *Pediatr Qual Saf*. 2021;6(4):E440.

Lee GA, Freedman D, Beddoes P, Lyness E, Nixon I, Srivastava V. Can we predict Acute Medical readmissions using the BOOST tool? A retrospective case note revi. *Acute Med*. 2016;15(3):119-123.

Lee KK, Yang J, Hernandez AF, Steimle AE, Go AS. Post-discharge follow-up characteristics associated with 30-day readmission after heart failure hospitalization. *Med Care*. 2016;54(4):365-372.

Managed Healthcare Executive. Younger Americans use ERs as their primary care provider. https://www.managedhealthcareexecutive.com/view/younger-americans-use-ers-their-primary-care-provider

Meo N, Cornia PB. Focusing on the medically ready for discharge patient using a reliable design strategy: a quality improvement project to improve length of stay on a medicine service. *Qual Manag Health Care*. 2022;31(1):14-21.

Meo N, Liao JM, Reddy A. Hospitalized after medical readiness for discharge: a multidisciplinary quality improvement initiative to identify discharge barriers in general medicine patients. *Am J Med Qual*. 2019;35(1):23-28.

Meo N, Paul E, Wilson C, Powers J, Magbual M, Miles KM. Introducing an electronic tracking tool into daily multidisciplinary discharge rounds on a medicine service: a quality improvement project to reduce length of stay. *BMJ Open Qual*. 2018;7(3):174.

Naylor MD. Advancing high value transitional care: the central role of nursing and its leadership. *Nurs Adm Q*. 2012;36(2):115-126.

Naylor MD, Bowles KH, McCauley KM, et al. High-value transitional care: translation of research into practice. *J Eval Clin Pract*. 2013;19(5):727-733.

Naylor MD, Brooten DA, Campbell RL, Maislin G, McCauley KM, Schwartz JS. Transitional care of older adults hospitalized with heart failure: a randomized, controlled trial. *J Am Geriatr Soc*. 2004;52(5):675-684.

Naylor MD, Hirschman KB, Hanlon AL, et al. Comparison of evidence-based interventions on outcomes of hospitalized, cognitively impaired older adults. *J Comp Eff Res*. 2014;3(3):245-257.

Naylor MD, Hirschman KB, Toles MP, Jarrín OF, Shaid E, Pauly MV. Adaptations of the evidence-based Transitional Care Model in the U.S. *Soc Sci Med*. 2018;213:28-36.

Oduyebo I, Lehmann CU, Pollack CE, et al. Association of self-reported hospital discharge handoffs with 30-day readmissions. *JAMA Intern Med*. 2013;173(8):624-629.

Office of the Assistant Secretary for Planning and Evaluation, U.S. Department of Health and Human Services. Trends in the utilization of emergency department services, 2009-2018. 2021. https://aspe.hhs.gov/pdf-report/utilization-emergency-department-services

Parry C, Coleman EA, Smith JD, Frank J, Kramer AM. The care transitions intervention: a patient-centered approach to ensuring effective transfers between sites of geriatric care. *Home Health Care Serv Q*. 2003;22(3):1-17.

Parry C, Min SJ, Chugh A, Chalmers S, Coleman EA. Further application of the care transitions intervention: results of a randomized controlled trial conducted in a fee-for-service setting. *Home Health Care Serv Q*. 2009;28(2-3):84-99.

Patel H, Yirdaw E, Yu A, et al. Improving early discharge using a team-based structure for discharge multidisciplinary rounds. *Prof Case Manag*. 2019;24(2):83-89.

Pauly MV, Hirschman KB, Hanlon AL, et al. Cost impact of the transitional care model for hospitalized cognitively impaired older adults. *J Comp Eff Res*. 2018;7(9):913-922.

Penn Nursing. NewCourtland Center for Transitions and Health. Transitional care model. https://www.nursing.upenn.edu/ncth/transitional-care-model/

Reinke CE, Kelz RR, Baillie CA, et al. Timeliness and quality of surgical discharge summaries after the implementation of an electronic format. *Am J Surg*. 2014;207(1):7-16.

Rodziewicz TL, Houseman B, Hipskind JE. Medical error reduction and prevention. *StatPearls*. NCBI Bookshelf. https://www.ncbi.nlm.nih.gov/books/NBK499956/

Romano MJ, Segal JB, Pollack CE. The association between continuity of care and the overuse of medical procedures. *JAMA Intern Med*. 2015;175(7):1148-1154.

Salmasian H, Freedberg DE, Abrams JA, Friedman C. An automated tool for detecting medication overuse based on the electronic health records. *Pharmacoepidemiol Drug Saf*. 2013;22(2):183-189.

Sharma G, Kuo YF, Freeman JL, Zhang DD, Goodwin JS. Outpatient follow-up visit and 30-day emergency department visit and readmission in patients hospitalized for chronic obstructive pulmonary disease. *Arch Intern Med*. 2010;170(18):1664-1670.

Silvestri D, Goutos D, Lloren A, et al. Factors associated with disparities in hospital readmission rates among US adults dually eligible for Medicare and Medicaid. *JAMA Health Forum*. 2022;3(1):E214611.

Smith M, Saunders R, Stuckhardt L, McGinnis JM. *Best Care at Lower Cost: The Path to Continuously Learning Health Care in America*. The National Academies Press; 2013.

Stevens JP, Nyweide DJ, Maresh S, Hatfield LA, Howell MD, Landon BE. Comparison of hospital resource use and outcomes among hospitalists, primary care physicians, and other generalists. *JAMA Intern Med*. 2017;177(12):1781-1787.

The Commonwealth Fund. CareMore: improving outcomes and controlling health care spending for high-needs patients. Published March 28, 2017. https://www.commonwealthfund.org/publications/case-study/2017/mar/caremore-improving-outcomes-and-controlling-health-care-spending

Upadhyay S, Stephenson AL, Smith DG. Readmission rates and their impact on hospital financial performance: a study of Washington Hospitals. *Inquiry*. 2019;56:1-10.

US Department of Health and Human Services. Reduce the proportion of emergency department visits with a longer wait time than recommended—AHS-09. Healthy People 2030 | health.gov. https://health.gov/healthypeople/objectives-and-data/browse-objectives/health-care-access-and-quality/reduce-proportion-emergency-department-visits-longer-wait-time-recommended-ahs-09

Uscher-Pines L, Pines J, Kellermann A, Gillen E, Mehrotra A. Deciding to visit the emergency department for non-urgent conditions: a systematic review of the literature. *Am J Manag Care*. 2013;19(1):47.

Vargas Bustamante A, Fang H, Garza J, et al. Variations in healthcare access and utilization among Mexican immigrants: the role of documentation status. *J Immigr Minor Health*. 2012;14(1):146-155.

Vaughn VM, Gandhi TN, Chopra V, et al. Antibiotic overuse after hospital discharge: a multi-hospital cohort study. *Clin Infect Dis*. 2021;73(11):e4499-e4506.

Voss R, Gardner R, Baier R, Butterfield K, Lehrman S, Gravenstein S. The care transitions intervention: translating from efficacy to effectiveness. *Arch Intern Med*. 2011; 171(14):1232-1237.

Williams MV, Li J, Hansen LO, et al. Project BOOST implementation: lessons learned. *South Med J*. 2014;107(7):455-465.

Xu S, Hom J, Balasubramanian S, et al. Prevalence and predictability of low-yield inpatient laboratory diagnostic tests. *JAMA Netw Open*. 2019;2(9).

5

Postacute Care

Clinical Case

After having returned to the hospital due to an unsuccessful recovery at home, Jessica and her husband Daniel decided that she will go to whichever facility her insurance will cover and that the medical team recommends. The social worker Lynn returns to Jessica's room and Jessica asks about what the different facility options are for her recovery.

During her previous hospital stay, the patient had a strong preference to return home after hospital discharge. However, due to challenges encountered recovering at home, along with her need to return to the hospital, she is now open to going to dedicated facilities where she can continue her recovery after her acute care needs are addressed in the hospital. However, she is unfamiliar with these posthospital—termed "postacute" care options. This is a commonly encountered situation among hospitalized patients.

There are several options for dedicated postacute care services that are intended to support patients after their acute care needs are addressed during hospitalization. Providing more support than hospital discharge to home with regular clinic follow-up, these postacute options include home health agencies (HHAs), inpatient rehabilitation facilities (IRFs), long-term care hospitals (LTCHs), and skilled nursing facilities (SNFs). Factors contributing to the choice of postacute care services include care needs, patient preference, service availability, and insurance coverage. Because they can play roles in how and where patients receive care across the continuum, dedicated postacute care facilities and services are important systems factors in US health care.

SYSTEMS FACTOR: POSTACUTE CARE FACILITIES AND SERVICES

Dedicated postacute care facilities and services represent a large and growing category of care for patients and spending for the US health care system.

Between 2001 and 2013, spending on postacute care doubled, and was the fastest growing category of Medicare spending in that time period. Approximately 22% of all hospital discharges nationally were to postacute care facilities (SNF, IRF, LTCH) or to home with dedicated postacute services (HHA), with an even higher proportion among Medicare patients (estimated at 42% of all hospital discharges in 2013). It is important to understand the role of major facility and service types given their prevalence and impact on patients' health care experiences.

Home Health Agencies

Home health services are a set of services that can be delivered to patients in their homes. These services are provided by agencies and can involve a combination of nursing care, physical and occupational therapy, speech therapy, social work, durable medical equipment and home supplies, and home health aide support.

Home health services are intended for patients who have part-time or intermittent need for skilled nursing care, rather than around-the-clock care needs—a distinction that differentiates individuals who would be good candidates for home health services from individuals who would require more complex and intense supports at dedicated postacute care facilities. Patients also need to qualify for home health services. For instance, Medicare will only cover home health services if a patient is considered "homebound," meaning that the patient:

- Has difficulty leaving home without mobility or disability (eg, needs a wheelchair or walker) due to an illness or injury
- Is not recommended to leave home due to a medical condition
- Is unable to leave home because it's a major effort

To qualify for home health services under the Medicare program, homebound patients must be under the care of a clinician and have a face-to-face visit with that clinician related to their need for home health services, during which the clinician determines that the patient has one or more of the following needs:

- Intermittent skilled nursing care
- Physical therapy
- Occupational therapy
- Speech therapy

In addition to the abovementioned requirements, patients are expected to have a condition that should improve in a reasonable amount of time.

Even for patients who qualify, home health services may not be all inclusive. Services do not include meal delivery, assistance with activities of daily living (ADLs; eg, toileting, bathing) solely, or assistance with household tasks that are not specifically related to illness (eg, cooking, cleaning).

The diagnoses that are most commonly discharged for home health services are chronic obstructive pulmonary disease, cellulitis, heart failure, shock, and total hip/knee joint replacement. The average length of stay for home health services among Medicare patients is approximately 45 days, and the average number of visits per admission is 33.

As entities delivering home health services, HHAs must be certified by Medicare. Some of the central certification requirements include physician and nursing oversight over the services the agency provides, maintenance of records on all patients, and receipt of a license in their respective state to operate and practice.

In sum, postacute home health services are intended for patients who are homebound and require a combination of nursing, speech therapy, physical therapy, and/or occupational therapy delivered episodically over a defined period, rather than around-the-clock and indefinitely.

Inpatient Rehabilitation Facilities

IRFs are facilities where patients can receive ongoing hospital-level care in conjunction with more intensive physical rehabilitation. After hospitalization for acute illness or injury, patients could be considered for transfer or discharge from the hospital to an IRF in order to receive higher intensity physical therapy, occupational therapy, speech therapy, and other rehabilitation services. Historically, the most common conditions for which patients are admitted to an IRF are stroke (most common, 20% of admissions), debility, brain injury, lower extremity fracture, cardiac conditions, spinal cord injuries, joint replacement of lower extremity, and other orthopedic and neurologic conditions.

To qualify for a stay in an IRF, a patient must be evaluated by a clinician who specializes in rehabilitation medicine, as opposed to a clinician from other specialties. The evaluating rehabilitation medicine clinician must attest that the patient needs face-to-face supervision by a rehabilitation clinician. The patient must also meaningfully participate in and stand to benefit from at least two types of intensive levels of therapy, at least one of which must be physical therapy or occupational therapy. The patient is expected to participate in a minimum of 3 hours of therapy per day, 5 days per week.

During the patient's IRF stay, their care must be supervised by a rehabilitation clinician, who is required to have face-to-face visits with the patient at least 3 times per week. Lastly, the patient is expected to need the services of an intensive interdisciplinary and coordinated team approach to their care. A small proportion of patients (1.6% of all hospitalized patients) are discharged to IRFs. Nearly 60% of patients who are discharged to IRFs are insured through Medicare.

IRFs can be freestanding facilities or can be dedicated units with a hospital. In 2019, three-quarters of IRFs were specialized units within a hospital, and one-quarter were freestanding facilities. Hospital-associated IRFs tend to have fewer beds than their freestanding counterparts and provide care to patient populations with greater clinical complexity. Facilities have to meet several requirements in order to be considered an IRF. To qualify as an IRF that is eligible for Medicare payment, IRFs must have the following:

- Rehabilitation nursing, physical therapy, occupational therapy, speech therapy, psychological services, social services, and orthotic and prosthetic services
- Medical director trained in rehabilitation medicine who is either in the facility full time at a freestanding IRF or at least 20 hours per week at a hospital-affiliated IRF
- Dedicated interdisciplinary approach that includes a physician, social worker, and therapist in every discipline treating the patient
- Treatments made by the physician and in collaboration with the licensed therapists on the team
- Admission diagnosis mix wherein 60% of all admissions are from 1 of 13 diagnoses determined by the Centers for Medicare and Medicaid Services (CMS)

To summarize, IRFs provide postacute services to a small subset of patients who require short-duration, high-intensity, and frequent rehabilitation services from a multidisciplinary team that includes nursing, allied health therapy services, as well as care from a rehabilitation physician. IRFs can be freestanding or attached to a hospital, with the two types of IRFs varying with respect to facility size and patient case-mix.

Long-Term Care Hospitals

LTCHs were first acknowledged as a postacute care entity in the 1980s, when CMS created and implemented the Inpatient Prospective Payment System. At the time, there were approximately 40 LTCHs—formerly, primarily tuberculosis and chronic disease facilities caring for patients during prolonged hospital stays—that were excluded from the Inpatient Prospective Payment System and reimbursed using preexisting reimbursement approaches. These exclusions were based on considerations that these hospitals took care of more complex cases at a higher cost.

Since then, the number of LTCHs and reimbursement system for LTCHs have changed. As of 2023, there are more than 300 LTCHs reimbursed in a prospective payment system that is distinct from and typically reimburses at higher rates than the Inpatient Prospective Payment System. These facilities can be freestanding or affiliated with a larger hospital.

LTCHs are used by a small subset of patients, with just 0.5% of hospital discharges resulting in LTCH admission. In order for a patient to qualify for a stay at an LTCH, they must have an anticipated length of stay of 25 days or longer. The most common conditions admitted to LTCHs are pulmonary edema and respiratory failure (24%), respiratory system diagnoses requiring a ventilator for 96+ hours (18%), and sepsis (6%).

In sum, LTCHs are a postacute care option for a small subset of patients who have highly complex care needs and require prolonged hospitalization, such as those suffering from chronic respiratory illness requiring a ventilator or recovering from sepsis.

Skilled Nursing Facilities

SNFs are the most commonly utilized postacute care option among Medicare patients, and the second most commonly utilized option (after home health services) among patients overall in the United States. Nine percent of all hospital discharges and 40% of discharges to postacute care are to SNFs, and there are more SNFs in the United States than other postacute care options.

To be discharged to a SNF after a hospitalization, patients must need skilled nursing (eg, wound care, medication management) and/or short-term rehabilitation services (eg, physical therapy, occupational therapy, speech therapy). Importantly, although facilities can serve as both SNFs and "nursing homes," a SNF designation is different from a "nursing home" designation in that the latter refers to long-term custodial services and supports for patients.

Patients needing SNF care generally require around-the-clock nursing care and supervision, as opposed to intermittent supports for patients discharged home with home health services. SNFs commonly provide services to patients after orthopedic procedures and to those recovering after sepsis, kidney, and urinary tract infections, pneumonia, heart failure, or shock.

Comparisons of Postacute Care Facilities and Services

In sum, each postacute care option not only has features in common with other postacute care options but also has features that differentiate themselves to help address the needs of patients with different circumstances. For instance,

SNF services are distinct from those offered through other postacute care options. Patients needing SNF care generally require around-the-clock nursing care and supervision, as opposed to intermittent supports for patients discharged home with home health services. SNFs and IRFs also differ in nature. While SNFs and IRFs are similar with respect to the types of services they can provide, the two differ with respect to the intensity of services (eg, hours of therapy per day) and supervision. In contrast to diagnoses typically requiring more time and intensive rehabilitation at IRFs, SNFs more commonly provide services to patients after orthopedic procedures and those recovering after sepsis, kidney and urinary tract infections, pneumonia, heart failure, or shock. LTCHs differ significantly from other postacute care options as they focus on treating chronic critical illness, whereas other options (HHAs, IRFs, SNFs) focus on postillness rehabilitation. Table 5.1 provides an overview of similarities and differences between the core postacute care options.

Table 5.1 Postacute Care Facilities and Services

	HHAs	IRF	LTCH	SNF
Common hospital discharge diagnoses	■ COPD ■ Cellulitis ■ Heart failure and shock ■ Hip/knee joint replacement	■ Stroke ■ Debility ■ Brain injury ■ Lower extremity fracture ■ Cardiac conditions ■ Spinal cord injuries ■ Other orthopedic and neurologic conditions	■ Pulmonary edema and respiratory failure ■ Respiratory diagnoses requiring a ventilator 96+ h ■ Sepsis	■ Joint replacement ■ Hip and femur procedure ■ Sepsis ■ Kidney and urinary tract infections ■ Pneumonia ■ Heart failure ■ Shock
Focus of care	■ Postillness rehabilitation	■ Intra- and postillness rehabilitation	■ Chronic critical illness care, including ventilator management	■ Postillness rehabilitation
Health professions caring for patients	■ Nursing ■ PT ■ OT ■ Speech ■ Social services ■ Coordinate with off-site physician	■ Nursing ■ PT ■ OT ■ Speech ■ Social services ■ Physicians involved in medical and rehabilitative care	■ Nursing ■ PT ■ OT ■ Speech ■ Social services ■ Physicians involved in medical and rehabilitative care	■ Nursing ■ PT ■ OT ■ Speech ■ Social services ■ Physicians involved in medical care

	HHAs	IRF	LTCH	SNF
Hours of care	Non-24/7 care, home visit based	24/7 care, minimum of 3 h of therapy 5 d a wk	24/7 care	24/7 care
Duration of care	Episodic, average LOS ~45 d	Episodic, average LOS ~13 d	Episodic or indefinite, minimum LOS 25 d	Episodic, average LOS ~28 d
Percentage of total hospital discharges to post-acute care	50.2%	7.2%	2.2%	40.4%

COPD, chronic obstructive pulmonary disease; HHAs, home health agencies; IRF, inpatient rehabilitation facility; LOS, length of stay; LTCH, long-term care hospital; OT, occupational therapy; PT, physical therapy; SNF, skilled nursing facility.

Source: Data from Agency for Healthcare Research and Quality. An all-payer view of hospital discharge to postacute care, 2013 #205. May 2016. https://hcup-us.ahrq.gov/reports/statbriefs/sb205-Hospital-Discharge-Postacute-Care.jsp

Back to the Clinical Case

In this patient's case, she has recovered from her medical condition and would not need the services of an LTCH. She did not suffer a higher acuity, intense medical event such as a stroke, spinal cord injury, or new severe fracture that would involve the intensive therapies provided through an IRF. Nonetheless, she could likely benefit from physical therapy, occupational therapy, and nursing in a SNF setting rather than a home setting with home health services.

TAKEAWAYS

- Options for postacute care, either via a facility or a set of services, for patients differ depending on patient need and other factors.
- Home health is the most common type of postacute care and involves frequent but not around-the-clock services including nursing, physical therapy, occupational therapy, and speech therapy, delivered in patients' home settings.
- IRFs provide the highest intensity of rehabilitative services, including physical therapy, occupational therapy, speech therapy, social services, and physician services, around the clock via a coordinated multidisciplinary team led by a physician with expertise in rehabilitative medicine.

- LTCHs are facilities concentrated in certain areas of the country that provide around-the-clock highly complex medical care, including ventilator management, for patients with prolonged critical illness.
- SNFs are the most common postdischarge postacute care setting for Medicare patients, and provide episodic, around-the-clock nursing services and therapy services that are more intense than home health, but less intense than those provided in IRFs.

Clinical Case Continued

At multidisciplinary discharge rounds, Jessica's clinical care team discusses several postacute care facility options. The team believes that Jessica would benefit from further rehabilitation at a SNF, which is discussed with and agreed upon with Jessica and her husband. The discharge planner, Patrick, begins the referral process by gathering key pieces of Jessica's clinical information, checks her insurance status, and asks for her preferences with regard to different SNFs.

To receive care at a SNF—the most commonly utilized postacute care facility—a patient must be placed through a referral process. The SNF referral process considers whether a patient is a good match for the facility according to its clinical, financial, or operational factors. The referral process is often complex and represents a key systems factor that determines a patient's access to postacute care.

SYSTEMS FACTOR: SKILLED NURSING FACILITY REFERRAL PROCESS

For a patient to receive care in a SNF after hospitalization, the patient must have needs related to skilled nursing (eg, wound care, medication management) and/or short-term rehabilitation services (eg, physical therapy, occupational therapy, speech therapy). The hospital care team considers a patient's needs for skilled nursing and/or rehabilitation services in the context of their physical function, social support, cognition, pain, home environment, insurance status, and medical readiness (Table 5.2). When these patient needs are identified, for instance, through discussion during multidisciplinary discharge rounds, clinicians can begin the SNF referral process.

The referral process (Figure 5.1) generally begins while the patient is still in the hospital, where clinical and financial information about the patient is sent to a hospital team member (often a social worker and/or a case manager) who serves as a discharge planner. The discharge planner then discusses SNF options with the patient and the family by providing a list of SNF facilities that are available.

In identifying facilities of interest, patients consider factors such as location, prior experience, the experience of family and friends, and reported quality of the facilities. Once patients narrow down the list, the discharge planner prepares to send referrals to SNF admissions coordinators at candidate facilities. Preparation can involve checking patient records (eg, to gather hospital progress notes, consultation notes, medication lists, contacts for hospital clinicians), and insurance eligibility (eg, referral authorizations).

Table 5.2 Considerations During the SNF Referral Process

	Primary Individual(s) Involved	Factors to Consider for SNF
Physical function	Physical therapist	Whether a patient is functioning below their prior baseline status
Social support	Nurse	Whether a patient lives alone or lives with family and friends
Cognition	Physical therapist	For a patient with dementia, whether a patient can safely learn new skills, improve balance, and progress with rehabilitation
Pain	Physical therapist	Whether a patient has achieved pain control at baseline and during rehabilitation
Home environment	Physical therapist	Whether a patient has stable housing, and if housing is conducive to ongoing rehabilitation (stairs, durable medical equipment, etc)
Insurance status	Nurse	Whether a patient is covered by insurance, and, if so, which type of insurance
Medical readiness	Physician	Whether a patient's acute conditions are stabilized

SNF, skilled nursing facility.

Source: Adapted from Burke RE, Lawrence E, Ladebue A, et al. How hospital clinicians select patients for skilled nursing facilities. *J Am Geriatr Soc*. 2017;65(11):2466-2472.

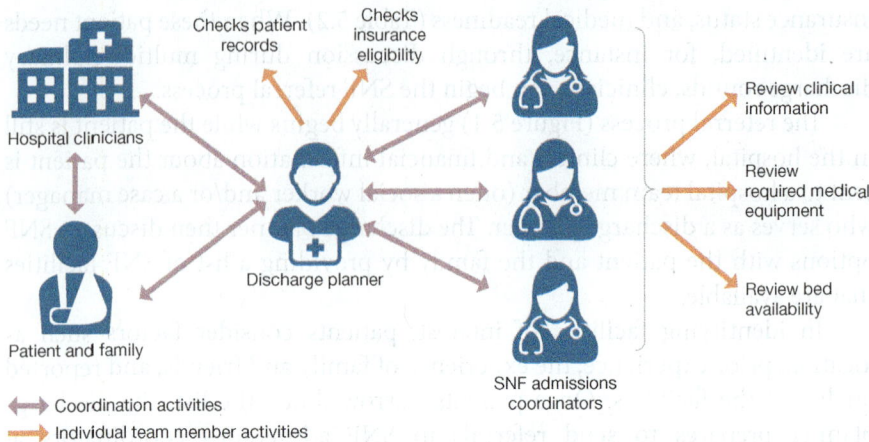

Figure 5.1 SNF Referral Process. SNF, skilled nursing facility. (Source: Data from Strickland C, Chi N, Ditz L, et al. Factors influencing admission decisions in skilled nursing facilities: retrospective quantitative study. *J Med Internet Res.* 2023;25:e43518.)

SNF admissions coordinators then review referrals with an eye toward patients' clinical information, required medical equipment, and bed availability. After reviewing available information, admissions coordinators can deny a referral if they believe a patient is not a good match at their facility. The patient may decide to accept or decline any SNF admission offer that is made.

For patients who do not have prior experience at SNFs, proximity close to home and family can be the most important deciding factor in choosing a facility. Patients are also likely to choose SNFs at which their family and friends have received care. For those with prior experience at SNFs, patients are likely to choose the SNF with which they are already familiar. Patients also factor in quality in choosing SNFs, as defined by factors such as cleanliness, amenities, indicators of clinical quality, and staff availability and friendliness. To assist and better inform patients regarding how to choose SNFs, the CMS developed a website called the Nursing Home Compare. The website uses a Five-Star Quality Rating System to classify the quality of care in a given Medicare-participating SNF and allows patients to compare SNFs in a given location.

Clinical Factors That Affect the Skilled Nursing Facility Referral Process

Patients' clinical diagnoses play a role in determining whether they are likely to receive SNF admission offers. Some of the most common hospital discharge diagnoses associated with patients accepted to SNFs include joint replacement surgery, sepsis, kidney and urinary tract infection, and pneumonia. These diagnoses are associated with, on average, shorter patient stays at SNFs; in turn, SNFs are more inclined to accept referrals with these diagnoses to increase bed turnover and availability.

Conversely, the hospital diagnoses associated with the least number of patients accepted to SNFs include psychiatric and substance use–related diagnoses. These diagnoses represent conditions that are often challenging to treat in SNFs as patients with psychiatric and substance use–related diagnoses often require additional staffing. Patients admitted to SNFs with these conditions are associated with longer stays.

Financial Factors That Affect the Skilled Nursing Facility Referral Process

Patients' insurance types play a role in determining whether they are likely to receive SNF admission offers. In 2022, Medicaid and Medicare paid for 62% and 13% of patient stays at SNFs, respectively. The remaining 25% of patient stays at SNFs were paid through private insurance.

Studies have shown that the odds of a SNF referral acceptance are lower when patients are covered by Medicaid as opposed to Medicare or private insurance. Specifically, studies have found that patients covered under private insurance have the highest odds of being accepted to SNFs, followed by patients covered by Medicare, and then, lastly, patients covered by Medicaid.

Operational Factors That Affect the Skilled Nursing Facility Referral Process

SNFs' nurse staffing levels and geographic area play a role in determining bed availability and whether patients are likely to receive SNF admission offers. Numerous studies have shown that inadequate staffing levels and day-to-day variations in staffing levels can negatively affect the quality of SNF care. Higher numbers of nurse staffing have been associated with fewer patient pressure ulcers, decreased infections, and lower mortality rates.

In 2023, the CMS proposed a rule to address the inadequate staffing levels in SNFs. The rule proposed an increase in minimum patient-facing hours for nurses and required facilities to have a registered nurse around the clock. Furthermore, the rule created new reporting requirements regarding Medicaid payments for institutional long-term services and supports (LTSS) and provided $75 million for training for nursing aides. At the time of the rule proposal, studies showed that more than 80% of SNFs would need to hire more nursing staff to meet the proposed minimum requirements.

There are also notable and persistent geographic variations in the availability of SNF care. Facilities located in urban areas are nearly 20% more likely to deny a referral than those located in rural areas. As facilities in urban areas receive referrals more regularly, the SNF admissions coordinators have more to review and choose from than those in rural areas.

Back to the Clinical Case

The discharge planner, patient, and patient's husband together would review a list of potential SNFs. The patient's primary hospital diagnosis is a knee infection associated with recent total knee arthroplasty, one of the most common hospital discharge diagnoses for patients at SNFs. The patient has Medicare insurance that would cover her upcoming SNF stay, which could affect her ability to be placed in a SNF, as compared to other insurance types. The next steps in the SNF referral process for this patient would be for the discharge planner to send SNF referrals to the admissions coordinators at nearby SNFs with bed availability, who would then evaluate the patient for fit. While these referrals are being processed, the hospital discharge planner would also check insurance eligibility for the patient's SNF stay.

TAKEAWAYS

- To receive care at a SNF, patients must go through a referral process that involves patients and loved ones, hospital clinicians, discharge planners, and SNF admissions coordinators.
- Some of the most common hospital discharge diagnoses associated with patients accepted to SNFs include joint replacement surgery, sepsis, kidney and urinary tract infection, and pneumonia.
- Compared to patients covered under Medicare, patients covered under Medicaid have lower odds of a SNF referral being accepted, whereas patients covered under private insurance have higher odds of being accepted.
- Clinical, financial, and operational factors play a role in whether patients are likely to be accepted to SNFs.

Clinical Case Continued

After waiting several days, Jessica learns from the discharge planner that there are two SNFs, Skilled Nursing A and Skilled Nursing B, that have an available bed for her and are willing to admit her from the hospital tomorrow. Each of the SNFs is located similarly close to her home, possesses services she will need, and is covered by her insurance. Given these similarities, Jessica is not sure which to choose and asks the discharge planner about the safety and quality of care at each facility.

This patient is faced with a common decision of choosing a SNF facility from available options for postacute care. While there are approximately 6000 hospitals in the United States, there are more than 15 000 SNFs, and comparatively less is known about safety—a critical component of quality—in SNFs than in hospitals. Approximately one in five Medicare patients experience harm from the care they receive at a SNF, and more than half of those adverse events are preventable and related to inadequate patient monitoring, treatment that did not meet standard of care, or a delay in providing necessary care.

In addition to safety and other components of care quality (eg, staffing levels, health outcomes), patients might make other special considerations when choosing a SNF. For instance, approximately 4% of SNF beds in the United States are located in special care units, which have expertise in caring for certain populations such as individuals with dementia. More personal experience–related factors can also play a role, such as quality of food or communal atmosphere of the facility.

Given how common it is for hospitalized patients to require postacute services in SNFs, and the implications for subsequent care (eg, impacts on readmissions, outpatient follow-up, future hospital care), policies governing SNF quality is a health systems factor to understand.

HEALTH SYSTEMS FACTOR: POLICIES GOVERNING SKILLED NURSING FACILITY QUALITY

As noted, SNFs have grown in numbers in the United States over time. Since their early emergence, however, there has been public sentiment about poor quality of care at SNFs and these facilities being institutions or options of last resort. Patient sentiment, and willingness to use SNFs, has only grown in salience as some facilities have evolved and adopted a dual role by providing long-term custodial care as well as shorter term nursing and rehabilitation care for people recovering after hospitalization. Collectively, these dynamics underscore the importance of policies that have been implemented to ensure the quality of care at SNFs, a health systems factor that can impact Americans requiring care at such facilities.

1940s to 1980s: Nursing Home Standards Through the Hill-Burton Act, Medicare, and Medicaid

Much of the growth in SNFs in the United States can be traced to the Hill-Burton Act of 1946. This law introduced massive amounts of investment in the growth and development of health care facilities, including SNFs.

However, while this law supported the growth in SNFs (by 1954, there were 9000 SNFs in the United States), assuring quality was a challenge, with very few states requiring that facilities be licensed. Although Congress passed legislation in 1950 requiring states to create SNF licensing programs, it did not specify any standards for how SNFs should be licensed, or any enforcement procedures for assuring quality.

This resulted in wide between-state variation in what constituted a SNF, and enforcement measures were rarely taken. The combination of heavy investment in the growth of SNFs as health care facilities, coupled with limited quality standards or enforcement, created national concerns surrounding the quality of care delivered at SNFs. In 1960, nearly half of all SNF beds did not meet fire and health standards, and many facilities were found to have untrained staff and offered limited services.

The passage of Medicare and Medicaid in 1965 created a new opportunity to set standards and enforcement for SNF quality. The Medicare program provided funding for patients to receive care after hospitalization at SNFs (then referred to as Extended Care Facilities), and the Medicaid program was able to provide funding for skilled nursing services. New funding created an opportunity to set care standards for SNFs interested in participating in Medicare and Medicaid.

However, very few SNFs—only 740 of the initial 6000 applicants to the Medicare and Medicaid programs—were able to meet standards in the first year, and many facilities that failed to do so faced the prospect of closure. In turn, out of concern for creating bed shortages from SNF closures, the Medicare and Medicaid programs reimbursed SNFs, even if they failed to meet quality criteria. Medicare and Medicaid did this by creating a category of SNFs that were deemed to be "in substantial compliance," even if they never met preestablished standards. More than half of the initial 6000 SNF applicants received funding based on the "substantial compliance" designation.

In the 1960s, the number of SNF beds more than doubled and government spending on SNFs in the 1970s quadrupled. At the same time, concerns about poor quality, neglect, and abuse persisted, and several regulatory efforts were made to strengthen quality standards at SNFs with limited effect.

1980s to 2000s: Nursing Home Reform Act of 1986

National momentum to meaningfully address quality in SNFs, growing over several decades, led to a landmark Institute of Medicine report in 1986. The report called for increased regulation of SNF quality after it concluded that care was "shockingly deficient," outlining concerns related to neglect and abuse, poor quality of life, and poor and unstandardized information surrounding SNF care. This report, in addition to a 1987 report by the Government Accountability Office finding that more than one-third of SNFs did not meet minimum federal standards, precipitated the passing of the landmark legislation called the Omnibus Budget Reconciliation Act of 1987, more commonly referred to as the Nursing Home Reform Act.

The Nursing Home Reform Act put in place a number of measures aimed at improving quality and protecting patients at SNFs. The legislation had the following areas of focus:

Established patient-centered standards. The Nursing Home Reform Act created a set of higher and more patient-centered standards than those previously established. For example, the Act created quality-of-life rights including freedom from abuse, mistreatment, and neglect, as well as protections for patients to voice concerns without retaliation. It also restricted the use of physical restraints, which were previously more commonplace, except under very specific circumstances.

Improved staffing. The Nursing Home Reform Act also increased staffing requirements for SNFs, focusing on improving coverage and training of SNF staff. Specifically, the law required SNFs to have a registered nurse as director of nursing, as well as licensed practical nurses at the facility around the clock. The Act also created new standards for nursing aides, including a requirement for at least 75 hours of training and passing a competency test.

Stricter compliance and enforcement measures. The Nursing Home Reform Act created new stipulations to monitor for compliance with standards, and more tools for enforcing compliance. For example, the Act required states to make unannounced visits to SNFs at least once every 15 months, where they would directly observe care delivered to patients and interview patients on their care experience. SNFs that were found to be falling short of expectations would face enforcement actions proportionate to the degree of their infractions. Enforcement measures ranged from fines, creating corrective plans of action, putting in place new temporary managers, or payment denial for all new or existing Medicare or Medicaid patients.

Created a single national certification system. Prior to the Nursing Home Reform Act, there were disparate expectations and certification systems. There were standards and certifications that differed state by state and between the Medicaid and Medicare programs. The Act merged Medicare and Medicaid standards and processes into a single system, creating an understanding of uniform minimum expectations from SNFs nationally.

Created minimum expectations for patient assessment. The Act led to the development and required implementation of a clinical assessment tool for patients called the Minimum Data Set. These data were intended to constitute a system for assessing individual patient's functional status and detecting changes in their condition. SNFs were required to fill out the full Minimum

Data Set annually, which was 6 pages long and contained 18 sections, and to conduct shorter versions of the assessment on a quarterly basis.

After initially raising the alarm about quality of care at SNFs and contributing to the impetus for the passing of the Nursing Home Reform Act, the Institute of Medicine subsequently concluded that SNF quality improved overall since the law's passing.

Still, while the Act may have helped raise the overall standard of care, research suggested that wide variation in quality of care persisted. For instance, after implementation of the Act, there was greater than 3-fold variation in pressure sore incidence across facilities, ranging from 7% of patients in some facilities to 23% in others. In addition, similar challenges existed in other elements of SNF care, including malnutrition, dehydration, incontinence care, pain management, rehospitalization, overall quality of life, and other elements of quality.

2000s to Present: Five-Star Quality Rating System and Nursing Home Compare

The next major development in policies governing SNF quality came from a CMS program. Faced with public concern about SNF quality and evidence of between-facility variation, CMS established the Five-Star Quality Rating System in 2008. After collaborating with experts from patient advocacy groups, SNFs, and academic researchers, CMS created a rating system for SNF quality of care, ranking each SNF from one star (much below average quality) to five stars (much above average quality).

In doing so, CMS built on similar star programs in place for other medical care facility types, such as hospitals and HHAs. Under the Five-Star Quality Rating System, patients were able to directly compare SNFs in their area using Medicare's "Nursing Home Compare," a tool hosted on a publicly available website and included information about quality performance that could be compared across multiple SNFs. The program, therefore, based its star ratings on the following three core components:

Health inspection survey results. As required initially by the Nursing Home Reform Act, every year state and federal surveyors make unannounced visits to perform on-site assessments of SNF services. The assessments focus on patient health, rights, and quality of life, and incorporate direct observation of care and patient interviews. The results of these assessments are incorporated into the Five-Star Quality Rating System.

Quality measure performance. On the Nursing Home Compare site, CMS collects and reports on 19 SNF-related quality measures that patients can use.

A subset of those measures is incorporated into the SNF's official star rating. Some of those measures focus on patients at a SNF for a short stay, and some are focused on patients at a SNF for a longer term stay.

The measures focus on a variety of components of quality care, such as changes in a patient's mobility or need for assistance with ADLs, the percentage of patients who develop new or developing ulcers while at a SNF, the percentage of patients who experience a urinary tract infection or have a urinary catheter placed for several days, the percentage of patients who were put in physical restraints, and other quality measures. Measures related to mobility and assistance with ADLs have the strongest weight, and for some of the measures SNFs are compared to other facilities in the state, and for some measures SNFs are ranked against other facilities throughout the country.

Staffing information. This component of the Five-Star Quality Rating System reports and compares SNFs based on the number of hours of nursing and other health care staff a facility employs per patient per day. This measure is adjusted on the basis of overall clinical complexity of a SNF's patient population.

CMS gives every SNF a star rating for each of the three core components individually, as well as a composite score across all three. When the program was first implemented, 12% of the country's SNFs received a full five-star rating, 22% received a one-star rating, and the remaining facilities were relatively evenly distributed among two- to four-star ratings. Smaller SNFs with fewer beds have been found to have higher overall star ratings, on average, than larger SNFs. As another way of educating patients, CMS also publishes a list of SNFs with consistently poor performance, called "Special Focus Facilities." These facilities have twice as many annual inspections as other SNFs, and the designation is clearly marked on the Nursing Home Compare site.

The Nursing Home Compare website and Five-Star Quality Rating System have been updated since their inception. For instance, studies found that star ratings had limited correlation with rates of preventable hospital readmissions. In response, preventable readmissions are now reported on the Nursing Home Compare site.

Back to the Clinical Case

In this patient's case, she is able to review quality of care at her two candidate SNFs using the Nursing Home Compare website, as well as put that information into context through information provided through the Five-Star Quality Rating System. While this information is not perfect, it can still inform the patient's choice about where to receive SNF care. In addition, she could also benefit from inquiring about whether either of the candidate facilities has a special care unit for people with dementia.

TAKEAWAYS

- Large-scale public investment through the Hill-Burton Act and passage of Medicare and Medicaid led to the rapid growth of SNFs. However, variable standards and certification processes with limited enforcement contributed to early SNF quality concerns and public mistrust.
- The Nursing Home Reform Act of 1986 established more rigorous uniform standards regulating SNF quality, protecting patient rights, and included meaningful enforcement measures that supported improvements in quality of care delivered at SNFs nationally.
- The Five-Star Quality Rating System published on Nursing Home Compare gives patients a tool to compare the quality of care delivered at individual SNFs based on performance on select quality measures, health inspections, and staffing data.

Clinical Case Continued

Review of the two SNF options reveals that Skilled Nursing A has higher overall and component star ratings, as well as a dementia unit. Jessica selects Skilled Nursing A, where she is discharged 2 days later. Over the next 2 weeks, Jessica works with the physical and occupational therapists 1 to 2 hours per day, for 5 days a week. After this period, she progresses to being able to get out·of bed, to the bathroom, and back to bed without difficulty, and is able to dress herself and shower independently.

However, she still is not able to get up and down the stairs due to challenges with strength and stability. This limitation is concerning to Jessica because she lives on the third floor of an apartment building without an elevator. Jessica is also worried about how long she'll be able to stay at Skilled Nursing A to work on strength and functioning goals— an issue she brings up with Skilled Nursing A's lead administrator.

The patient faces a common situation and is seeking to determine when she would be ready to discharge home from the SNF. Many factors can influence this determination, including the variation in care needs, primary reasons for SNF stay (shorter term recovery, longer term custodial care), and progress from therapies. Realistically, another consideration is financial: how and to what extent SNF care is covered by the patient's insurance. In fact, care coverage and reimbursement is a health systems factor that affects the postacute care received by patients in SNFs.

SYSTEMS FACTOR: SKILLED NURSING FACILITY CARE COVERAGE AND REIMBURSEMENT

Out-of-pocket costs for SNF care can vary widely. While nearly a third of patients will not have to pay for any care out of pocket, patients in the 95th percentile for out-of-pocket expenditures on SNF care will spend approximately $50 000 on SNF care in their lifetime. This is a salient issue at a national level, given that more than half of older US adults are expected to stay overnight at a SNF at some point in their life, with an average length of stay of 28 days. An important consideration for SNF care coverage and reimbursement is the fact that SNFs can provide long-term custodial care and/or short-term rehabilitative care, and that coverage and reimbursement differ for these situations across insurers.

Skilled Nursing Facility Care Coverage: Examples From Medicare and Medicaid

For instance, consider Medicare and Medicaid, the country's major public health insurance programs. These two programs have different policies in the types of care they will cover and reimburse for patients receiving care at SNFs, and how long coverage lasts.

In general, Medicare is designed mostly to cover short-term rehabilitative stays at SNFs, with nearly half of all hospital discharges to postacute options in 2013 being to SNFs among Medicare patients.

Medicare organizes its SNF coverage based on benefit periods—periods of time that begin the day a patient is admitted to a hospital or a SNF and ends when that patient has not received any hospital or SNF care for 60 days in a row. There is no limit to the number of benefit periods a patient can have.

To qualify for a SNF stay, a patient must be enrolled in Medicare Part A and have a qualifying 3-day inpatient hospitalization. Once a patient qualifies for their SNF stay, Medicare activates that benefit period's SNF coverage. In a given benefit period, Medicare offers the following SNF coverage:

- Days 1 through 20: Medicare pays for 100% of SNF costs.
- Days 21 through 100: Patients with Traditional Medicare insurance pay $200 out of pocket per day, and Medicare pays the rest.

■ Days 101 and beyond: Patients with Traditional Medicare and no other source of health insurance coverage pay for 100% of the SNF costs.

For days that Medicare covers, SNF benefits include a patient's room, meals, skilled nursing care, physical therapy, occupational therapy, speech therapy, social services, medications and supplies, dietary counseling, and ambulance transportation if needed. Due to the duration of these benefits, Medicare can be considered a payer of short-term rehabilitative stays at SNFs, but not long-term stays. Therefore, for patients insured through Traditional Medicare, the duration of the benefits coupled with the nature of reimbursement could influence a SNF's prioritization of discharge planning.

In contrast, Medicaid is designed to pay for short-term or long-term stays, including custodial care, through its broader LTSS benefits. While Medicaid programs can pay for SNF services that are similar to those covered by Medicare, the LTSS benefit in state Medicaid programs can also pay for long-term assistance with ADLs (eating, bathing, dressing) and instrumental ADLs (managing medications, housekeeping) for patients who need assistance with these activities due to age, illness, or disabilities.

To that end, Medicaid is the country's largest payer of long-term care services at SNFs, with LTSS benefits accounting for approximately 30% of Medicaid expenditures nationally. More than 60% of residents at SNFs nationally have their stays primarily reimbursed by Medicaid. For patients who are dually eligible for Medicare and Medicaid, their SNF stay would first be covered by Medicare until the benefit period expires, at which point Medicaid benefits would initiate.

Skilled Nursing Facility Care Reimbursement

1965 to 1997: Reimbursement on a "Reasonable Cost" Basis

Similar to how hospitals were initially reimbursed in the Medicare program before the introduction of the diagnosis-related group (DRG) system, SNFs were initially reimbursed by Medicare on a retrospective, reasonable cost basis; SNFs provided the services they felt were indicated and Medicare paid for those services afterward, with little regulation. As a result of retrospective payments, reimbursement varied depending on the care already provided.

During this time, Congress was concerned about growing hospital costs. In 1983, it passed the Inpatient Prospective Payment System for hospitals, the consequences of which include decreases in hospital length of stay and increases in patients being discharged to SNFs (in some cases, with greater degrees of medical service needs). This environment—defined by rising numbers of higher complexity patients moving through a system with limited cost oversight contributed to a rapid rise in SNF-related health care costs. Between

1990 and 1998, Medicare and Medicaid expenditures on SNF care increased from less than $2 billion to more than $10 billion.

1997 to 2019: The First Skilled Nursing Facility Prospective Payment Model and Per Diem Payment

In response to increases in SNF spending, Congress in 1997 passed the Balanced Budget Act, which introduced a new payment system for SNF care that remains the foundation for SNF reimbursement. In particular, the Act also introduced prospective payments for SNFs and ended retrospective reasonable cost reimbursement. This Skilled Nursing Facility Prospective Payment System (SNF PPS) was defined by several features. First, it paid facilities on a prospective per diem (ie, per day) basis, thereby creating incentives to manage costs per day of a SNF stay, but not necessarily to manage costs associated with total lengths of stay.

Second, the SNF PPS created different levels of per diem payments based on the resource or staffing needs of each patient. Resource needs were based on the Resource Utilization Group-III (RUG-III) system, which was developed in the early 1990s using staff-time information from SNFs in six states. In this system, patients are first classified into 7 categories, and ultimately 1 of 44 more granular levels of payment based on their disease severity and care needs (Table 5.3). Patients who meet the criteria for multiple categories are grouped depending on the category with the highest payment rate.

For instance, within the rehabilitation category, additional classification is heavily influenced by the number of weekly therapy minutes received (eg, physical therapy, occupational therapy, speech). Different RUG-III classifications have a range of total therapy time assigned to them, with the highest level being 720+ weekly minutes of therapy. Patients can move from one RUG-III classification to another, meaning that SNF reimbursement can vary depending on what services patients receive and their ability to meet minimum criteria of different RUG-III classifications.

Overall, this system has created a number of economic incentives around SNF care. First, guaranteed per diem rates across a defined benefit period mean that SNFs are not necessarily incentivized to actively manage SNF length of stay. Second, the payment system can influence SNF admission decisions. In particular, SNFs may be more hesitant to admit patients who they perceive to be highly complex, likely to require SNF resources exceeding the reimbursement rate, or having needs that aren't captured by the RUG-III reimbursement system. Third, a RUG-III system that involve ranges and levels may distort facilities' incentives to deliver care: some may be prompted to expend fewer resources on patients' care (eg, if a range of expenses fall within

Table 5.3 Core Categories of the RUG-III in the SNF Prospective Payment System

Category	Typical Needs
Rehabilitation	Physical therapy, occupational therapy, speech therapy
Extensive services	Complex clinical needs such as intravenous nutrition or medication, ventilatory/airway support, or other major comorbidities
Special care	Care for medical conditions such as multiple sclerosis, cerebral palsy, stage 3 or 4 pressure ulcers, radiation, surgical wounds or open lesions, tube feeding, pneumonia
Clinically complex	Care requiring skilled nursing management such as burns or wound care, transfusions, chemotherapy, oxygen therapy, or pneumonia
Impaired cognition	Additional assistance due to cognitive impairment
Behavior problems	Additional assistance due to behavior challenges such as wandering, refusal of care, hallucinations
Reduced physical function	Primarily need assistance with ADLs

ADLs, activities of daily living; RUG-III, Resource Utilization Group-III; SNF, skilled nursing facility.

Source: Adapted from Provider Policy Manual. Division of Medicaid, state of Mississippi. https://sos.ms.gov/ACProposed/00017429b.pdf

a RUG-III classification) or commit more resources to patients' care (eg, if increasing expenses crosses a threshold for a new RUG-III classification, and, in turn, greater reimbursement).

In its first 2 years of the SNF PPS's implementation, SNF expenditures decreased by 14% nationwide. However, evidence suggested that under the payment system, SNFs reduced staffing levels, provided fewer therapy services overall, and avoided admitting higher risk patients. Other evidence suggested that some SNFs exhibited high rates of thresholding—delivering services to meet thresholds for higher RUG-III classifications and receiving greater reimbursements. Collectively, these dynamics raised concerns that SNF care could be driven more by financial motivation than patient care needs.

2019 to Present: Per Diem Payment Under the Patient-Driven Payment Model

In response to such limitations, Medicare replaced the RUG-III system with the Patient-Driven Payment Model (PDPM) in 2019. While the PDPM still operates under a per diem reimbursement structure, it reflects three main changes from the initial SNF PPS system:

De-emphasize volume of therapy services. Instead of assigning reimbursement based on the number of therapy minutes provided, the PDPM focuses on patient-level clinical and functional characteristics at the time of admission when assigning reimbursement. This is intended to address possible thresholding behavior.

Change per diem rate from fixed to variable. In the initial PPS structure, SNFs received the same per diem reimbursement rate each day. Medicare found that actual service needs tended to be higher earlier in a SNF stay and then decrease over time. In the PDPM, Medicare includes a variable per diem adjustment, comparatively raising the per diem rate for earlier components of the stay and decreasing reimbursement for subsequent days.

Balance reimbursement based on therapy and nontherapy needs. Whereas the previous reimbursement system heavily weighted therapy services provided in reimbursement, the new system aims to reward SNFs for providing a wider variety of services. This is intended to address the concern that SNFs were providing high levels of therapy services independent of need and avoiding patients with higher medical or social complexity. The PDPM does so by adding a separate reimbursement adjustment for each of the following factors: physical therapy, occupational therapy, speech therapy, nursing, and nontherapy ancillary services. Each has its own criteria for classification and its own contribution to final reimbursement.

The impacts of this payment model remain unclear given implementation in 2019 immediately preceding the COVID-19 pandemic. Nonetheless, commonalities in different iterations of SNF reimbursement systems include the following:

- Reimbursement is provided prospectively via per diem payments.
- Reimbursement is related to care delivered at the SNF rather than based on systems-level outcomes, such as readmissions, care coordination, or cost reduction.

2013 to Present: Large-Scale Experiments With Episode-Based Payments

Recognizing the importance of care coordination across hospital and postacute care settings such as SNFs, Medicare has tested several episode-based payment models meant to encompass and create financial incentives for hospitals, clinicians, and SNFs to improve coordination, quality, and cost-efficiency across defined surgical or medical episodes of care.

These episode-based payments, also referred to as bundled payments, served as potential alternatives to per diem reimbursement. Through bundled payments, clinicians assume accountability for the quality and cost of care delivered during a predetermined episode of care. Clinicians or medical care organizations that achieve cost savings get to keep a portion of those savings, and those who do not may face financial penalties.

The first Medicare episode-based payment model that included SNFs in care episodes was the Bundled Payments for Care Improvement (BPCI) initiative, a voluntary model launched in 2013 that lasted through 2016. The BPCI created episode-based payment options for 48 different clinical episodes, including episodes focused on the following:

- Cardiac care (eg, congestive heart failure, myocardial infarction)
- Cardiac procedures (eg, pacemaker placement, stent placement)
- Gastrointestinal surgery (eg, bariatric surgery)
- Gastrointestinal care (eg, gastrointestinal obstruction or hemorrhage)
- Neurologic care (eg, seizures or stroke)
- Medical or critical care (eg, pneumonia, urinary tract infections)
- Spinal procedures (eg, spinal fusion)
- Other orthopedic care (eg, femur or hip fractures, joint replacements)

There were four different models for care episodes in which clinicians and medical care organizations could choose to participate. One of these focused strictly on care delivered in postacute care settings such as SNFs and one focused on care delivered in both hospital and postacute settings in the 90 days after hospital discharge. In these models, clinicians and medical care organizations were paid on a fee-for-service basis throughout the episode, and costs were reconciled after the episode concluded.

Research has demonstrated associations between bundled payments and cost savings with stable quality for surgical and medical episodes, with one study of a high performer observing a 20% reduction in Medicare expenditures for joint replacement episodes driven in part by reduced postacute care spending. Building on findings from this model, Medicare launched a similar successor model encompassing SNFs and postacute care, called BPCI Advanced, which runs through 2025.

The main potential benefit of including SNFs within episode-based payment models is the added incentive for postacute care facilities to communicate, coordinate, and collaborate with hospitals and clinicians to deliver high quality, cost-efficient care. Strategies for doing so have included informal hospital-postacute care facility networks and formalized financial relationships between hospitals and SNFs.

Back to the Clinical Case

In this case, because the patient is insured through Medicare and is within her first 20 days of a SNF stay, Medicare would pay for the entirety of her SNF care without patient cost sharing. If this patient's SNF stay were to exceed 100 days, her long-term care at the SNF would be covered through Medicaid since she is dually eligible for Medicaid as well as Medicare. If the SNF accepting the patient participated in an episode-based payment model, such as BPCI Advanced, it might coordinate the patient's care with the discharging hospital and clinicians to address quality and cost outcomes.

> ### TAKEAWAYS
>
> - Medicare and Medicaid have different SNF benefits: Medicare typically covers up to 100 days of SNF care focused on short-term rehabilitation; Medicaid covers both short-term rehabilitation stays and long-term custodial care at SNFs.
> - SNFs historically are paid predominantly by Medicare on a per diem basis with emphasis on therapy minutes, creating incentives related to provision of therapy minutes, management of daily expenses, and management of SNF length of stay.
> - Over the past decade, Medicare has implemented large-scale episode-based payment models that encompass the care that patients receive across hospital and SNF settings, with evidence demonstrating cost savings and stable quality for surgical and medical episodes of care.

Implications

The systems factors in this chapter have implications for access to postacute care. The types of postacute care options are organized on the basis of patient need, but such care options are not distributed uniformly. For instance, approximately 95% of LTCHs are concentrated in urban areas and in the south, which may make this care site less of an accessible option elsewhere.

When patients plan to discharge from a hospital to a SNF, the SNF referral process also has access implications. This process, where SNFs can consider whether a patient is a good match based on clinical, financial, or operational factors, gives SNFs considerable agency in which patients are offered admission. Studies show that patients with lower overall medical or social complexity are more likely to be offered SNF admission.

There are also differences in accessibility to SNFs based on whether the patient is in an urban or a rural community. For example, SNFs in urban areas generally receive more referrals to admit patients than in rural areas. Consequently, SNFs in urban areas are approximately 20% more likely to deny a patient referral than a rural SNF. In addition, availability of SNFs in the west and east regions was lower than in the central region, which could reflect higher labor costs not covered by CMS reimbursements. Further, with the advent of the Five-Star Quality Rating System, more information is known about the quality of SNFs that patients have access to in addition to the availability of SNFs for patient placement. One study found that between 2011 and 2019, availability of SNF beds per population declined overall, declined more so in urban than nonurban areas, and that the share of available SNF beds that had four- or five-star ratings also declined.

The systems factors also have implications for quality of care. Statutory and regulatory efforts have had an impact on quality of care. For instance, enactment of the Nursing Home Reform Act was found to be associated with lower use of physical (eg, hand ties) and chemical (eg, antipsychotic medication) restraints on patients. In particular, these practices decreased by more than 40% in the decade after the law was implemented, with many attributing the improvement to the law and educational initiatives that took place in individual SNFs. Similarly, the incidence of pressure sores (eg, breakdown of the skin that can lead to infection, usually the result of prolonged immobility and neglect) also decreased after implementation of the law.

The Five-Star Quality Rating System also has quality implications, including in how patients view quality of care at SNFs and in how SNFs focus quality improvement efforts. After implementation of the program, demand grew for higher quality SNFs (gained, on average, an 8% market share) and decreased for lower quality counterparts (lost 6% market share). SNFs reportedly pay close attention to their star ratings and develop strategies to improve their ratings. Evidence suggests that quality of care on a number of SNF quality components improved after implementation of the Five-Star Quality Rating System, although few studies have been able to discern the relationship between the star system and observed improvements.

The nature of SNF reimbursement also has quality implications, as it may influence care delivery patterns based on financial rather than quality motivations. For example, one concern about RUG-III assignment methods was the potential incentive for thresholding behavior. One study found that higher thresholding was associated with lower overall quality outcomes, including lower functional improvement and higher rates of 30-day readmissions.

The systems factors also have implications for health care costs. For instance, the relative supply of particular types of postacute care settings, and their cost compared to one another, have implications for the costs to US health care overall. LTCHs are the most expensive postacute care settings, with an average length of stay of 26 days and average cost of admission of more than $50 000 for ventilated patients. However, since LTCHs are relatively concentrated in urban areas and in the south, the impact on total US health care costs may be less than if they were more widely distributed.

The per diem nature of SNF reimbursement also poses cost implications. One concern about this type of approach is that it may conceivably create incentives for longer SNF lengths of stay, which could in turn increase costs of care. Despite the fact that longer SNF length of stay is associated with a small, reduced risk of short-term hospital readmission for some complex cases, one study found that staying 1 additional day in a SNF added over $300 to the average total cost of care.

In addition, de-emphasizing the role of therapy minutes in determining reimbursement may have cost implications. In particular, after implementation of the PDPM, therapy minutes decreased by 19% from 2019 to 2022. This reduction in therapy minutes occurred without changes in overall length of stay, functional status at discharge, or readmission to the hospital.

Lastly, systems factors discussed in this chapter have important equity implications. In the SNF referral process, patient diagnoses that are most commonly denied admission to SNFs are those related to mental illness and substance use disorders, which underscores inequities related to people living with mental health conditions. Further, patients with Medicaid insurance are more likely to be denied admission to a SNF than those with Medicare or private insurance. Even among patients admitted to SNFs, there can be inequities in the quality of care received. After the implementation of the Five-Star Quality Rating System, patients shifted from lower star rating SNFs to higher star rating SNFs; however, this shift was greater among patients enrolled in Medicare compared to those dually enrolled in Medicare and Medicaid. Furthermore, another study found that the strongest predictor of being admitted to a one-star facility was being dually eligible for Medicare and Medicaid health insurance. Identifying as Black or Hispanic was also associated with increased odds of being admitted to a one-star facility.

Multiple-Choice Questions

1. Lisette is a 76-year-old woman who lives alone and is admitted to the hospital after a fall from feeling generalized weakness. Her hospital evaluation found no fractures, but she did have pneumonia. She was treated over the course of 3 days under inpatient status with intravenous antibiotics, fluids, and oxygen. She is medically ready for discharge and will need to finish oral antibiotics after she leaves the hospital. The hospital physical therapist and occupational therapist recommend against a discharge to

home because they do not think it's a safe environment for her given her weakness and inability to take her medications every day without help. Based on her needs, what is the most appropriate postacute care setting for Lisette?

   A. Home health
   B. SNF
   C. IRF
   D. LTCH

2. Which of the following is least likely to affect the SNF referral process and the likelihood of a patient's acceptance to a SNF?

   A. The patient's insurance type
   B. Star ratings of the hospital where the patient is admitted
   C. Star ratings of SNF
   D. Geographic location of SNF

3. Which of the following are components of quality for which SNFs receive a star rating on the Nursing Home Compare site?

   A. Health inspections
   B. Patient loneliness
   C. Staffing
   D. A and C

4. Sylvia is a 77-year-old woman insured through Traditional Medicare and admitted to a SNF after a hospitalization for COVID-19 pneumonia. She was admitted for 28 days. What is Sylvia's out-of-pocket cost sharing responsibility for this SNF stay?

   A. $0 out of pocket
   B. $100 a day for all 28 days
   C. The entire cost
   D. $0 out of pocket for the first 20 days and $200 daily for days 21 through 28

Answers

1. The correct answer is B. SNF is the most appropriate for this patient since it will be able to provide around-the-clock care, help manage the patient's medications and meals, and she will receive regular rehabilitation services to help her regain her strength until she can go home. She qualifies for a SNF stay in the Medicare program, since she's been hospitalized under inpatient status at least 3 days.

2. The correct answer is B. The SNF star ratings, not the hospital star ratings, directly inform patients and the multidisciplinary care team on where to send SNF referrals. The SNFs with higher star ratings are likely to receive more referrals from hospitals.

3. The correct answer is D. Nursing Home Compare reports a star rating for health inspections, staffing, and other individual components, as well as a star rating for overall performance.

4. The correct answer is D. Since Sylvia is covered by Medicare, reimbursement for her care is governed by Medicare benefits, where she has $0 of cost sharing for the first 20 days and pays $200 daily out of pocket for days 21 to 100.

Bibliography

Agarwal R, Liao JM, Gupta A, Navathe AS. The impact of bundled payment on health care spending, utilization, and quality: a systematic review. *Health Aff (Millwood)*. 2020;39(1): 50-57.

Agency for Healthcare Research and Quality. An all-payer view of hospital discharge to postacute care, 2013 #205. Published May 2016. https://hcup-us.ahrq.gov/reports/statbriefs/sb205-Hospital-Discharge-Postacute-Care.jsp

American Hospital Association. Fact sheet: inpatient rehabilitation facilities—a unique and critical service: new COPs proposed for IRFs. https://www.aha.org/system/files/media/file/2019/07/fact-sheet-irf-0719.pdf

American Hospital Association. Fast facts on U.S. hospitals, 2023. https://www.aha.org/statistics/fast-facts-us-hospitals

American Hospital Association. Study downplays vital role of long-term care hospitals in patient care. *AHA News*. https://www.aha.org/news/blog/2021-05-26-study-downplays-vital-role-long-term-care-hospitals-patient-care

Barnett ML, Wilcock A, McWilliams JM, et al. Two-year evaluation of mandatory bundled payments for joint replacement. *N Engl J Med*. 2019;380(3):252-262.

Bartlett VL, Ross JS, Balasuriya L, Rhee TG. Association of psychiatric diagnoses and Medicaid coverage with length of stay among inpatients discharged to skilled nursing facilities. *J Gen Intern Med*. 2022;37(12):3070.

Bostick JE. Relationship of nursing personnel and nursing home care quality. *J Nurs Care Qual*. 2004;19(2):130-136.

Burke RE, Lawrence E, Ladebue A, et al. How hospital clinicians select patients for skilled nursing facilities. *J Am Geriatr Soc*. 2017;65(11):2466-2472.

Carter C, Garrett AB, Wissoker D. Reforming Medicare payments to skilled nursing facilities to cut incentives for unneeded care and avoiding high-cost patients. *Health Aff (Millwood)*. 2012;31(6):1303-1313.

Center for Medicare Advocacy. CMS confirms steep decline in therapy at nursing facilities. https://medicareadvocacy.org/cms-confirms-steep-decline-in-therapy-at-nursing-facilities/

Center for Medicare Advocacy. Discharge planning: tips for evaluating a hospital's skilled nursing facility placement choices. https://medicareadvocacy.org/discharge-planning-tips-for-evaluating-a-hospitals-skilled-nursing-facility-placement-choices/

Centers for Medicare and Medicaid Services. BPCI advanced. https://www.cms.gov/priorities/innovation/innovation-models/bpci-advanced

Centers for Medicare and Medicaid Services. Brief explanation of five-star rating methodology. https://www.cms.gov/medicare/provider-enrollment-and-certification/certification andcomplianc/downloads/brieffivestartug.pdf

Centers for Medicare and Medicaid Services. Bundled payments for care improvement (BPCI) initiative: general information. https://www.cms.gov/priorities/innovation/innovation-models/bundled-payments

Centers for Medicare and Medicaid Services. CMS issues historic star quality rating system for nursing homes. https://www.cms.gov/newsroom/press-releases/cms-issues-historic-star-quality-rating-system-nursing-homes

Centers for Medicare and Medicaid Services. Dually eligible individuals—categories. https://www.cms.gov/medicare-medicaid-coordination/medicare-and-medicaid-coordination/medicare-medicaid-coordination-office/downloads/medicaremedicaidenrolleecategories.pdf

Centers for Medicare and Medicaid Services. Five-star quality rating system. https://www.cms.gov/medicare/health-safety-standards/certification-compliance/five-star-quality-rating-system

Centers for Medicare and Medicaid Services. Home health providers. https://www.cms.gov/medicare/health-safety-standards/guidance-for-laws-regulations/home-health-agencies/home-health-providers

Centers for Medicare and Medicaid Services. Home health services. https://www.medicare.gov/coverage/home-health-services

Centers for Medicare and Medicaid Services. Long-term care hospital—general information. Provider Data Catalog. https://data.cms.gov/provider-data/dataset/azum-44iv

Centers for Medicare and Medicaid Services. *Medicare and Home Health Care.* 2003. https://www.cms.gov/Medicare/Quality-Initiatives-Patient-Assessment-Instruments/HomeHealthQualityInits/Downloads/HHQIHHBenefits.pdf

Centers for Medicare and Medicaid Services. Medicare and Medicaid Programs: minimum staffing standards for long-term care facilities and Medicaid institutional payment transparency reporting (CMS 3442-P). https://www.cms.gov/newsroom/fact-sheets/medicare-and-medicaid-programs-minimum-staffing-standards-long-term-care-facilities-and-medicaid

Centers for Medicare and Medicaid Services. Medicare skilled nursing facility (SNF) transparency data (CY2013). https://www.cms.gov/newsroom/fact-sheets/medicare-skilled-nursing-facility-snf-transparency-data-cy2013

Centers for Medicare and Medicaid Services. Patient driven payment model. Fact sheet: variable per diem adjustment. https://www.cms.gov/Medicare/Medicare-Fee-for-Service-Payment/SNFPPS/Downloads/PDPM_Fact_Sheet_VPD_v3_508.pdf

Centers for Medicare and Medicaid Services. Skilled nursing facility (SNF) care. https://www.medicare.gov/coverage/skilled-nursing-facility-snf-care

Chidambaram P, Burns A. 10 things about long-term services and supports (LTSS). *Kaiser Family Foundation.* Published September 15, 2022. https://www.kff.org/medicaid/issue-brief/10-things-about-long-term-services-and-supports-ltss/

Chidambaram P, Burns A. A look at nursing facility characteristics between 2015 and 2023. *Kaiser Family Foundation*. Published January 5, 2024. https://www.kff.org/medicaid/issue-brief/a-look-at-nursing-facility-characteristics/

Chidambaram P. What share of nursing facilities might meet proposed new requirements for nursing staff hours? *Kaiser Family Foundation*. Published September 18, 2023. https://www.kff.org/medicaid/issue-brief/what-share-of-nursing-facilities-might-meet-proposed-new-requirements-for-nursing-staff-hours/

Division of Medicaid, State of Mississippi. Provider policy manual. https://sos.ms.gov/ACProposed/00017429b.pdf

Einav L, Finkelstein A, Mahoney N. Long-term care hospitals: a case study in waste. RePEc: research papers in economics. Published online August 1, 2018. https://siepr.stanford.edu/publications/working-paper/long-term-care-hospitals-case-study-waste

Fries BE, Schneider DP, Foley WJ, Gavazzi M, Burke R, Cornelius E. Refining a case-mix measure for nursing homes: Resource Utilization Groups (RUG-III). *Med Care*. 1994;32(7):668-685.

Fuller RL, Goldfield NI, Hughes JS, McCullough EC. Nursing home compare star rankings and the variation in potentially preventable emergency department visits and hospital admissions. *Popul Health Manag*. 2019;22(2):144-152.

Gadbois EA, Tyler DA, Mor V. Selecting a skilled nursing facility for postacute care: the patient and family perspective running title: skilled nursing facility selection. *J Am Geriatr Soc*. 2017;65(11):2459.

Grabowski DC, Chen A, Saliba D. Paying for nursing home quality: an elusive but important goal. *J Am Geriatr Soc*. 2023;71(2):342-348.

Harrington C, Edelman TS. Failure to meet nurse staffing standards: a litigation case study of a large US nursing home chain. *Inquiry*. 2018;55:46958018788686.

Hurd MD, Michaud PC, Rohwedder S. Distribution of lifetime nursing home use and of out-of-pocket spending. *Proc Natl Acad Sci U S A*. 2017;114(37):9838-9842.

Institute of Medicine (US) Committee on Improving Quality in Long-Term Care; Wunderlich GS, Kohler PO, eds. *Improving the Quality of Long-Term Care: State of Quality of Long-Term Care*.: National Academies Press (US); 2001. https://www.ncbi.nlm.nih.gov/books/NBK224503/

Institute of Medicine (US) Committee on Nursing Home Regulation. Appendix A, history of federal nursing home regulation. *Improving the Quality of Care in Nursing Homes*. National Academies Press (US); 1986. https://www.ncbi.nlm.nih.gov/books/NBK217552/

Joyce NR, McGuire TG, Bartels SJ, Mitchell SL, Grabowski DC. The impact of dementia special care units on quality of care: an instrumental variables analysis. *Health Serv Res*. 2018;53(5):3657-3679.

Kaiser Family Foundation. Distribution of certified nursing facility residents by primary payer source. https://www.kff.org/other/state-indicator/distribution-of-certified-nursing-facilities-by-primary-payer-source/

Kaiser Family Foundation. Total number of certified nursing facilities. https://www.kff.org/other/state-indicator/number-of-nursing-facilities/

Keehan SP, Fiore JA, Poisal JA, et al. National health expenditure projections, 2022-31: growth to stabilize once the COVID-19 public health emergency ends. *Health Aff (Millwood)*. 2023;42(7):886-898.

Konetzka RT, Yi D, Norton EC, Kilpatrick KE. Effects of Medicare payment changes on nursing home staffing and deficiencies. *Health Serv Res*. 2004;39(3):463.

Levinson DR. *Adverse Events in Skilled Nursing Facilities: National Incidence Among Medicare Beneficiaries (OEI-06-11-00370; 02/14).* Office of the Inspector General, US Department of Health and Human Services; 2014.

Liao JM, Navathe AS, Werner RM. The impact of Medicare's alternative payment models on the value of care. *Annu Rev Public Health.* 2020;41:551-565.

McGarry BE, White EM, Resnik LJ, Rahman M, Grabowski DC. Medicare's new patient driven payment model resulted in reductions in therapy staffing in skilled nursing facilities. *Health Aff (Millwood).* 2021;40(3):392-399.

McWilliams JM, Hatfield LA, Landon BE, Hamed P, Chernew ME. Medicare spending after 3 years of the Medicare Shared Savings Program. *N Engl J Med.* 2018;379(12):1139-1149.

Medicare Payment Advisory Commission. Inpatient rehabilitation facility services (March 2022 Report). Published March 2022. https://www.medpac.gov/document/chapter-9-inpatient-rehabilitation-facility-services-march-2022-report/

Medicare Payment Advisory Commission. Long-term care hospitals payment system. Payment basics. Published November 2021. https://www.medpac.gov/wp-content/uploads/2021/11/medpac_payment_basics_21_ltch_final_sec.pdf

Medicare Payment Advisory Commission. Skilled nursing facility services (March 2022 Report). https://www.medpac.gov/document/chapter-7-skilled-nursing-facility-services-march-2022-report/

Miller KEM, Chatterjee P, Werner RM. Trends in supply of nursing home beds, 2011-2019. *JAMA Netw Open.* 2023;6(3):e230640.

Mukamel DB, Saliba D, Ladd H, Konetzka RT. Daily variation in nursing home staffing and its association with quality measures. *JAMA Netw Open.* 2022;5(3):e222051.

National Academies of Sciences, Engineering, and Medicine; Health and Medicine Division; Board on Health Care Services; Committee on the Quality of Care in Nursing Homes. Introduction. *The National Imperative to Improve Nursing Home Quality: Honoring Our Commitment to Residents, Families, and Staff.* National Academies Press (US); 2022. https://www.ncbi.nlm.nih.gov/books/NBK584662/

Navathe AS, Troxel AB, Liao JM, et al. Cost of joint replacement using bundled payment models. *JAMA Intern Med.* 2017;177(2):214-222.

O'Connor M, Hanlon A, Naylor MD, Bowles KH. The impact of home health length of stay and number of skilled nursing visits on hospitalization among Medicare-reimbursed skilled home health beneficiaries. *Res Nurs Health.* 2015;38(4):257-267.

Prusynski R. Medicare payment policy in skilled nursing facilities: Lessons from a history of mixed success. *J Am Geriatr Soc.* 2021;69(12):3358-3364.

Prusynski RA, Frogner BK, Dahal AD, Skillman SM, Mroz TM. Skilled nursing facility characteristics associated with financially motivated therapy and relation to quality. *J Am Med Dir Assoc.* 2020;21(12):1944-1950.e3.

Prusynski RA, Frogner BK, Dahal AD, Skillman SM, Mroz TM. Skilled nursing facility characteristics associated with financially motivated therapy and relation to quality. *J Am Med Dir Assoc.* 2020;21(12):1944-1950.e3.

Rahman M, White EM, McGarry BE, et al. Association between the patient driven payment model and therapy utilization and patient outcomes in US skilled nursing facilities. *JAMA Health Forum.* 2022;3(1):E214366.

Reaves EL, Musumeci M. Medicaid and long-term services and supports: a prime. *Kaiser Family Foundation.* Published December 15, 2015. https://www.kff.org/medicaid/report/medicaid-and-long-term-services-and-supports-a-primer/

Rivera-Hernandez M, Rahman M, Mor V, Trivedi AN. Racial disparities in readmission rates among patients discharged to skilled nursing facilities. *J Am Geriatr Soc*. 2019; 67(8):1672.

Rolnick JA, Liao JM, Emanuel EJ, et al. Spending and quality after three years of Medicare's bundled payments for medical conditions: quasi-experimental difference-in-differences study. *BMJ*. 2020;369:m1780.

Schumacher RC, Chiu M, de Leon J, Krause K, Makam AN. Appropriateness of long-term acute care hospital transfer: a multicenter study of Medicare ACO beneficiaries. *J Am Med Dir Assoc*. 2021;22(8):1767-1771.e5.

Seneff MG, Wagner D, Thompson D, Honeycutt C, Silver MR. The impact of long-term acute-care facilities on the outcome and cost of care for patients undergoing prolonged mechanical ventilation. *Crit Care Med*. 2000;28(2):342-350.

Shang J, Needleman J, Liu J, Larson E, Stone PW. Nurse staffing and healthcare-associated infection, unit-level analysis. *J Nurs Adm*. 2019;49(5):260-265.

Shen K, McGarry BE, Grabowski DC, Gruber J, Gandhi AD. Staffing patterns in US nursing homes during COVID-19 outbreaks. *JAMA Health Forum*. 2022;3(7):e222151.

Shield R, Winblad U, McHugh J, Gadbois E, Tyler D. Choosing the best and scrambling for the rest: hospital–nursing home relationships and admissions to postacute care. *J Appl Gerontol*. 2018;38(4):479-498.

Strickland C, Chi N, Ditz L, et al. Factors influencing admission decisions in skilled nursing facilities: retrospective quantitative study. *J Med Internet Res*. 2023;25:e43518.

Tamara Konetzka R, Yan K, Werner RM. Two decades of nursing home compare: what have we learned? *Med Care Res Rev*. 2021;78(4):295-310.

Turcotte LA, Poss J, Fries B, Hirdes JP. An overview of international staff time measurement validation studies of the RUG-III case-mix system. *Health Serv Insights*. 2019;12: 1178632919827926.

Wang Y, Zhang Q, Spatz ES, et al. Persistent geographic variations in availability and quality of nursing home care in the United States: 1996 to 2016. *BMC Geriatr*. 2019;19(1):1-11.

Waters K, Handa L, Caballero B, Telahun A, Bann M. Substance use disorder as a predictor of skilled nursing facility referral failure. *J Gen Intern Med*. 2022;37(13):3506-3508.

Werner RM, Bressman E. Trends in postacute care utilization during the COVID-19 pandemic. *J Am Med Dir Assoc*. 2021;22(12):2496-2499.

Werner RM, Coe N, Qi M, Konetzka RT. The value of an additional day of postacute care in a skilled nursing facility. *Am J Health Econ*. 2023;9(1):1-21.

Werner RM, Konetzka RT, Polsky D. Changes in consumer demand following public reporting of summary quality ratings: an evaluation in nursing homes. *Health Serv Res*. 2016;51 (Suppl 2):1291-1309.

White C. Medicare's prospective payment system for skilled nursing facilities: effects on staffing and quality of care. *Inquiry*. 2005;42(4):351-366.

White C, Pizer SD, White AJ. Assessing the RUG-III resident classification system for skilled nursing facilities. *Health Care Financ Rev*. 2002;24(2):7-15.

Wiener JM, Freiman MP, Brown D. *Nursing Home Care Quality Twenty Years After The Omnibus Budget Reconciliation Act of 1987*. Kaiser Family Foundation; 2007.

Winzelberg GS. The quest for nursing home quality: learning history's lessons. *Arch Intern Med*. 2003;163(21):2552-2556.

Zhang W, Luck J, Patil V, Mendez-Luck CA, Kaiser A. Changes in therapy utilization at skilled nursing facilities under Medicare's patient driven payment model. *J Am Med Dir Assoc*. 2022;23(11):1765-1771.

Zhu JM, Patel V, Shea JA, Neuman MD, Werner RM. Hospitals using bundled payment report reducing skilled nursing facility use and improving care integration. *Health Aff (Millwood)*. 2018;37(8):1282-1289.

Zuckerman RB, Wu S, Chen LM, Joynt Maddox KE, Sheingold SH, Epstein AM. The five-star skilled nursing facility rating system and care of disadvantaged populations. *J Am Geriatr Soc*. 2019;67(1):108-114.

6

Urgent Care

> ## Clinical Case
>
> Because of the number of days remaining in her Medicare skilled nursing facility benefit period, Jessica is able to stay at skilled nursing facility A for a few more days. During this period, she gets stronger and then is discharged home from the skilled nursing facility. A few days later, on a Saturday, Jessica starts to feel light-headed, dizzy, confused, and sweaty. Her husband, Daniel, takes her blood sugar reading and sees that her blood sugar is low. He provides her some glucose tablets.
>
> Jessica starts to feel better a half hour later, and when they recheck Jessica's blood sugar, it has improved back to normal range. Jessica has never experienced hypoglycemia before, and she is worried about what to do. Jessica and her husband decide they should seek some medical attention for assessment and advice about how to manage insulin dosing. They call her primary care clinician, Dr Jackson, but learn that the office closed for the day without available after-hours clinicians. The office voicemail recommends going to the emergency room (ER) for any medical emergencies.
>
> Jessica and her husband consider going to the ER but decide not to because they are worried about long wait times. They wonder if there are any other care options.

This situation is common and potentially difficult to navigate. In this instance, the patient had a symptomatic medical issue from hypoglycemia that appears to be resolving but could recur, with serious or potentially life-threatening consequences. Unfortunately, the patient's options for seeking care are limited, in part due to challenges in ambulatory and ER settings.

These challenges emanate from several systems factors discussed in Chapter 1: Ambulatory Care and in Chapter 2: Emergency Care. In particular, the patient's inability to see her primary care clinician on a Saturday is driven by the hours of operation in ambulatory settings, a systems factor that restricts patient access outside regular weekday daytime hours. Unfortunately, the options that ambulatory practices can adopt to address hours of operation (eg, making primary care clinicians available by telephone at all times, having clinicians within a given practice share after-hours responsibilities, creating nurse triage lines, or implementing freestanding after-hours clinics as part of a larger integrated health system) do not appear to be available in this patient's case. Retail clinics provide additional ways for patients to access ambulatory care. But these facilities generally have narrow focuses (eg, treating minor conditions such as ear infections or bronchitis) that may not provide the care that patients need.

In the absence of ambulatory care options, patients in these circumstances might instead turn to ERs as an alternative. Since ERs are always open and access to emergency care is protected by the Emergency Medical Treatment and Active Labor Act, going to the ER is certainly a possible care option. However, in this case, the patient's care may not qualify for emergency stabilization services as her symptoms and hypoglycemia have improved. In addition, under ER triage methods, such as the Emergency Severity Index system, she would likely be designated as lower acuity. In turn, her emergency care would be affected by patient flow management as a systems factor that underlies the work in ERs to manage the influx, throughout, and outflow of patients. Given widespread challenges with crowding, patient flow management would likely result in considerable wait times for patients in this case.

The convergence of these ambulatory and emergency care systems factors ultimately creates a gap for patients seeking care for urgent, but not necessarily emergent, medical needs. Urgent care centers have emerged to fill this gap.

Urgent Care Centers: A Product of Ambulatory and Emergency Care Systems Factors

Urgent care centers are freestanding medical facilities that provide timely outpatient medical services for acute illnesses or injuries that would not likely result in death or severe disability if not treated immediately but have the potential to evolve into more serious medical emergencies if care is delayed more than 24 hours.

These facilities typically evaluate and treat illnesses that are beyond the capabilities of ambulatory and retail clinics but may not require the emergency stabilization expertise and capabilities of a full-scale ER. That is ostensibly part of the value proposition for urgent care centers: offering another site of care on the continuum between ambulatory and emergency care, with capacity and hours of operation that go beyond the former and services that can be delivered more conveniently and cheaply than the latter.

The Rise and Initial Fall of Urgent Care Centers: 1970s to the Early 1990s

Urgent care centers first emerged in the United States in 1973 in Rhode Island and Delaware. Clinicians, mostly those trained in emergency medicine and family medicine, noticed that patients were often seeking care in hospital ERs for urgent, but nonlife-threatening complaints. As an alternative to the hospital ER and typical ambulatory care clinics, these clinicians opened what, at the time, was referred to as freestanding ERs—what would later be referred to as urgent care centers.

These facilities were not physically connected to any hospital, and its clinicians cared for urgent, but not imminently life- or limb-threatening medical problems. Clinicians who operated these facilities used advertising and marketing techniques to generate business from patients with acute care needs, paying particular attention to make the experience of care more convenient than care received in ERs. Advertising efforts were directed at patients with health insurance, and people were typically required to provide payment or proof of insurance when they first arrived. Patients who sought care at these early urgent care centers typically saw a clinician within 15 to 30 minutes of arrival, and the facilities were typically open 15 hours a day, 7 days a week.

After the initial success of the first urgent care centers, they began to grow in number. In 1980, there were just 180 urgent care centers in the United States. By 1985, there were more than 3000 throughout the country. Going beyond the concept of a freestanding ER, hospitals began to purchase existing urgent centers or build their own.

However, after this initial rise, urgent care centers experienced a stark decline in the mid-1980s and early 1990s due to a few factors. First, given the entrepreneurial environment contributing to the growth of urgent care centers, there was concern about quality of care, and whether the clinicians who staffed these facilities were appropriately trained to provide the care being advertised. Clinicians at urgent care facilities were frequently and derogatorily referred to as a "doc in the box," a term that appeared in a 1982 article called "Shopping Mall Medicine." One physician was quoted in the article as saying that "[urgent care centers are] not out to improve the quality of medicine; they're looking at another form of revenue…They want to put up a 'Doc in the Box' sign every place there's a McDonald's."

Second, poor profitability prompted hospitals that purchased urgent care centers to shutter them. In part, closures were believed to result from higher overhead costs (eg, driven by union wages and additional management and nursing staff) for centers associated with a hospital, compared to freestanding centers. Third, even though many individual urgent care centers advertised themselves, there was not a consistent marketing strategy for urgent care as a concept and care setting. Patients, therefore, often did not know exactly what urgent care was, the services offered, or how it differentiated from other care settings.

A Resurgence of Urgent Care: Mid-1990s to the Present

Urgent care centers experienced a resurgence beginning in the mid-1990s. This rebound was thought to be driven largely by increasing acceptance of the concept of urgent care as a viable alternative to frustrations with ambulatory and emergency care. Those frustrations were grounded in real challenges. In 2002, fewer than 60% of US adults who had an urgent medical need felt they could have their needs addressed as soon as they wanted.

In response to these circumstances, urgent care centers grew once again—and rapidly. By the mid-2000s, there were as many as 20 000 centers throughout the United States, with approximately two new centers opening every week. Between 2008 and 2015, visits to urgent care centers grew 115%, and accounted for nearly $50 billion in annual revenue by 2023. This growth occurred unevenly across geographic areas, with approximately half of all centers located in suburban, rather than in urban or rural, locations. Growth in urgent care centers also varied across states, with some growing to possess higher concentrations of these facilities (for instance, with 1 center per 25 000 people in Tennessee) than others (for instance, with 1 center per 42 000 people in California and Illinois).

Services and Workforce at Urgent Care Centers

Urgent care exists on the care continuum between ambulatory and emergency care (Figure 6.1).

On one side of the continuum, ambulatory care tends to provide services ranging from preventive care (eg, cancer screening, vaccinations, healthy life-style counseling) to chronic disease management (eg, diabetes, hypertension, chronic obstructive pulmonary disease management), management of nonurgent minor acute conditions (eg, upper respiratory infections), minor injuries (eg, laceration repair), and basic diagnostic laboratory and imaging tests.

However, access to ambulatory clinics is often limited by hours of operation. While retail ambulatory clinics can provide expanded after-hours options, these sites often offer more narrowly focused services that encompass some preventive care (eg, vaccinations) and management of simple acute conditions, but not management of more moderate acute illnesses (eg, moderate or severe asthma exacerbations).

On the other side of the care continuum, emergency care offer services not generally managed by ambulatory care, including management of moderate

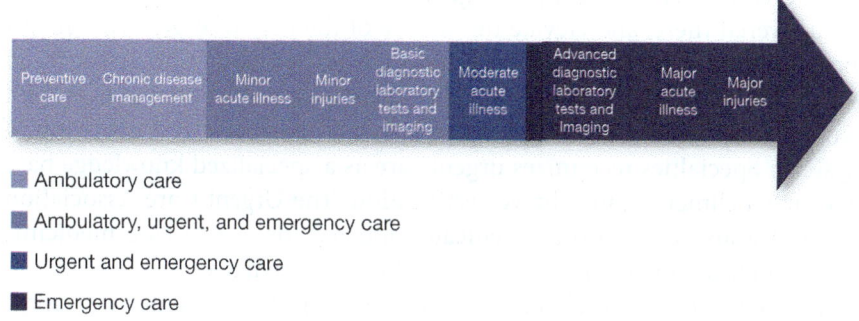

- ▥ Ambulatory care
- ▥ Ambulatory, urgent, and emergency care
- ▥ Urgent and emergency care
- ▥ Emergency care

Figure 6.1 Continuum of Ambulatory Care, Urgent Care, and Emergency Care Services. This figure depicts a general range of services provided in ambulatory, urgent, and emergency care settings. Specific services may vary at specific care sites along the continuum. (Source: Data from American Academy of Urgent Care Medicine. What is urgent care medicine. Accessed October 24, 2023. https://aaucm.org/what-is-urgent-care-medicine/)

and major acute conditions (eg, myocardial infarction, cerebrovascular accident, sepsis) and major injuries (eg, gunshot wounds), as well as advanced diagnostic laboratory and imaging tests (eg, magnetic resonance imaging).

Urgent care bridges ambulatory and emergency care. On one level, these centers provide services that can be otherwise offered in either ambulatory or emergency care settings, such as treatment of minor injuries and basic diagnostic laboratory and imaging studies. On another level, urgent care centers also provide services that otherwise might only be offered by emergency care, such as the management of moderate acute illnesses. In some cases, urgent care centers can provide advanced diagnostic studies, such as computed tomography (CT) imaging.

Ultimately, urgent care represents another setting where patients can receive services that would otherwise be delivered in ambulatory or emergency care settings, rather than a site for unique services not provided at other sites. In this way, urgent care centers fill a void in access and service convenience, emphasizing timely service while also accepting high volumes of patients (~70 patients per day on average).

Urgent care centers are usually staffed by physicians, nurse practitioners, and physician assistants. A 2009 research study found that family medicine was the most common specialty among the physician workforce, with family medicine doctors staffing nearly 75% of all urgent care centers at that time. Other common physician specialties staffing urgent care centers include emergency medicine, internal medicine, and pediatrics.

Since clinicians can spend their careers in urgent care settings, dedicated training and professional development programs have emerged to meet the needs of clinicians practicing in urgent care centers, increase the quality of care delivered there, and elevate the stature of the field of urgent care medicine. For instance, national organizations such as the Urgent Care Association of America offer online and in-person trainings, national conferences, and even a 1-year urgent care fellowship program. The American Association of Physician Specialties recognizes urgent care as a specialized knowledge base for which a clinician can achieve certification. The Urgent Care Association of America also cosponsors a dedicated journal for urgent care medicine, focused on teaching urgent care–related clinical knowledge.

At the same time, the composition of the urgent care center workforce is changing, with nurse practitioners and physician assistants making up an increasing percentage of the workforce. In 2009, it was estimated that 70% of clinicians working in urgent care centers were physicians. In 2022, that number decreased to 16%, with the remainder of clinicians represented by nurse practitioners and physician assistants.

Regulation of Urgent Care Centers

Care provided at urgent care centers varies in part due to limited certification and regulation, with 80% of US states, as of 2019, opting not to create dedicated licensing requirements for these facilities. Most often, urgent care centers operate under an individual physician's license or under a hospital license. When operating under a physician license, urgent care centers are overseen by state medical boards, which focus on misbehavior of individual clinicians rather than facilities. When operating under a hospital license, urgent care centers are viewed as extensions of a hospital, which limits oversight over the centers themselves.

One consequence of the latter is that centers can be built without the need to undergo the certificate of need process—one by which states consider need in order to review and approve the building of new medical facilities. This review and approval oversight only occurs when urgent care centers are licensed as their own entities—a rarity—and not when they are licensed under hospitals.

Even among states that do require dedicated licensure for urgent care centers, there is considerable variation in what that licensure entails. New York, for instance, uses more stringent licensure for urgent care centers that offer a large number of services while allowing smaller urgent care centers to be considered physician practices and, in turn, subject to less stringent licensure requirements. Also, unlike ERs associated with a hospital, urgent care centers do not have state or federal requirements to treat or stabilize patients who are unable to pay for care.

Outside of state-level licensure, multiple national trade groups have implemented accreditation programs to guide care delivery at urgent care centers. A small percentage of centers have achieved the accreditation through the Urgent Care Association of America. Some of the requirements in the Association's accreditation program include that the urgent care center must do the following:

- Accept walk-in patients of all ages for a broad spectrum of illness and injury.
- Provide x-ray, electrocardiogram (ECG), and many types of laboratory tests on site.
- Administer oral, intramuscular, and intravenous medications and fluids.
- Perform minor procedures (eg, cyst removals, incision and drainage, suture lacerations) when indicated.
- Be open 7 days a week, except for national holidays.
- Have a physician medical director.
- Be able to provide advanced cardiac life support services in case of an emergency while 9-1-1 is called, and have oxygen, a drug cart with emergency medications, and a defibrillator available with trained staff who know how to use the equipment.

Achieving accreditation can confer certain benefits. One is the ability for a center to differentiate itself from others in the community. Another is an advantage in achieving designation as in-network facilities for insurance plans.

Back to the Clinical Case

While the patient's needs could potentially be addressed by her primary care clinician, hours of operation preclude that option. Her lower acuity condition may not be suited for the broader range of ER capabilities. Assuming there is an urgent care center in the patient's neighborhood, the wait time and individual costs of her care could be considerably lower at an urgent care center than they would be in an ER.

In contrast to care the patient would receive in the ER, the patient would benefit from recognizing that urgent care centers would not necessarily be required to provide medical care. In addition, although clinicians at an urgent care center could address her acute concern (low blood sugar), they are not involved in decisions related to the patient's ongoing chronic disease management (diabetes), such as longer term changes to her insulin regimen.

TAKEAWAYS

- Urgent care centers have emerged and grown in number over time, driven in part by systems factors in ambulatory and emergency care that have created a gap in convenient options for urgent care needs.
- Urgent care centers provide services that are otherwise available at ambulatory care, emergency care settings, or both, but do so via added access and convenience.
- Urgent care centers are disproportionately located in suburban, higher income areas with a high percentage of privately insured populations and are increasingly staffed by nurse practitioners and physician assistants.
- Although there is limited direct licensure of urgent care centers, there have been increasing efforts to recognize high-quality care at urgent care centers through accreditation programs by national trade organizations.

Implications

The modern reemergence of urgent care centers has implications for access to care. At present, 80% of Americans live within 10 minutes of an urgent care center, a reality that is based in part in patients having difficulty accessing care in ambulatory settings due to hours of operation and challenges in ER settings due to the need for patient flow management and potentially long wait times. Wait times are generally considered shorter at urgent care centers than ERs. As of 2017, the wait time at 90% of urgent care centers was estimated to be 30 minutes or less, while in some ERs, the median wait time is nearly 2.5 hours.

In addition to being a potential alternative to ERs as a site of care, urgent care centers may directly affect nearby ERs. A research study found that the presence of an urgent care center in the same zip code as an ER reduced the total number of ER visits by residents of that zip code by nearly 20%, largely due to reduction in ER visits for lower acuity issues that had the longest ER wait times.

The rise of urgent care centers can also pose implications for quality of care. Although research in this area is limited, one 2018 study evaluating antibiotic prescription patterns in different care settings found that a higher percentage of patients received inappropriate antibiotic prescriptions for respiratory conditions in urgent care centers, compared to other sites of care. In particular, patients received antibiotics inappropriately in 46% of urgent care visits, compared to 25% of ER visits, 17% of medical office visits, and 14% of retail clinic visits.

Additional quality concerns can arise from the variability in services offered at urgent care centers, and the possibility that patients inappropriately seek care at urgent care centers when other sites (ambulatory or emergency care) might be more appropriate. For this reason, the American College of Emergency Physicians has advocated that urgent care centers should not be permitted to use the word "emergency" or "ER" in their names or advertising materials. Other studies have raised concerns that access to urgent care centers may come at the expense of patient care continuity with their usual or regular ambulatory clinicians, which can negatively impact the quality of preventive care and chronic disease management.

Urgent care centers also pose cost implications. On a per visit basis, the use of urgent care can reduce the cost of care for patients that would have otherwise visited an ER. Costs for an ER visit have been estimated to be approximately 10 times the cost of an urgent care visit. However, at the population level, substituting ER for urgent care visits may contribute to overall increases in total costs of care. A 2021 study found that for a reduction in one low-acuity ER visit, there were approximately 37 additional visits to urgent care centers. In turn, the $1646 saved, on average, from one less ER visit led to an average of $6327 in additional costs from more urgent care visits.

Lastly, urgent care centers can affect health equity. In particular, although these centers may improve access to care, the benefit may not been uniform across communities. A 2016 study found that nonhospital-associated urgent care centers were located in 38.6% of the highest income communities but only 16.4% of the lowest income communities; and in 29.6% of communities with the highest percentage of privately insured individuals but only 19.4% of communities with the lowest percent of privately insured individuals. Another potential equity concern is that, unlike ERs, urgent care centers are not required to care for patients if they're unable to pay for services. Instead, centers can turn patients away or could potentially engage in patient dumping.

Multiple-Choice Questions

1. Nina, a 73-year-old woman, trips over her bathroom rug at home and hits her shoulder but does not sustain any other injuries. Over the course of the day, her shoulder pain is persistent and impeding her ability to perform activities of daily living. Two weeks ago, she was diagnosed with an upper respiratory infection, but over the past few days her symptoms have worsened, and she has developed a new wheeze. It is the weekend, and her primary care clinician's office is closed. She would benefit from evaluation with basic diagnostic laboratory tests and imaging and potential treatment

based on those findings. Based on the information presented in Figure 6.1, which of the following care settings would generally be equipped to evaluate and treat this patient?

A. A retail clinic

B. An urgent care center

C. An ER

D. A, B, and C

2. Which of the following is *not* an Urgent Care Association of America accreditation criterion for urgent care centers?

A. Administer oral, intramuscular, and intravenous medications and fluids

B. Open 7 days a week, including on national holidays

C. Provide x-ray, ECG, and many types of laboratory tests on site.

D. Provide advanced cardiac life support services in case of an emergency while 9-1-1 is called, and have oxygen, a drug cart with emergency medications, and a defibrillator available with trained staff who know how to use the equipment.

3. As of 2019, what percentage of US states have dedicated licensing requirements for urgent care centers?

A. 20%

B. 40%

C. 60%

D. 80%

Answers

1. The correct answer is D. The patient is experiencing a minor acute illness, for which she'll need basic diagnostic laboratory tests and imaging, and treatment of a minor injury. As shown in Figure 6.1, this is likely in the scope of services that can be provided at a retail clinic, urgent care center, and an ER.

2. The correct answer is B. Urgent care centers are required to be open 7 days a week; however, they are not required to be open on national holidays.

3. The correct answer is A. In the remaining states, urgent care centers most often operate under an individual physician's license or under a hospital license.

Bibliography

AAUCM. What is urgent care medicine. Accessed October 24, 2023. https://aaucm.org/what-is-urgent-care-medicine/

Allen L, Cummings JR, Hockenberry JM. The impact of urgent care centers on nonemergent emergency department visits. *Health Serv Res*. 2021;56(4):721-730.

American College of Emergency Physicians. Policy statement: urgent care centers. January 2022. Accessed October 23, 2023. https://www.acep.org/siteassets/new-pdfs/policy-statements/urgent-care-centers.pdf

Ayers AA. Why private equity and other 'smart money' is bullish on brick-and-mortar urgent care. *J Urgent Care Med*. Published May 31, 2022. Accessed October 24, 2023. https://www.jucm.com/why-private-equity-and-other-smart-money-is-bullish-on-brick-and-mortar-urgent-care/

Barlow B, Sandler M, Ayers A. How urgent care can address its degrading scope of practice. *J Urgent Care Med*. Published November 30, 2022. Accessed October 24, 2023. https://www.jucm.com/how-urgent-care-can-address-its-degrading-scope-of-practice/

Bates DDB, Vintonyak A, Mohabir R, et al. Use of a portable computed tomography scanner for chest imaging of COVID-19 patients in the urgent care at a tertiary cancer center. *Emerg Radiol*. 2020;27(6):597-600.

Cision PR Newswire. The Urgent Care Association of America unveils new accreditation program. Published March 20, 2014. Accessed October 23, 2023. https://www.prnewswire.com/news-releases/the-urgent-care-association-of-america-unveils-new-accreditation-program-251207411.html

Fahimi J, Larimer E, Hamud-Ahmed W, et al. Long-term mortality of patients surviving firearm violence. *Inj Prev*. 2016;22(2):129-34.

Freudenheim M. Shopping mall medicine. New York Times. Published December 5, 1982. Accessed October 24, 2023. https://www.nytimes.com/1982/12/05/magazine/shopping-mall-medicine.html

Gray BK, Janiak B. Urgent care centres. *Arch Emerg Med*. 1985;2(4):197-199.

Le ST, Hsia RY. Community characteristics associated with where urgent care centers are located: a cross-sectional analysis. *BMJ Open*. 2016;6(4):e010663.

LI Urgent Care. What is the UCAOA accreditation designation. Accessed October 24, 2023. https://li-urgent-care.com/accreditation/ucaoa-2/

Mcneely S. Urgent care centers: an overview. *Am J Clin Med*. 2012;9(2):80-81. Accessed October 24, 2023. http://aapsus.org/wp-content/uploads/ucc80.pdf

Memmel J, Spalsbury M. Urgent care medicine and the role of the APP within this specialty. *Dis Mon*. 2017;63(5):105-114.

Meyersohn N. Why urgent care centers are popping up everywhere. CNN. Published January 28, 2023. Accessed October 24, 2023. https://www.cnn.com/2023/01/28/business/urgent-care-centers-growth-health-care/index.html

National Conference of State Legislatures. Certificate of need laws. Accessed October 24, 2023. https://www.ncsl.org/health/certificate-of-need-state-laws

National Urgent Care Center Accreditation. National Urgent Care Center Accreditation. Accessed October 23, 2023. http://ucaccreditation.org/

Palms DL, Hicks LA, Bartoces M, et al. Comparison of antibiotic prescribing in retail clinics, urgent care centers, emergency departments, and traditional ambulatory care settings in the United States. *JAMA Intern Med.* 2018;178(9):1267-1269.

Physicians Immediate Care Blog. Physicians Immediate Care achieves UCA accreditation. Published January 19, 2022. Accessed October 23, 2023. https://physiciansimmediatecare.com/physicians-immediate-care-achieves-ucaoa-accreditation/

Pollart SM, Compton RM, Elward KS. Management of acute asthma exacerbations. *Am Fam Physician.* 2011;84(1):40-47.

Poon SJ, Schuur JD, Mehrotra A. Trends in visits to acute care venues for treatment of low-acuity conditions in the United States from 2008 to 2015. *JAMA Intern Med.* 2018;178(10):1342-1349.

Ramgopal S, Karim SA, Subramanian S, Furtado AD, Marin JR. Rapid brain MRI protocols reduce head computerized tomography use in the pediatric emergency department. *BMC Pediatr.* 2020;20(1):14.

Sax DR, Warton EM, Mark DG, et al. Evaluation of the Emergency Severity Index in US emergency departments for the rate of mistriage. *JAMA Netw Open.* 2023;6(3):e233404.

Solomon T, Popkin KJ, Chen A, Uttley L, Baruch S. Making convenient care the right care for all: improving state oversight of urgent care centers and retail clinics. Community Catalyst. Accessed October 23, 2023. https://www.communitycatalyst.org/wp-content/uploads/2022/11/Urgent-Care-Center-BriefAppendix-2.pdf

Urgent Care Association. Accreditation. Accessed October 23, 2023. https://urgentcareassociation.org/quality/accreditation/

Villaseñor S, Krouse HJ. Can the use of urgent care centers improve access to care without undermining continuity in primary care? *J Am Assoc Nurse Pract.* 2016;28(6):335-341.

Wang B, Mehrotra A, Friedman AB. Urgent care centers deter some emergency department visits but, on net, increase spending. *Health Aff (Millwood).* 2021;40(4):587-595.

Weinick RM, Betancourt RM. No appointment needed: the resurgence of urgent care centers in the United States. California Healthcare Foundation. Published September 2007. Accessed October 24, 2023. https://www.chcf.org/wp-content/uploads/2017/12/PDF-NoAppointmentNecessaryUrgentCareCenters.pdf

Weinick RM, Bristol SJ, DesRoches CM. Urgent care centers in the U.S.: findings from a national survey. *BMC Health Serv Res.* 2009;9:79.

7

Home-Based and Virtual Care

Clinical Case

Jessica seeks care at the local urgent care center. While there, her vital signs and repeat blood glucose are within normal limits. The urgent care center gives her some crackers, instructions to check her blood glucose every 4 hours for the rest of the day, and discharges her home.

Two weeks later, Jessica has a follow-up visit with her primary care clinician, Dr Jackson, where she explains the events leading up to her urgent care visit. Jessica shares that she's frustrated that she needed to seek care outside the home during this episode, and that she did not have tools to more closely monitor her blood glucose at home that do not require frequent finger-stick measurements. She asks Dr Jackson if there are any resources that would enable her to treat herself at home if she has a mild hypoglycemia episode rather than seek attention in urgent care or emergency care.

This situation, where the patient felt she did not have the resources to manage an acute or a chronic medical condition at home, is common. Typically, patients seek medical care for acute and chronic needs at facilities (eg, primary care clinician's office, urgent care center, hospital). However, many patients would likely choose to receive care in home settings, including for chronic, acute, and postacute care, if there were resources to make it safe and feasible. The ability to access home-based care—or care delivered at home focused specifically on treating medical conditions—is particularly important for people who are considered homebound (ie, those who need supportive devices such as crutches or a wheelchair to leave the home, have a condition that would make leaving the home difficult, or for whom leaving home could worsen their medical condition). In the Medicare population, approximately

7.5 million patients are either completely homebound or need assistance to leave their homes.

Despite the potential benefits to patients, home-based care has been historically limited. For instance, between 2011 and 2017, only 5% of Medicare patients received any home-based care, most of whom were considered homebound. Still, even among homebound Medicare patients, only 11% received any home-based care.

However, this dynamic appears to be changing. Patients have increasingly been able to safely administer more of their health care in the comfort of their own homes, including for chronic, acute, and postacute medical needs. Between 2022 and 2025, the percentage of total Medicare expenditures spent on home-based care is expected to triple or quadruple, with the possibility that approximately 25% of total Medicare expenditures being delivered in the community in 2022 could shift to the home by 2025.

An important facilitator of whether patients can safely receive home-based care is access to virtual solutions, such as different forms of telemedicine, and certain treatment technologies. In this patient's case, access to telemedicine or treatment technology that would enable her to more closely monitor her blood glucose without the need for intermittent finger sticks may have obviated the need to seek attention at urgent care. In this way, telemedicine and treatment technologies are collectively a systems factor that can affect if and how Americans can receive health care at home.

SYSTEMS FACTOR: TELEMEDICINE AND TREATMENT TECHNOLOGY

Virtual solutions such as telemedicine can enable patients to safely receive home-based care by allowing them and their clinicians to evaluate, communicate, and monitor their medical conditions. Certain treatment technologies enable patients to receive care at home—another facilitator of home-based care and complement to virtual telemedicine services.

Telemedicine

There are two general types of telemedicine. The first type, asynchronous telemedicine, refers to technologies that enable a patient and clinician to communicate health information with one another, but not necessarily in real time. The second type, synchronous telemedicine, refers to technologies that enable a patient and clinician to communicate with one another specifically in real time.

Asynchronous Telemedicine

Remote patient monitoring. The first type of asynchronous telemedicine is remote patient monitoring, which encompasses devices that allow patients to directly gather health information without the need for in-person testing and then communicate that information virtually to clinicians for evaluation and analysis. Some common remote patient monitoring technologies and their uses are shown in Figure 7.1.

Remote patient monitoring can focus on cardiovascular health, including blood pressure or heart rhythm monitoring. Remote blood pressure monitoring allows patients to measure their blood pressure at home with a device that sends measurements to the clinician.

A second cardiovascular remote patient monitoring technology is heart rhythm monitoring, which allows patients to monitor their heart rhythm continuously at home with a device that sends data to the clinician. Some remote heart rhythm monitoring devices, for example, send real-time and summary data including average heart rate and variability, ST-segment analysis, QTc interval data, information about ventricular ectopy, and presence of bundle branch blocks or atrial arrhythmias. Patients are also able to inform some

Blood pressure monitoring
• Allows patients to measure their blood pressure at home with a device that sends measurements to the clinician

Heart rhythm monitoring
• Allows patients to monitor their heart rhythm continuously at home with a device that sends data to the clinician

Continuous glucose monitoring
• Allows patients to measure blood glucose continuously at home with a device that does not require finger sticks and sends measurements to the clinician

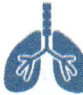
Pulse oximetry monitoring
• Allows patients to measure their blood oxygen saturation and heart rate continuously with a device that sends measurements to the clinician

Weight monitoring
• Allows patients to measure their weight at home with a device that sends measurements to the clinician

Figure 7.1 Remote Patient Monitoring.

heart rhythm monitoring devices when they are experiencing any symptoms (eg, chest pain, palpitations), and clinicians can then correlate those symptoms with any abnormalities found in heart rhythm data.

A third common remote patient monitoring technology is the continuous glucose monitor (CGM). This technology allows patients to measure blood glucose continuously at home with a device that does not require finger sticks and sends measurements to the clinician.

A fourth common remote patient monitoring technology is pulse oximetry monitoring, which allows patients to measure their blood oxygen saturation and heart rate continuously with a device that sends measurements to the clinician.

Finally, weight monitoring is a remote patient monitoring technology that allows patients to measure their weight at home with a device that sends measurements to the clinician.

Store-and-forward. A second type of asynchronous telemedicine is store-and-forward. This involves the use of technology for secure electronic sharing of medical information, such as photographs, videos, data collected from remote patient monitors, or direct questions that can be reviewed and responded to at a later time. One way store-and-forward can be used is for patients to communicate virtually with their clinician, usually through an electronic health record's secure messaging portal.

Store-and-forward can also be used for clinicians to communicate with one another, a practice often referred to as an e-consult. In an e-consult, the receiving and referring clinicians communicate asynchronously through the electronic health record and no direct visit takes place between the patient and the receiving clinician.

Together, remote patient monitoring and store-and-forward telemedicine provide ways patients can use virtual methods to share medical information with their clinicians, ask questions of their clinicians, and receive medical advice based on that information without necessarily needing to leave home.

Synchronous Telemedicine

The first type of synchronous telemedicine is audiovisual telemedicine, which includes the use of virtual conferencing technology for a real-time interactive health care visit, where the patient and clinician are in different locations. The second type, audio-only telemedicine, refers to the use of phone or other audio technology for a real-time interactive health care visit, where the patient and clinician are also in different locations. Audiovisual and audio-only telemedicine can facilitate real-time visits between clinicians and patients for acute or chronic illnesses that do not require hands-on physical examination, without needing to leave home.

Treatment Technologies

Beyond the ability to evaluate and monitor patients' medical conditions using asynchronous and synchronous telemedicine, another component of home-based care is the ability to treat or manage conditions and related health needs from home. A range of treatment technologies can help, facilitating the treatment of acute and chronic medical conditions at home of varying degrees of complexity. Three examples of treatment technologies for home-based care are described in Figure 7.2 and in subsequent text.

Smart medication dispensers. They are specialized devices that can remind patients to take medication, organize and dispense medication, track medication adherence, and communicate adherence information with the patient's clinician. Patients with multiple chronic conditions and who take several medications each day may have difficulties taking their medications appropriately and consistently. Incomplete medication adherence can also be associated with poor health outcomes, including hospitalization and death. Therefore, smart medication dispensers represent a potential tool that can support home-based care.

Home infusions. They are another type of treatment technology that can support home-based care. Infusion devices are long-existing technologies for delivering intravenous medications that can be made available outside of dedicated facilities, hospitals, and clinics, for use at home for certain ambulatory medications (eg, chemotherapy) or for hospital medications (eg, intravenous

Smart medication dispensers
- Specialized devices that can remind patients to take medication, organize and dispense medication, track medication adherence, and communicate adherence information with the patients' clinician

Home infusion
- Intravenous medication administration systems made available for use at home for certain ambulatory medications (eg, chemotherapy) or for hospital medications (eg, intravenous fluids or antibiotics)

Home dialysis
- Machines that guide patients through the process of receiving dialysis from home rather than in a specific dialysis facility

Figure 7.2 Treatment Technologies.

fluids or antibiotics). Therefore, home infusions represent an important deployment of technology to facilitate home-based care.

Home dialysis. They are machines that can guide patients through the process of receiving hemodialysis from home rather than in a dialysis facility. Peritoneal dialysis, which requires patients to infuse dialysis solution into the lining of their abdomen, has been historically done at home for decades. Home hemodialysis is an additional advancement that can help patients circumvent facility-based hemodialysis in which they travel multiple times a week to facilities for 3- to 5-hour dialysis sessions.

Integrating Telemedicine and Treatment Technologies for Home-Based Care

Together, the combination of asynchronous and synchronous telemedicine and treatment technologies enables patients to receive home-based care (Figure 7.3). These three tools can be applied to address patients' chronic, acute, and postacute care needs.

Chronic Care Needs

When integrated, telemedicine and treatment technologies can be used to address patients' chronic care needs. For instance, consider a patient with diabetes and end-stage kidney disease on dialysis. A patient with these conditions has extensive ongoing care needs, including dialysis possibly several times per week, adjustments to diabetes medication such as insulin in response to fluctuations in blood glucose, and ongoing visits with their clinician team. In the absence of telemedicine and treatment technologies at home, a patient living with these conditions would need to leave home, possibly several times per week, to meet many or all their chronic care needs.

In contrast, telemedicine and certain treatment technologies can allow for a patient such as this to receive all or most of their care from home. For example, the patient with end-stage kidney disease can accumulate extra fluid, gain weight, and potentially require hospitalization if these developments are not managed in a timely manner. Remote weight monitoring can enable a clinician and patient to more closely assess and act on weight information, for instance, by titrating diuretic medications, adjusting salt and fluid intake, or changing someone's dialysis plan. Similarly, a patient with end-stage kidney disease can be prone to blood pressure fluctuations, including having blood pressures that are particularly hypertensive or hypotensive. Remote blood pressure monitoring can allow for the patient to asynchronously share their blood pressure information (and fluctuations) with their clinician, and synchronous telemedicine visits can provide opportunities for the patient to discuss treatment plans from home.

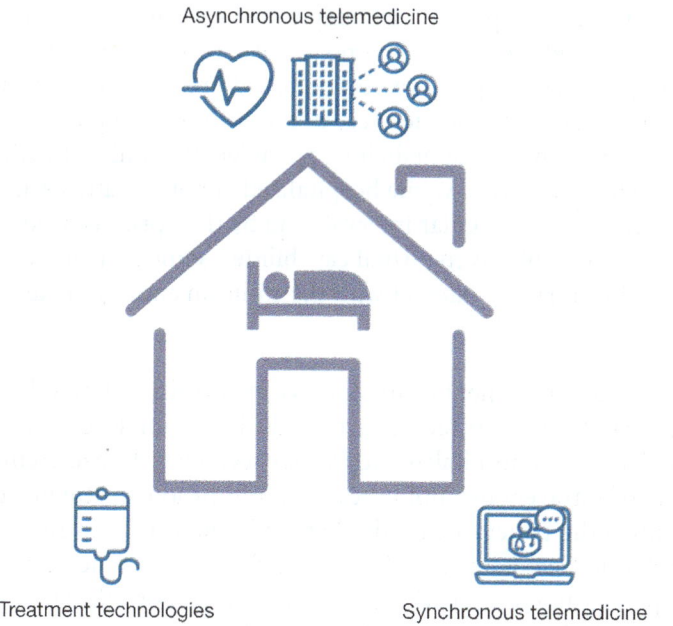

Asynchronous telemedicine

Treatment technologies   Synchronous telemedicine

Figure 7.3 Integrating Telemedicine and Treatment Technologies for Home-Based Care.

When incorporated in the home environment, treatment technologies can also facilitate home-based care for chronic care needs. For example, this hypothetical patient with diabetes may have to balance multiple medications taken several times per day. Smart medication dispensers, in their capacity to organize, dispense, and remind patients to take their medications, represent a potential tool that can support chronic home-based care. Similarly, both peritoneal dialysis and hemodialysis would enable this patient to receive dialysis from home. In the absence of these treatment technologies, the patient would likely have to leave home approximately for several hours at a time multiple times per week.

Acute Care Needs

Telemedicine and treatment technologies can also enable patients to manage more acute care needs from home. For instance, one model that seeks to integrate telemedicine and treatment technology is Hospital at Home. In this model, patients are first identified in the emergency room or by a clinician in the community as being sick enough to require hospital-level care, but able to be safely treated at home. Patients who are able to be treated via defined treatment protocols, such as for congestive heart failure or chronic obstructive pulmonary disease exacerbations, pneumonia, or cellulitis, are often considered a good fit for the Hospital at Home model.

Under this model, patients are assigned a care team that can include physicians, nurses, and therapists. Patients are also provided with remote patient monitoring (eg, remote pulse oximetry, blood pressure, heart rhythm monitoring), treatment technologies (eg, home infusion supplies), and devices capable of synchronous telemedicine (eg, tablets that link with clinicians via audiovisual telemedicine). While hospitalized at home, patients are visited in person by clinicians at regular intervals and by therapists as needed or as determined by protocol. Given virtual capabilities, some patients receiving care under Hospital at Home interact with the clinician entirely via telemedicine.

Postacute Care Needs

Telemedicine and treatment technologies can also enable home-based care in ways that may address postacute care needs. For example, consider a patient who may have been hospitalized for sepsis secondary to bacteremia, requiring weeks of intravenous antibiotics. Home infusion treatment technology may facilitate the patient being discharged home earlier to receive intravenous antibiotic treatment from home. Synchronous telemedicine could enable the patient to connect with their primary care or other clinicians for a posthospital discharge visit. Asynchronous telemedicine such as remote pulse oximetry could provide clinicians with early signs of clinical worsening, such as hypoxemia or tachycardia, and prompt subsequent action. In these ways, telemedicine and treatment technologies could remove barriers to patients receiving postacute services at home.

Back to the Clinical Case

In this patient's case, telemedicine could have enabled her to receive care at home rather than at urgent care. For example, a CGM would enable this patient to have real-time measurements of her blood glucose level without the need for finger sticks, offering insight into her response to home treatments for hypoglycemia and providing information about further changes in her blood glucose levels. In addition, information from remote monitoring could be sent to her clinician to then asynchronously provide advice on medication regimen and disease management. Treatment technology such as a smart medication dispenser could help the patient organize and take her medications at home in a way that supports safety and adherence.

TAKEAWAYS

- Asynchronous and synchronous telemedicine can facilitate evaluation and monitoring of medical conditions from home.

- Treatment technologies (eg, smart medication dispensers, home infusion, home dialysis) can enable patients to treat their medical conditions from home.
- Together, the combination of telemedicine and treatment technologies can facilitate patients receiving health care in home settings for chronic, acute, and postacute care needs.

Clinical Case Continued

Jessica's primary care clinician prescribes her a CGM and explains that she and her husband will be able to use it to check her blood glucose levels throughout the day. The primary care clinician also explains that she will be able to access Jessica's CGM measurements through the electronic health record.

   The primary care clinician also schedules a video telemedicine visit with Jessica to discuss the results of her CGM. Jessica's husband is relieved and feels comfortable with a video visit, as both he and Jessica have been using Zoom to connect with their grandchildren for years. The patient and her husband were not aware of video visits as an option and ask the primary care clinician if they are a new feature to the clinic.

In this situation, the patient needs a way to access care and address care needs (eg, insulin administration, monitoring glucose levels) while facing difficulties leaving home. The two telemedicine solutions proposed by the primary care physician are designed to help. In particular, CGM can generate the information needed to guide the patient's care while reducing the burden of checking and reporting these data to the primary care clinician. An audiovisual visit can enable the patient to stay connected with her clinicians while remaining at home. Beyond technologic advances and regulatory approval, adoption of telemedicine requires a payment system that incentivizes its use. In this way, reimbursement for telemedicine is a health systems factor driving its incorporation into patient care at scale.

HEALTH SYSTEMS FACTOR: REIMBURSEMENT FOR TELEMEDICINE

Telemedicine has been rapidly growing in US health care. In 2018 and 2019, just 15% of clinicians used telemedicine. By 2021, that number had increased to nearly 90%. Much of that change took place during the COVID-19 pandemic, and three-quarters of US adults who were asked indicated that they would want to continue using telemedicine after the pandemic ended.

Setting aside restrictions for in-person contact in the earliest phases of the pandemic, this rapid scaling up of telemedicine use by clinicians and patients was not driven primarily by technology, which existed for synchronous and asynchronous telemedicine modalities before COVID-19. Instead, one major difference and driver of rapid telemedicine adoption was a collection of changes in reimbursement policy.

Reimbursement for Asynchronous Telemedicine

Reimbursement for remote patient monitoring. From a technology perspective, remote patient monitoring, including for remote blood glucose, weight, pulse oximetry, and blood pressure, has been available for decades. However, before 2019, uptake of remote patient monitoring was not widespread, and mostly centered on CGM, as it was already reimbursable via existing billing codes. In 2019, Medicare introduced broader codes that enabled reimbursement for other types of remote patient monitoring.

Initial uptake was modest, as billing codes involved limitations and restrictions, such as minimum number of days clinicians needed to monitor patient data using the technology in order to be reimbursed. In addition, clinicians were required to have established relationships with the patient to be reimbursed for the use of remote patient monitoring. In response to the COVID-19 Public Health Emergency, Medicare and private payers loosened many of their restrictions on clinician reimbursement for the use of remote patient monitoring.

Subsequently, during the first year of the COVID-19 pandemic, billing for remote patient monitoring more than quadrupled. Among patients being remotely monitored, approximately half were still using it 6 months after initiation, and the estimated annual charges per patient using these technologies were approximately $700.

Reimbursement for store-and-forward. Historically, Medicare did not directly reimburse store-and-forward interactions such as secure messaging in most instances, and Medicaid reimbursement varied significantly state by state. These realities made the use of secure messaging between a clinician and patient via store-and-forward uncompensated care.

Still, the use of store-and-forward was relatively prevalent, as 6 in 10 patients prior to the pandemic had access to an electronic health record secure messaging portal that was capable of store-and-forward, and 6 in 10 patients who had access to store-and-forward technology on a secure messaging portal reported using the technology. This widespread use was facilitated in part by the Meaningful Use of Certified Electronic Health Records Program, a component of the Health Information Technology for Economic Clinical Health Act. This policy at first financially rewarded clinicians for having electronic health records with this technology and later penalized clinicians if they did not have a portal capable of secure messaging or if they had it but it was not sufficiently used. Therefore, despite no direct reimbursement for store-and-forward telemedicine, underlying financial incentives played a role in facilitating its scaling.

During the COVID-19 pandemic, patients' secure messages to clinicians increased by more than 50%, and to make the use of store-and-forward sustainable, reimbursement policy changed. In response to this increase in secure messaging use during the pandemic, Medicare made a particular type of store-and-forward interaction, called e-visits, reimbursable. An e-visit is an asynchronous interaction between a clinician and patient conducted via an electronic health record's secure messaging portal. In order to be eligible for reimbursement, an e-visit must be initiated by the patient, and must require at least 5 minutes of a clinician's time for medical decision-making.

Reimbursement for Synchronous Telemedicine

Reimbursement prior to the COVID-19 Public Health Emergency. Before the COVID-19 Public Health Emergency, synchronous telemedicine was reimbursable by Medicare for approximately 100 different services under limited circumstances and included numerous restrictions. Office visits, psychotherapy, and preventive health screenings were reimbursable under certain circumstances, but clinicians could not be reimbursed by Medicare for using synchronous telemedicine during emergency room visits, physical or occupational therapy, or many other types of care. Medicare reimbursement for telemedicine was contingent on whether the visit was occurring at an eligible "originating site" (or physical location of the Medicare patient at the time of service) and eligible "geographic site" (representing the rurality or urbanicity of the patient and clinician). Prior to the Public Health Emergency, only medical facilities were eligible originating sites, and so patients could not have a reimbursed telemedicine visit from home. In addition, eligible geographic sites were restrictive, and typically reserved for isolated rural areas. Clinicians also could not be reimbursed for telemedicine visits under any circumstance when they were located in a different state than their patient.

In addition, synchronous telemedicine could only be reimbursed if it was delivered via real-time audiovisual technology that met specific data security requirements and was not reimbursed if it was delivered via audio-only methods (eg, telephone visits). The clinician billing for synchronous telemedicine needed to have an established relationship, defined as having seen the patient in person within the past 3 years.

Even when synchronous telemedicine was reimbursed, rules existed limiting the amount a clinician could be paid for a telemedicine service and was generally paid a lower rate than if that service was provided in person. As a result, telemedicine use was relatively low. In 2016, telemedicine accounted for less than half a percent of Medicare Part B spending. Similarly, in February of 2020, at the beginning of the COVID-19 Public Health Emergency, one-tenth of a percent of primary care visits were delivered via telemedicine. Patients who did use telemedicine overall had positive experiences—appreciated the ease of use, reduced travel time, and improved communication—and some patients preferred telemedicine over face-to-face visits.

Reimbursement during and after the COVID-19 Public Health Emergency. When COVID-19 first arrived in the United States, people were encouraged to quarantine at home, making in-person visits for nonemergent health care needs a less viable option for care. This created the necessity for telemedicine to scale and expand within health systems.

To facilitate this, Congress gave Medicare the authority to change telemedicine reimbursement policy through the Coronavirus Preparedness and Supplemental Appropriations Act and the Coronavirus Aid, Relief, and Economic Security Act. In addition, when the President declared a national emergency, the Secretary of Health and Human Services was empowered to make temporary changes to Medicare and Medicaid program requirements under the authority of an 1135 Waiver of the Social Security Act. With this authority, Medicare made the following major changes to telemedicine reimbursement policy:

- Any clinician can bill Medicare for telemedicine services.
- Clinicians did not need to have a preexisting relationship with a patient to bill for telemedicine services.
- Clinicians and patients each can be at home when billing for telemedicine services.
- Telemedicine can be provided to patients who are in a different state.
- Security standards for which platforms could be used for telemedicine visits were loosened, and platforms commonly used in non–health care settings (eg, FaceTime, Skype, and Zoom) were reimbursable for health care services.
- Audiovisual and audio-only services were both reimbursable by Medicare.
- Clinicians can waive patient cost sharing for visits paid for by federal programs.
- All telemedicine visits, including audiovisual and audio-only visits, would be reimbursed at the same rate as in-person care.

These changes to reimbursement policy had a profound impact on the use of telemedicine in health care. Although the use of in-person ambulatory health care services overall decreased, the use of telemedicine among Medicare patients increased more than 60-fold between 2019 and 2020. Audio-only and audiovisual telemedicine use were both prevalent in 2021 and 2022; one study found that about 40% of adult telemedicine visits were audio-only visits, while the remainder were audiovisual visits.

In addition to medical care organizations that previously saw patients in person increasingly adopting telemedicine, reimbursement changes facilitated the growth of clinicians who provided care exclusively through telemedicine. One such company, Teladoc, provided 10 million visits in 2020, more than double the number it provided in 2019.

However, since the regulatory authority for many of the changes to telemedicine reimbursement was predicated on the COVID-19 Public Health Emergency, questions remain for how telemedicine would be reimbursed and what role synchronous telemedicine will have in US health care after the Public Health Emergency was declared over in May of 2023.

While permanent reimbursement changes were still in flux as of January 2024, many have at least been temporarily continued. For instance, through the Consolidated Appropriations Act of 2023, many telemedicine reimbursement flexibilities have been extended through the end of 2024; audio-only and audiovisual telemedicine are being paid for at parity with in-person services, and patients are able to receive telemedicine services from their home.

Back to the Clinical Case

In this patient's case, reimbursement would help enable home-based care via processes that involve her sending blood glucose levels to her clinician asynchronously via store-and-forward and interacting with her clinician via a synchronous telemedicine visit.

TAKEAWAYS

- Before the COVID-19 Public Health Emergency, use of asynchronous and synchronous telemedicine was not widespread.
- The scaling and adoption of asynchronous and synchronous telemedicine in the health care system was driven in part by reimbursement policy changes prompted by the COVID-19 Public Health Emergency.

Clinical Case Continued

In their video telemedicine visit, Jessica shares that she and her husband have had a challenging time managing Jessica's medical conditions in general the past several months. Jessica's memory has continued to decline, sometimes causing her to forget to administer her medications, despite her smart medication dispenser reminders helping to prompt her each day. In addition, due to neuropathy that's developed in her feet from her diabetes, Jessica's developed diabetic foot ulcers that need monitoring for infection control, and she also feels unsteady on her feet when trying to shower or get dressed. The patient's husband explains that he helps as much as he can when he's at home, but that it's challenging to keep up with all of Jessica's care since he works full time. Although telemedicine and treatment technologies have helped them in being able to receive their medical care from home, they inquire about additional supports.

This situation underscores potential patient needs—and particular needs in home settings—that can exist despite excellent medical care facilitated by telemedicine and other technologies. Even after receiving home-based care via telemedicine and treatment technology, the patient has medical needs that require in-person assistance. For instance, her medical and cognitive illnesses impacted her ability to safely administer medications and monitor diabetic foot ulcers for infection control. In addition to direct home-based care needs, the patient also can use assistance in caring for her functional needs. These functional needs include performing activities of daily living (ADLs) such as showering and dressing, and instrumental activities of daily living (IADLs), such as managing money and shopping for groceries. This circumstance is common, with approximately 10% of Americans older than age 75 needing assistance with at least one ADL and nearly 20% requiring assistance with at least one IADL.

Addressing medical and functional needs can be an important part of home-based care. In turn, a workforce that can deliver home-based care and provide functional supports represents a systems factor in US health care.

SYSTEMS FACTOR: HOME-BASED CARE AND FUNCTIONAL SUPPORT WORKFORCE

Of the more than 20 million Americans who need assistance with caring for themselves, 17 million are living at home and in the community. With an aging population, the home-based care and functional support workforce has grown considerably and is expected to continue to grow in coming years. Between 2008 and 2018, the number of home-based care and functional support workers doubled from 2.9 million to 5.8 million. Between 2018 and 2028, an additional 1.3 million new home-based care and functional support jobs are expected, making home-based care and functional support workers the fastest growing position in the US economy.

Home-Based Care and Functional Support Workforce Members

A number of groups and individuals form the home-based care workforce, including those working for Home Health Agencies (eg, occupational therapists, physical therapists, speech therapists, nurses). Services delivered by these individuals working for Home Health Agencies are typically time limited and aimed at addressing postacute care needs after hospitalization, rather than long-term medical needs. In addition, there are ongoing functional needs that other workers can address. There are different types of workers that form this expanded home-based care and functional support workforce, with distinct but overlapping responsibilities and training (Table 7.1).

Nursing aides. These individuals work in several care settings (eg, hospitals, skilled nursing facilities, assisted living facilities) as well as in people's personal or group homes. They help patients with some home-based care needs such as blood pressure measurement, range of motion exercises, infection control (eg, wound monitoring), and also assist patients with ADLs. In some cases, nursing aides may also help with household tasks and IADLs. Nursing aide certifications are implemented by individual states, but each certification program must follow minimum federal standards. Specifically, the federal training program requirements for a certified nursing aide include the following:

- A minimum of 75 hours of training, and the overall training must be under the general supervision of a nurse with at least 2 years' experience, of which at least 1 year must be in a long-term care facility.
- A minimum of 16 hours of their training must be in a laboratory or other controlled environment where the nursing aide student demonstrates knowledge while performing tasks under the direct supervision of a nurse.
- Before the nursing aide student ever takes care of a patient, they must receive 16 hours of training on the following topic areas:
  - Communication and interpersonal skills
  - Infection control
  - Safety and emergency procedures (eg, Heimlich maneuver)
  - Promoting patients' independence
  - Respecting patient rights

Table 7.1 Home-Based Care and Functional Support Workforce

Role	Typical Work Settings	Care Typically Provided	Federal Training Requirements
Nursing aides	<ul><li>Hospitals</li><li>Skilled nursing facilities</li><li>Assisted living facilities</li><li>Personal homes</li><li>Group homes</li></ul>	<ul><li>Clinical care</li><li>Activities of daily living</li><li>Limited household tasks</li></ul>	<ul><li>Training and certification required always</li></ul>
Home health aides	<ul><li>Assisted living facilities</li><li>Personal homes</li><li>Group homes</li></ul>	<ul><li>Clinical care</li><li>Activities of daily living</li><li>Instrumental activities of daily living</li><li>Household tasks</li></ul>	<ul><li>Training and certification required if billing to Medicare</li></ul>
Personal care aides	<ul><li>Assisted living facilities</li><li>Personal homes</li><li>Group homes</li></ul>	<ul><li>Limited clinical care</li><li>Activities of daily living</li><li>Instrumental activities of daily living</li><li>Household tasks</li><li>Facilitate patient engagement with community</li></ul>	<ul><li>None</li></ul>
Family and friends	<ul><li>Hospitals</li><li>Skilled nursing facilities</li><li>Assisted living facilities</li><li>Personal homes</li><li>Group homes</li></ul>	Varies, but may provide any of the following:<ul><li>Clinical care</li><li>Activities of daily living</li><li>Instrumental activities of daily living</li><li>Household tasks</li><li>Facilitate patient engagement with community</li></ul>	<ul><li>None</li></ul>

Source: Data from Kaiser Family Foundation. In response to home-care workforce shortages, most states report increasing Medicaid's payment rates and expanding worker opportunities. https://www.kff.org/medicaid/press-release/in-response-to-home-care-workforce-shortages-most-states-report-increasing-medicaids-payment-rates-and-expanding-worker-opportunities/

■ Additional required curricula include:
  ■ Basic nursing skills (eg, taking vital signs)
  ■ Personal care skills (eg, assistance with ADLs)
  ■ Mental health and social services needs (how to respond to patients, how to partner with family members)
  ■ Care of patients with cognitive disorders
  ■ Basic restorative services (eg, how to turn and position patients in bed, use of orthotic and prosthetic devices)
  ■ Resident rights (eg, maintaining privacy, avoiding use of restraints)

Of note, if a nursing aide student is employed or has an employment offer when they begin training, the training must be provided at no cost to the student. Similarly, if a student is not employed at the time of the start of the training, but receives employment within 12 months of the training, then the states must cover the cost of the training.

Home health aides. Home health aides are similar to nursing aides, with a few key differences. First, while nursing aides can work in many medical care facilities and individuals' homes, home health aides strictly work in patients' homes (eg, personal or group homes, assisted living facilities). Second, in addition to the services that nursing aides provide, home health aides may assist with some light household tasks such as preparing meals or changing linens. Third, no formal training is federally required to become a home health aide.

However, home health aides who work for a Home Health Agency that is Medicare certified (and therefore can bill Medicare for services) must follow federal training and certification standards. Individual states can also institute home health aide certifications that can vary in requirements so long as they meet minimum federal standards. The federal training requirements for Medicare certification for home health aides include 75 hours of training, and 16 of those hours must be spent in a laboratory or other controlled environment where the home health aide student demonstrates knowledge while performing tasks under the direct supervision of a nurse. The content of the federally required curriculum for Medicare-certified home health aides is similar to that for nursing aides. In addition to the baseline curriculum, for a Home Health Agency to maintain Medicare certification, all home health aides must receive an additional 12 hours of continuing education each year.

Personal care aides. Personal care aides may help with medication management, but they generally do not provide home-based medical care beyond this. Instead, personal care aides mostly assist patients with functional supports and other household tasks. They also help patients go to work and remain engaged in their communities. As of 2023, personal care aides do not need to follow federal training or certification standards, although some states or employers may require they complete a training program. In addition to working for agencies, personal care aides are increasingly self-employed or employed directly by patients themselves. Personal care aides usually work in personal or group homes or assisted living facilities.

Family and friends. The majority of older adults who receive assistance with home-based care and functional supports report receiving some help from family and friends. For instance, in 2016, approximately 75% of adults with disabilities received home-based care and functional support from family or friends, approximately 40% received assistance from paid workforce members (ie, nursing aide, home health aide, personal care aide), and approximately 30% received home-based care and functional support from a combination of the two. While family and friends continue to be the most common source of home-based care, between 2004 and 2016, care from other home-based care and functional support workforce members grew at twice the rate as home-based care from family and friends.

Since care from family and friends is delivered informally, there are no specific training requirements. However, if desired, the federal government does offer training programs on home-based care that family members can access. In addition, the specific nature of care may vary from person to person, but friends and family may assist directly with home-based care or functional support needs. They can provide care not only in personal homes but also in assisted living facilities, skilled nursing facilities, and hospitals. In some states, Medicaid programs will pay family members or friends to care for loved ones with disabilities.

In 2020, 85% of the home-based care and functional support workforce (other than family and friends) were female, more than 50% of the workforce had a high school education or less, more than 30% immigrated to the United States, and more than 60% identified as being members of Black, Indigenous, and People of Color (BIPOC) communities. Nearly 40% of this workforce lives in or near poverty and their overall median annual income in 2021 was $23 688.

In part due to the low compensation, there is an overall shortage in the paid home-based care and functional support workforce (other than family and friends) and a high number of vacancies for home-based care positions in skilled nursing facilities, assisted living facilities, and private homes. It's estimated that approximately one in five Medicare beneficiaries have unmet home-based or functional support needs, which is thought to be explained in part by home-based care and functional support workforce shortages.

Financing the Home-Based Care and Functional Support Workforce

Services delivered by the home-based care and functional support workforce are predominantly financed through Medicare and Medicaid; nearly 75% of the home-based care industry's annual revenue comes from these public payers.

Medicare will cover home-based care services from nursing aides and home health aides as part of its Home Health Services benefit. However, it will only pay for services from this workforce if a patient is also receiving skilled nursing services. In addition, Medicare will only pay for these services part time or intermittently, rather than on a long-term basis, and it never pays for assistance with household tasks (eg, cleaning).

Medicaid will cover home-based care services through Home and Community-Based Services (HCBS) benefits—a term used to refer to medical and supportive services to assist with ADLs and IADLs. A 2023 report estimated that more than 4 million Americans receive home-based care through Medicaid benefits. Individual states run their own Medicaid program and can develop their own criteria for eligibility. Generally, individuals must have limited financial resources and high levels of disability to qualify for Medicaid home-based care benefits.

Outside of Medicare and Medicaid, individuals may finance home-based care services by purchasing private long-term care insurance. Private long-term care insurance is uncommon; in 2014, approximately 11% of older adults had long-term care insurance. For those who do not receive their health insurance benefits through Medicare, Medicaid, or private long-term care insurance, home-based care services from home-based care and functional support workforce members are paid for out of pocket.

Back to the Clinical Case

Although she has received assistance through family and friends (in this case, her husband), the patient has additional medical and functional support needs. In particular, she could potentially benefit from the services delivered by nursing aides, home health aides, or personal care aides. Because she is dually eligible for Medicare and Medicaid, the patient could be eligible for long-term financial assistance for her home-based care needs through Medicaid HCBS benefits. In addition, the Medicaid program could potentially directly reimburse her husband to provide home-based care and functional support.

TAKEAWAYS

- Members of the home-based care and functional support workforce—nursing aides, home health aides, and personal care aides—can provide assistance with some medical care, ADLs, and IADLs.
- The different types of workers in the home-based care and functional support workforce have distinct but overlapping responsibilities and training.
- Most patients receive home-based care and functional support services from family and friends.
- Financing of home-based care and functional support services varies by insurance types.

Implications

The systems factors in this chapter have implications for patients' access to care in home settings. An example is telemedicine, whose adoption increased rapidly during the COVID-19 Public Health Emergency. One analysis reported that between January and June of 2020, in-person clinic visits among patients with commercial or Medicare Advantage insurance decreased by 30%. At the same time, telemedicine visits increased by more than 2000%, helping to mitigate the impact of reduced in-person care on overall health care accessibility. A 2021 survey found that 50% of US households reported using telemedicine because they otherwise did not have access to in-person care, and that 85% of telemedicine users were satisfied with their care. While telemedicine can complement in-person care and increase access to care for patients, it does not always completely replace the importance of in-person care. One qualitative study of homebound patients found that a lack of baseline familiarity with technology, limited use of technology, and worry about capacity to learn how to use technology were barriers to telemedicine use; these patients placed a high value on face-to-face communication offered via in-person visits.

The way that the home-based care and functional support workforce is structured and financed also has implications for access to home-based care. Just over half of older US adults with significant long-term care needs felt that, if they liquidated all their assets, they could pay for 2 years of home-based care.

The systems factors discussed also have implications for quality of care. For example, studies have found that the use of remote patient monitoring can improve care quality for managing chronic diseases such as chronic obstructive pulmonary disease and heart failure by reducing emergency room visits and hospital readmissions. Remote patient monitoring for patients with heart failure has been reported to reduce all-cause mortality and hospitalizations related to heart failure.

Existing evidence also suggests quality benefits when telemedicine and treatment technology are organized under a care delivery model, such as Hospital at Home. For instance, compared to those receiving usual care, patients hospitalized through Hospital at Home had better experiences with their care team, better sleep and physical activity levels during their hospitalization, and better experience with the overall admission process.

The systems factors also have implications for health care costs. Telemedicine programs centered around delivering home-based care for patients with specific conditions (eg, heart failure, diabetes, chronic obstructive pulmonary disease) have been associated with reduced overall cost of care. This finding is also true for Hospital at Home, in part due to lower readmission rates. The use of telemedicine can also yield cost savings for individual patients. For example, studies have shown that using telemedicine for home-based care reduced costs for patients compared to in-person care, driven at least in part by money saved on travel-related expenses, time spent to get to a visit, and the absence of facility fees.

However, questions remain about whether patients should use telemedicine as a substitute to in-person care or as a complement to in-person care. For instance, one study of audio-only and audiovisual telemedicine visits for acute respiratory infections found that although the cost per visit was lower for telemedicine than in-person visits, the authors found that nearly 90% of telemedicine visits were new or additional visits rather than replacements for in-person care, leading to an overall higher cost of care. Whether telemedicine is used as a substitute or complement poses cost implications not only for patients but also for medical care organizations.

Lastly, systems factors described in this chapter have important equity implications. A systematic review found that among individuals receiving home-based care, racial disparities exist with respect to individuals' ability to administer to their own ADLs and IADLs, and in hospitalization rates. In addition, inequities have also been observed in the type of care patients receive. For instance, although Black and Hispanic patients are disproportionately impacted by kidney disease, they are less likely than White patients to begin home dialysis.

Inequities have also been associated with use of synchronous telemedicine. Synchronous telemedicine utilization has been lower among rural than urban households, among communities without high-speed internet, among lower income households, and among communities with limited English proficiency. To the extent that increased use of synchronous telemedicine can better facilitate home-based care, these observations suggest that certain groups may accrue disproportionately more benefits than others.

Inequities also exist for the home-based care and functional support workforce. A high proportion of workforce members, such as nursing aides, home health aides, and personal care aides, live in or near poverty and receive public assistance. There can also be inequities in the quality of home-based care received. For example, among patients receiving home-based care from a Home Health Agency, racial and ethnic minorities were less likely than White patients to receive care from a Home Health Agency with a high-quality rating from Medicare.

Multiple-Choice Questions

1. Toni is a 27-year-old woman who develops a rash on her arm. Because she otherwise feels well, she takes a picture of her rash and sends it to her clinician via the electronic health record's secure messaging platform, along with a question of whether she needs further evaluation or treatment. The next day, her clinician responds by noting a potential infection and prescribing an antibiotic. What type of telemedicine did Toni use to facilitate home-based care?

    A. Audio-only telemedicine

    B. Remote patient monitoring

    C. Audiovisual telemedicine

    D. Store-and-forward

2. Which of the following statements is true about Medicare policy changes for reimbursement for telemedicine during the COVID-19 Public Health Emergency?

    A. Audio-only telemedicine was temporarily reimbursable but not at parity with audiovisual telemedicine.

    B. Audiovisual telemedicine was temporarily reimbursable but not at parity with in-person care.

    C. Audio-only and audiovisual telemedicine were temporarily reimbursable at parity with in-person care.

    D. Audio-only and audiovisual telemedicine were permanently reimbursable at parity with in-person care.

3. Frank is a 74-year-old with dementia and chronic care needs (chronic wounds, paralysis from the waist downward) insured through Medicaid. In addition to a nurse who provides wound care, another home-based

care and functional support worker visits him at home several times a week. This worker helps Frank bathe and get dressed, arrange his medications, and measure vital signs, but does not help with meal preparation or household tasks. The home-based care and functional support worker is state certified and has previously completed at least 75 hours of federally mandated training. Frank is most likely receiving help from what kind of home-based care and functional support worker?

A. Nursing aide

B. Home health aide

C. Personal care aide

D. None of the above

Answers

1. The correct answer is D. By sending a photo via an electronic health record secure messaging platform and allowing the clinician to asynchronously use this data for medical decision-making and communication, the patient used store-and-forward.

2. The correct answer is C. During the COVID-19 Public Health Emergency, Medicare policy changes made audio-only and audiovisual telemedicine temporarily reimbursable at parity with in-person care. As of January 2024, permanent reimbursement changes for audio-only and audiovisual telemedicine are undergoing further consideration.

3. The correct answer is A. While home-based care and functional support workforce members can have overlapping responsibilities, a nursing aide is more likely to assist with home-based care needs (eg, medication management, measure vital signs) and with IADLs, but not household tasks. Compared to other workforce members, nursing aides must also complete a federally mandated training program in order to achieve their required certification.

Bibliography

Alboksmaty A, Beaney T, Elkin S, et al. Effectiveness and safety of pulse oximetry in remote patient monitoring of patients with COVID-19: Ahmed Alboksmaty. *Eur J Public Health*. 2022;32(suppl 3):ckac129.303.

Aldila F, Walpola RL. Medicine self-administration errors in the older adult population: a systematic review. *Res Social Adm Pharm*. 2021;17(11):1877-1886.

American Academy of Family Physicians. Telehealth policies after the COVID-19 PHE. https://www.aafp.org/pubs/fpm/blogs/inpractice/entry/covid-phe-end-telehealth.html

American Lung Association. Pulse oximetry. https://www.lung.org/lung-health-diseases/lung-procedures-and-tests/pulse-oximetry

American Medical Association. CARES Act: AMA COVID-19 pandemic telehealth fact sheet. https://www.ama-assn.org/delivering-care/public-health/cares-act-ama-covid-19-pandemic-telehealth-fact-sheet

American Medical Association. Telehealth resource center: definitions. https://www.ama-assn.org/practice-management/digital/telehealth-resource-center-definitions

American Medical Association. Telehealth up 53%, growing faster than any other place of care. https://www.ama-assn.org/practice-management/digital/telehealth-53-growing-faster-any-other-place-care

Ashwood JS, Mehrotra A, Cowling D, Uscher-Pines L. Direct-to-consumer telehealth may increase access to care but does not decrease spending. *Health Aff (Millwood)*. 2017;36(3):485-491.

Assistant Secretary for Planning and Evaluation. How many older adults can afford to purchase home care? https://aspe.hhs.gov/reports/how-many-older-adults-can-afford-purchase-home-care-0

Assistant Secretary for Planning and Evaluation. Updated national survey trends in telehealth utilization and modality (2021-2022). Published April 19, 2023. https://aspe.hhs.gov/sites/default/files/documents/7d6b4989431f4c70144f209622975116/household-pulse-survey-telehealth-covid-ib.pdf

Bose S, Dun C, Zhang GQ, Walsh C, Makary MA, Hicks CW. Medicare beneficiaries in disadvantaged neighborhoods increased telemedicine use during the COVID-19 pandemic. *Health Aff (Millwood)*. 2022;41(5):635-642.

Castle NG. The influence of consistent assignment on nursing home deficiency citations. *Gerontologist*. 2011;51(6):750-760.

Centers for Disease Control and Prevention. End of the federal COVID-19 public health emergency (PHE) declaration. https://archive.cdc.gov/www_cdc_gov/coronavirus/2019-ncov/your-health/end-of-phe.html#:~:text=May%2011%2C%202023%2C%20marks%20the,to%20the%20COVID%2D19%20pandemic

Centers for Medicare and Medicaid Services. 1135 waiver at a glance. https://www.cms.gov/Medicare/Provider-Enrollment-and-Certification/SurveyCertEmergPrep/Downloads/1135-Waivers-At-A-Glance.pdf

Centers for Medicare and Medicaid Services. Activities of daily living (ADLs): activities of daily living are activities related to personal care. https://www.cms.gov/research-statistics-data-and-systems/research/mcbs/downloads/2008_appendix_b.pdf

Centers for Medicare and Medicaid Services. CFR-2004-title42-vol3-sec484-36. https://www.govinfo.gov/content/pkg/CFR-2004-title42-vol3/pdf/CFR-2004-title42-vol3-sec484-36.pdf

Centers for Medicare and Medicaid Services. CMS Manual System Pub 100-08 Medicare Program Integrity. 2017. https://www.cms.gov/Regulations-and-Guidance/Guidance/Transmittals/2017Downloads/R704PI.pdf

Centers for Medicare and Medicaid Services. End-stage renal disease (ESRD). https://www.medicare.gov/basics/end-stage-renal-disease

Centers for Medicare and Medicaid Services. Home health services coverage. https://www.medicare.gov/coverage/home-health-services

Centers for Medicare and Medicaid Services. Medicare telemedicine health care provider fact sheet. https://www.cms.gov/newsroom/fact-sheets/medicare-telemedicine-health-care-provider-fact-sheet

Centers for Medicare and Medicaid Services. MLN Matters® articles. 2006. www.cms.hhs.gov/MLNMattersArticles

Centers for Medicare and Medicaid Services. Online training for self-directed HCBS. https://www.medicaid.gov/medicaid/long-term-services-supports/direct-care-workforce/online-training-for-self-directed-hcbs/index.html

Chari AV, Engberg J, Ray KN, Mehrotra A. The opportunity costs of informal elder-care in the United States: new estimates from the American time use survey. *Health Serv Res.* 2015;50(3):871-882.

Commonwealth Fund. "Hospital at Home" programs improve outcomes, lower costs but face resistance from providers and payers. https://www.commonwealthfund.org/publications/newsletter-article/hospital-home-programs-improve-outcomes-lower-costs-face-resistance

Congress.gov. Coronavirus Preparedness and Response Supplemental Appropriations Act, 2020. One Hundred Sixteenth Congress of the United States of America. https://www.congress.gov/116/bills/hr6074/BILLS-116hr6074enr.pdf

Datta P, Barrett W, Bentzinger M, et al. Ambulatory care for epilepsy via telemedicine during the COVID-19 pandemic. *Epilepsy Behav.* 2021;116:107740.

Diamant MJ, Harwood L, Movva S, et al. A comparison of quality of life and travel-related factors between in-center and satellite-based hemodialysis patients. *Clin J Am Soc Nephrol.* 2010;5(2):268-274.

Fashaw-Walters SA, Rahman M, Gee G, Mor V, White M, Thomas KS. Out of reach: inequities in the use of high-quality home health agencies. *Health Aff (Millwood).* 2022;41(2):247-255.

Fierce Healthcare. Teladoc's virtual visits reach 3M during Q4 as revenue grows to $383M. https://www.fiercehealthcare.com/tech/teladoc-s-virtual-visits-reach-3m-during-q4-as-revenue-grows-to-383m

Fierce Healthcare. Tyto Care telehealth platform adds a pulse oximeter to expand at-home health monitoring. https://www.fiercehealthcare.com/tech/tyto-care-telehealth-platform-adds-a-pulse-oximeter-to-expand-at-home-health-monitoring

Franklin SS, Thijs L, Hansen TW, O'Brien E, Staessen JA. White-coat hypertension: new insights from recent studies. *Hypertension.* 2013;62(6):982-987.

Fried TR, Van Doorn C, O'Leary JR, Tinetti ME, Drickamer MA. Older person's preferences for home vs hospital care in the treatment of acute illness. *Arch Intern Med.* 2000;160(10):1501-1506.

Health IT Buzz. Use of telemedicine among physicians and development of telemedicine apps. Office of the National Coordinator of Health Information Technology. https://www.healthit.gov/buzz-blog/health-data/use-of-telemedicine-among-physicians-and-development-of-telemedicine-apps

Health IT National Learning Consortium. Fact sheet: how to optimize patient portals for patient engagement and meet meaningful use requirements. 2013. https://www.healthit.gov/sites/default/files/nlc_how_to_optimizepatientportals_for_patientengagement.pdf

Health Resources and Services Administration. Leveraging remote patient monitoring in your practice. https://telehealth.hhs.gov/documents/Leveraging+Remote+Patient+Monitoring+In+Your+Practice.pdf

HealthIT.gov. Individuals' access and use of patient portals and smartphone health apps, 2020. Office of the National Coordinator of Health Information Technology. https://www.healthit.gov/data/data-briefs/individuals-access-and-use-patient-portals-and-smartphone-health-apps-2020

Holmgren AJ, Downing NL, Tang M, Sharp C, Longhurst C, Huckman RS. Assessing the impact of the COVID-19 pandemic on clinician ambulatory electronic health record use. *J Am Med Inform Assoc*. 2022;29(3):453-460.

Huang KTL, Lu TJ, Alizadeh F, Mostaghimi A. Homebound patients' perspectives on technology and telemedicine: a qualitative analysis. *Home Health Care Serv Q*. 2016; 35(3-4):172-181.

Inglis SC, Clark RA, Dierckx R, Prieto-Merino D, Cleland JGF. Structured telephone support or non-invasive telemonitoring for patients with heart failure. *Cochrane Database Syst Rev*. 2015;2015(10):CD007228.

Jabbarpour Y, Jetty A, Westfall M, Westfall J. Not telehealth: which primary care visits need in-person care? *J Am Board Fam Med*. 2021;34(Suppl):S162-S169.

Jaramillo N, Malkov D, Nikakis J, Arora US, Cohen TJ. At-home ECG monitoring with a real-time outpatient cardiac telemetry system during the COVID-19 pandemic. *J Osteopath Med*. 2022;122(10):503-508.

Kaiser Family Foundation. FAQs on Medicare coverage of telehealth. https://www.kff.org/medicare/issue-brief/faqs-on-medicare-coverage-of-telehealth/

Kaiser Family Foundation. In response to home-care workforce shortages, most states report increasing Medicaid's payment rates and expanding worker opportunities. https://www.kff.org/medicaid/press-release/in-response-to-home-care-workforce-shortages-most-states-report-increasing-medicaids-payment-rates-and-expanding-worker-opportunities/

Kaiser Family Foundation. Medicare and telehealth: coverage and use during the COVID-19 pandemic and options for the future. https://www.kff.org/medicare/issue-brief/medicare-and-telehealth-coverage-and-use-during-the-covid-19-pandemic-and-options-for-the-future/

Kaiser Family Foundation. Medicaid financial eligibility in pathways based on old age or disability in 2022: findings from a 50-state survey—issue brief—9965. https://www.kff.org/report-section/medicaid-financial-eligibility-in-pathways-based-on-old-age-or-disability-in-2022-findings-from-a-50-state-survey-issue-brief/

Kaiser Family Foundation. Pandemic-era changes to Medicaid home- and community-based services (HCBS): a closer look at family caregiver policies. https://www.kff.org/medicaid/issue-brief/pandemic-era-changes-to-medicaid-home-and-community-based-services-hcbs-a-closer-look-at-family-caregiver-policies/

Kaiser Family Foundation. PHI Facts 3: America's direct-care workforce. https://www.phinational.org/wp-content/uploads/legacy/phi-facts-3.pdf

Kreider AR, Werner RM. The home care workforce has not kept pace with growth in home and community-based services. *Health Aff (Millwood)*. 2023;42(5):650-657.

Kyle MA, Blendon RJ, Findling MG, Benson JM. Telehealth use and satisfaction among U.S. households: results of a national survey. *J Patient Exp*. 2021;8:23743735211052737.

Leong MQ, Lim CW, Lai YF. Comparison of hospital-at-home models: a systematic review of reviews. *BMJ Open*. 2021;11(1):e043285.

Levine DM, Pian J, Mahendrakumar K, Patel A, Saenz A, Schnipper JL. Hospital-level care at home for acutely ill adults: a qualitative evaluation of a randomized controlled trial. *J Gen Intern Med.* 2021;36(7):1965-1973.

Li J, Sawanoi Y. The history and innovation of home blood pressure monitors. Paper presented at: 2017 IEEE HISTory of ELectrotechnolgy CONference, HISTELCON 2017; August 07-08, 2017; Kobe, Japan.

Mayo Clinic. Hemodialysis. https://www.mayoclinic.org/tests-procedures/hemodialysis/about/pac-20384824

McKinsey & Company. From facility to home: how healthcare could shift by 2025. https://www.mckinsey.com/industries/healthcare/our-insights/from-facility-to-home-how-healthcare-could-shift-by-2025

Medicaid and CHIP Payment and Access Commission. State efforts to address Medicaid home- and community-based services workforce shortages. Published March 2022. https://www.macpac.gov/wp-content/uploads/2022/03/MACPAC-brief-on-HCBS-workforce.pdf

MedicaidLongTermCare.org. Getting paid as a caregiver by Medicaid. https://www.medicaid-longtermcare.org/benefits/getting-paid-as-a-caregiver/

Michaud TL, Zhou J, McCarthy MA, Siahpush M, Su D. Costs of home-based telemedicine programs: a systematic review. *Int J Technol Assess Health Care.* 2018;34(4):400-409.

Michigan Department of Health and Human Services. Reimbursement of costs for the Nurse Aide Training and Competency Evaluation Program (NATCEP) Frequently Asked Questions (FAQ). www.michigan.gov/medicaidproviders

Narayan MC, Scafide KN. Systematic review of racial/ethnic outcome disparities in home health care. *J Transcult Nurs.* 2017;28(6):598-607.

National Archives. eCFR:: 42 CFR 483.152—requirements for approval of a nurse aide training and competency evaluation program. https://www.ecfr.gov/current/title-42/chapter-IV/subchapter-G/part-483/subpart-D/section-483.152

National Public Radio. The pandemic proved hospitals can deliver care to seriously ill patients at home. Shots: Health News from NPR. https://www.npr.org/sections/health-shots/2021/05/20/998046711/sick-but-hate-hospitals-in-home-medical-care-is-a-growing-option

North S. These four telehealth changes should stay, even after the pandemic. *Fam Pract Manag.* 2021;28(3):9-11. https://www.aafp.org/pubs/fpm/issues/2021/0500/p9.html

Nouri S, Khoong EC, Lyles C, Karliner L. Addressing equity in telemedicine for chronic disease management during the Covid-19 pandemic. *NEJM Catal Innov Care Deliv.* 2020;1(3).

Novak JE, Ellison DH. Diuretics in states of volume overload: core curriculum 2022. *Am J Kidney Dis.* 2022;80(2):264-276.

Patel SY, Mehrotra A, Huskamp HA, Uscher-Pines L, Ganguli I, Barnett ML. Trends in out-patient care delivery and telemedicine during the COVID-19 pandemic in the US. *JAMA Intern Med.* 2021;181(3):388-391.

Patel T, Ivo J, Pitre T, Faisal S, Antunes K, Oda K. An in-home medication dispensing system to support medication adherence for patients with chronic conditions in the community setting: prospective observational pilot study. *JMIR Form Res.* 2022;6(5):e34906.

PHI. It's time to care: a detailed profile of America's direct care workforce. https://www.phina-tional.org/wp-content/uploads/2020/01/Its-Time-to-Care-2020-PHI.pdf

PHI. Key facts & FAQ: understanding the direct care workforce. https://www.phinational.org/policy-research/key-facts-faq/

Polinski JM, Kowal MK, Gagnon M, Brennan TA, Shrank WH. Home infusion: safe, clinically effective, patient preferred, and cost saving. *Healthc (Amst)*. 2017;5(1-2):68-80.

Polsky M, Moraveji N, Hendricks A, Teresi RK, Murray R, Maselli DJ. Use of remote cardio-respiratory monitoring is associated with a reduction in hospitalizations for subjects with COPD. *Int J Chron Obstruct Pulmon Dis*. 2023;18:219-229.

PSNet. Remote patient monitoring. https://psnet.ahrq.gov/perspective/remote-patient-monitoring

QuickStats: percentage of adults with activity limitations, by age group and type of limitation—National Health Interview Survey,† United States, 2014. *MMWR Morb Mortal Wkly Rep*. 2019;65(1):14.

Reckrey JM, Yang M, Kinosian B, et al. Receipt of home-based medical care among older beneficiaries enrolled in fee-for-service Medicare. *Health Aff (Millwood)*. 2020;39(8):1289-1296.

Richter KP, Shireman TI, Ellerbeck EF, et al. Comparative and cost effectiveness of telemedicine versus telephone counseling for smoking cessation. *J Med Internet Res*. 2015;17(5):e3975.

Ritchie C, Leff B. Home-based care reimagined: a full-fledged health care delivery ecosystem without walls. *Health Aff (Millwood)*. 2022;41(5):689-695.

Rusli KDB, Tan AJQ, Ong SF, Speed S, Lau Y, Liaw SY. Home-based nursing care competencies: a scoping review. *J Clin Nurs*. 2023;32(9-10):1723-1737.

Scales K. It's time to care a detailed profile of America's direct care workforce. PHI. Published January 2021. https://www.phinational.org/wp-content/uploads/2020/01/Its-Time-to-Care-2020-PHI.pdf

Shafiee MA, Chamanian P, Shaker P, Shahideh Y, Broumand B. The impact of hemodialysis frequency and duration on blood pressure management and quality of life in end-stage renal disease patients. *Healthcare (Basel)*. 2017;5(3):52.

Shaver J. The state of telehealth before and after the COVID-19 pandemic. *Prim Care*. 2022;49(4):517-530.

SOA Research Institute. Informal caregiving: measuring the cost and reducing the burden. 2023. https://www.soa.org/498ea3/globalassets/assets/files/resources/research-report/2023/informal-caregiving-reducing-burden.pdf

Tang M, Mehrotra A, Stern AD. Rapid growth of remote patient monitoring is driven by a small number of primary care providers. *Health Aff (Millwood)*. 2022;41(9):1248-1254.

Tang M, Nakamoto CH, Stern AD, Mehrotra A. Trends in remote patient monitoring use in traditional Medicare. *JAMA Intern Med*. 2022;182(9):1005-1006.

Telgener PC, Lowe S. A look at the current reimbursement environment for continuous glucose monitoring (CGM): understanding the fundamentals. *J Diabetes Sci Technol*. 2008;2(4):681-684.

The ALS Association. FYI: different types of home care workers. https://www.als.org/navigating-als/resources/fyi-different-types-home-care-workers

The New York Times. Can new technology make home dialysis a more realistic option? https://www.nytimes.com/2022/11/10/business/home-dialysis-tablo-outset.html

US Department of Health and Human Services. Asynchronous direct-to-consumer telehealth. https://telehealth.hhs.gov/providers/best-practice-guides/direct-to-consumer/asynchronous-direct-to-consumer-telehealth

US Department of Health and Human Services. E-consults. https://telehealth.hhs.gov/providers/best-practice-guides/telehealth-for-emergency-departments/e-consults

US Department of Health and Human Services. Medicaid and Medicare billing for asynchronous telehealth. https://telehealth.hhs.gov/providers/billing-and-reimbursement/medicaid-and-medicare-billing-for-asynchronous-telehealth

USAGov. Get paid as a caregiver for a family member. https://www.usa.gov/disability-caregiver

Value and Systems Science Lab. Appendix B: evidence assessment report. Audio-only telemedicine evaluation work. 2023. https://www.insurance.wa.gov/sites/default/files/documents/audio-only-telemed-appendix-b.pdf

Van Houtven CH, Konetzka RT, Taggert E, Coe NB. Informal and formal home care for older adults with disabilities increased, 2004–16. *Health Aff (Millwood)*. 2020;39(8):1297-1301.

Walsh CA, Cahir C, Tecklenborg S, Byrne C, Culbertson MA, Bennett KE. The association between medication non-adherence and adverse health outcomes in ageing populations: a systematic review and meta-analysis. *Br J Clin Pharmacol*. 2019;85(11):2464-2478.

Washington State Legislature. RCW 70.41.020: definitions. https://app.leg.wa.gov/rcw/default.aspx?cite=70.41.020

Wellness Pharmacy. Smart dispenser. https://www.wellpharmacy.com/smart-dispenser/

Wolff JL, Spillman BC, Freedman VA, Kasper JD. A national profile of family and unpaid caregivers who assist older adults with health care activities. *JAMA Intern Med*. 2016;176(3):372-379.

Ye S, Kronish I, Fleck E, et al. Telemedicine expansion during the COVID-19 pandemic and the potential for technology-driven disparities. *J Gen Intern Med*. 2021;36(1):256.

8

Community-Based Care

Clinical Case

After learning of home-based care options from their primary care clinician, Dr Jackson, Jessica and her husband Daniel decide that he will cut down on work hours and serve as an informal caregiver to Jessica. In their subsequent video telemedicine visit a few months later, Jessica and her husband share with her primary care clinician that, unfortunately, they've still had a challenging time managing Jessica's medical conditions. Jessica's memory has continued to decline, sometimes causing her to forget to administer her medications or pay the bills. In addition to helping to perform Jessica's activities of daily living, her husband also recently took on the responsibility of preparing their meals. But he is new to cooking and unsure how to prepare meals that are nutritious for diabetes and help control Jessica's blood sugar levels.

While they are grateful for her primary care clinician's guidance during in-person and virtual visits, Jessica and her husband ask whether she knows of any resources or community groups that could help them navigate Jessica's health on an ongoing basis in between visits.

This situation underscores that even if patients and clinicians create excellent care plans during visits, patients nonetheless need to implement such plans in the context of their lives and communities. Visits to a clinician or medical care organization make up a small fraction of patients' lives; even with high-frequency (eg, weekly) visits, patients spend the vast majority of their time managing their medical conditions and health in community rather than health care settings. Ultimately, efforts to manage care outside of visits play a key role in affecting patients' overall health.

Despite recognition of these issues, the health care system has not been traditionally designed to promote community-based health interventions. In particular, as discussed in other portions of this book, health care reimbursement in the United States has generally been "visit-based" and focused on care delivery inputs—that is, services provided to patients in the context of visits. However, this approach to reimbursement can fail to emphasize things happening in between visits in community settings and incompletely capture their impact on health outcomes. In these ways, there are limited financial incentives for clinicians and medical care organizations to engage with patients on community-based care.

Policymakers have increasingly worked over the past few decades to reorient health care payment and delivery away from a completely visit-based approach toward an outcome- and population-based approach. In particular, policy leaders have sought to test and scale value-based payment (VBP)—arrangements designed to reward clinicians and medical care organizations for high-quality, cost-efficient care and better patient outcomes.

This move toward VBP has been a major health systems factor, one consequence of which is greater focus on supporting patients outside the confines of individual visits. Such supports can include developing community-based care resources that help patients navigate their medical conditions in their community contexts.

SYSTEMS FACTOR: VALUE-BASED PAYMENT

The goal of VBP is to reorient how health care is paid for, moving from a focus on the volume of care delivered (ie, more payment for more care delivered) toward the value of care delivered (ie, the quality and cost-efficiency of care). In this context, value has been defined by a "value equation" (Figure 8.1).

The value equation frames how payment arrangements attempt to operationalize and improve value. One way is to improve the quality of care while maintaining costs; another is to reduce costs of care while maintaining quality; and yet another is to both improve quality and contain costs.

The Centers for Medicare and Medicaid Services has extensively tested VBP via a series of programs and models since the passage of the Patient Protection and Affordable Care Act (ACA). In turn, in subsequent years, value-based models and arrangements have grown to represent increasing proportions of all health care payment in the United States. In 2015, 38% of health care payments in the country was tied to some form of value-based arrangement, a figure that grew to approximately 60% in 2021. Although there

$$Value = \frac{Quality}{Costs}$$

Figure 8.1 The Value Equation.

are many different types of VBP arrangements, each with unique features, there are also a number of underlying, crosscutting elements.

Understanding these elements—which include how quality is defined and measured, types of models, and types of payments that can exist within models—is central to understanding VBP as a broader systems factor.

Defining and Measuring Quality

VBP aims to maintain or improve health care quality, which is a multidimensional concept. In 2001, the Institute of Medicine created a framework for defining quality based on six domains, which can be described and conceptualized as the following:

- *Safety.* Having a low likelihood that the care intended to help actually causes harm
- *Effectiveness.* Providing appropriate services to those who may benefit, and not to those who might not benefit
- *Patient centeredness.* Respectful of the preferences and values of individual patients
- *Timeliness.* Minimizing waits or potentially harmful delays
- *Efficiency.* Reducing waste of supplies, services, or human resources
- *Equity.* Consistent in overall quality regardless of a patient's gender, race, rurality, socioeconomic status, sexual orientation, or other personal characteristics (Figure 8.2)

Typically, quality is operationalized through a select set of quality measures, which the Centers for Medicare and Medicaid Services defines as "standards for measuring the performance and improvement of population health or of health plans, providers of services, and other clinicians in the delivery of health care." Quality measures can be derived from surveys of patients, from claims data, from medical charts, or from large data registries.

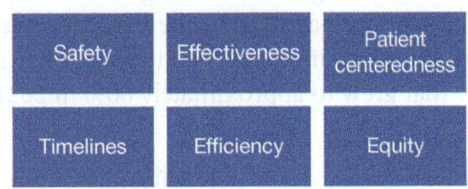

Figure 8.2 Components of Quality Care. (Adapted from Institute of Medicine. *Crossing the Quality Chasm: A New Health System for the 21st Century.* National Academy Press; 2001.)

These measures have become ubiquitous in health care. In 2020, the Centers for Medicare and Medicaid Services used 686 quality measures in measuring health care quality. Despite the large number of measures, they can be categorized in one of several measure types (Table 8.1).

Structural measures. These measures assess the features of a medical care organization's infrastructure and capacity to provide high-quality care. For example, structural measures can include the ratio of nurses to patients, or the presence and use of an electronic health record.

Process measures. These measures address actions or steps taken by medical care organizations or clinicians to improve quality. Examples of process measures include those related to preventive services (eg, the percentage of patients receiving an influenza vaccine) or chronic disease management (eg, the percentage of people with diabetes receiving a hemoglobin A_{1c} test).

Outcome measures. These measures focus on health endpoints and encompass clinical morbidity (eg, percentage of patients with a hospital-acquired infection) or mortality (eg, postoperative mortality rate) outcomes; patient-reported outcomes (eg, ability to complete activities of daily living, self-reported health status or pain levels).

Table 8.1 Types of Quality Measures

Type	Definition	Examples
Structural measures	Assess infrastructure and capacity to provide high-quality care	■ Presence and use of certified electronic health records ■ Nursing/patient ratios
Process measures	Assess actions or steps taken by medical care organizations or clinicians to provide high-quality care	■ Percentage of patients receiving an influenza vaccine ■ Percentage of patients with diabetes receiving a hemoglobin A_{1c}
Outcome measures	Assess clinical and patient-reported health endpoints that reflect high-quality care	■ Clinical (morbidity): Hospital-acquired infections ■ Clinical (mortality): Postoperative death rate ■ Patient reported: Self-reported health or pain status
Utilization measures	Assess resource utilization that reflects high-quality care	■ Hospitalization rates ■ Readmission rates ■ ER visit rates ■ Use of advanced diagnostic imaging

ER, emergency room.

Source: Donabedian A. Evaluating the quality of medical care. 1966. *Milbank Q.* 2005;83(4):691-729.

Utilization measures. These measures focus on the relationships between resource utilization and the quality of care provided. Some types of utilization can reflect lower quality care. For instance, emergency room (ER) visits and hospitalizations for many conditions may reflect lower quality ambulatory care, while hospital readmissions may reflect lower quality of care during posthospital discharges. In turn, ER visit, hospitalization, and readmissions rates can be used to measure quality. Similarly, on the premise that advanced diagnostic imaging may not be appropriate for some conditions, the frequency of imaging utilization could be used to capture quality of care.

While quality measures are not unique to VBP, they are incorporated into payment arrangements in an effort to create accountability for high-quality care among participating medical care organizations. Once quality measures are identified, participants' performance on those measures must be assessed in VBP programs. Performance assessment can occur in several ways:

Binary performance. In this approach, assessment is based on achieving—or not achieving—a discrete level of performance. This level can be defined on an absolute scale (eg, achieving a 90% preventive care screening rate among eligible patients) or comparative scale (eg, being in the top 50% of all organizations with respect to preventive care screening rates). In either case, participants either achieve or do not achieve a given performance level.

Relative performance. In this approach, performance is assessed depending on relative change compared to an initial performance level. This method acknowledges that medical care organizations may begin at different stages of performance or progress, and seeks to account for positive changes (ie, improvements) between starting and ending performance levels. For instance, assessment can be based on how well a medical care organization improves in measures of safety or patient experience relative to performance on the same measures in a prior baseline year.

These approaches of assessing quality performance do not need to be mutually exclusive. For instance, primary care VBP programs can couple the two approaches, first assessing medical care organizations' binary quality performance on a comparative scale (eg, placement in the top 50th percentile on a given quality measure) before using relative performance (eg, improvement in performance during the VBP program, as compared to baseline performance). As another example, hospital VBP programs can calculate two quality scores: those based on binary performance and those based on relative performance and use the higher of the two to determine hospital performance.

Rather than assess quality based on performance against measures, VBP programs also assess quality based on the activities that organizations complete, such as implementing practice improvements that engage community resources to address drivers of health, creating and implementing plans to improve access for patients who have limited English proficiency, or by obtaining or renewing a waiver to prescribe buprenorphine for opioid use disorder. While they cannot be directly tied to improvement in quality measures, such activities ostensibly seek to improve the quality of care and are therefore included in some value-based programs. In particular, medical care organizations can be credited for attesting to or providing other evidence of improvement activities that factor into VBP programs alongside performance assessment.

Types of Value-Based Payment Models

While value and VBP can be applied in multiple ways as theoretical constructs, VBP models are specific arrangements between a payer and medical care organizations that involve value-based incentives. Discrete rules govern the administration and conduct of each model, including those related to eligibility and participation (organizations that are eligible to, or must, join the model), performance assessment (ways in which organizations are assessed in the model), and financial incentives (the financial implications of different performance levels). A number of different VBP model types have been tested over the past two decades, most of which can be considered under one of two headings: episode-based and population-based models.

Episode-based models. In episode-based models, participating medical care organizations agree to assume accountability for the costs and quality of care for a defined episode of care. Episodes are defined by triggers (events that start an episode), duration and scope (the length of time and scope of services encompassed by the episode), and outcomes (episode-specific clinical, quality, utilization, or cost outcomes against which participants will be assessed).

For instance, in the episode-based Medicare Bundled Payments for Care Improvement model, hospitals and physician groups were eligible to assume quality and cost accountability for episodes involving medical conditions (eg, acute exacerbation of heart failure) or surgical procedures (eg, lower extremity joint replacement surgery). Episodes were triggered by hospitalization and spanned hospitalization and up to 90 days of postacute care. Participants were assessed on a range of episode-based outcomes, including total episode spending.

As another example, in the Medicare Oncology Care Model, physician groups were eligible to assume quality and cost accountability for patients with cancer undergoing chemotherapy. Episodes were triggered by the receipt of chemotherapy treatment and spanned 6 months. Participants were assessed on a range of quality- and cost-related outcomes, including total episode spending.

Population-based models: In population-based models, participating medical care organizations agree to assume accountability for the costs and quality of care for a defined patient population. Populations can be defined on the basis of individuals' health care use (eg, a group of patients receiving most of their care from a given medical care organization), the presence of specific medical conditions (eg, a group of patients with a given chronic disease), a particular site or type of care (eg, primary care for a group of patients), or a combination of factors.

A prevalent population-based model centers on organizations called Accountable Care Organizations (ACOs). ACOs define populations based on individuals' overall health care use, aligning patients with the clinicians and medical care organizations that either provide the most services or incur the most charges for those patients. Certain models, such as Medicare's Kidney Care First initiative, identify patients based on the presence of a chronic kidney disease diagnosis and align them with clinicians and medical care organizations that provide disease-related services. Yet other models, such as the Comprehensive Primary Care and Comprehensive Primary Care Plus programs, define patients based on primary care services, rather than all health care services, received through certain primary care groups.

Population-based models typically assess clinical, quality, and spending outcomes based on performance over a 1-year period. The exact outcomes vary depending on the nature of the populations encompassed, but generally emphasize preventive services (eg, immunization, cancer screening), chronic disease management (eg, glucose control for patients with diabetes) or disease progression (eg, progression of chronic kidney disease to end-stage kidney disease), and selected utilization measures (eg, hospitalization rates).

Types of Payment in Value-Based Payment Models

Although specifics vary by program, most VBP models involve a combination of up to four types of payments: population-based payments, infrastructure payments, reconciliation payments, and performance-based payments.

Population-based payments. These types of payments are provided to clinicians and medical care organizations participating in VBP models—generally population-based models—based on the nature of the population being cared for, rather than based on specific services or visits. Population-based payments are provided on a per-individual, per-time unit (eg, per month or per year) basis, and in turn may be referred to in different models as "per-member-per-month," "per-patient-per-month," or "per-beneficiary-per-year" payments.

Population-based payment amounts are guided by population sizes, with greater total payments to clinicians and medical care organizations caring for larger populations. The size of population-based payments also depends on a number of additional factors, including patient complexity (eg, clinical and other factors that affect a patient's health care use) and underlying intent (eg, whether population-based payments are designed to either partially or fully replace fee-for-service reimbursement).

Infrastructure payments. As the name suggests, these payments are intended to support infrastructure investments that enable clinicians and medical care organizations to successfully redesign and improve care within VBP models. This approach acknowledges that success in VBP models can require up-front investments in Health Information Technology, staffing, care management, coordination, and other capabilities.

For instance, in the Advanced Payment ACO Model, Medicare gave a select group of smaller physician-led ACOs a series of infrastructure payments—a flat up-front payment, another fixed up-front payment based on the number of patients in the ACO, and additional monthly payments intended to support infrastructure and care coordination. Policymakers extended this method via rule changes to the longest running Medicare ACO model, the Shared Savings Program. The Making Care Primary Model provides another example. In this model, participating practices that are new to VBP models receive a $145 000 up-front infrastructure payment, which can be used on staffing, addressing social determinants of health, or other infrastructure investments such as Health Information Technology that are relevant to population-based care delivery.

Reconciliation Payments. These payments reflect the overall performance of clinicians and medical care organizations in VBP models. In particular, performance on quality, spending, and other outcomes are "reconciled" at the end of a performance period. Based on that performance, participants may receive additional payments (for positive performance) or be subject to penalties (for negative performance). In episode-based models, reconciliation payments can be termed "net payment reconciliation amounts." In population-based models, such payments are often called "shared savings" (additional payments made to participants that achieve cost-efficiency and generate population savings; shared between participants and the payer) or "shared losses" (penalties levied on participants that fail to achieve cost-efficiency or population savings; shared between participants and the payer).

As an example of a population-based model, consider an ACO program that holds participating clinicians and medical care organizations accountable for quality (calculated based on performance on predetermined quality metrics) and expected costs of care (calculated based on total spending, compared against a predetermined benchmark spending target) over a 1-year period. At the end of the year, if its population-wide observed spending is less than the benchmark, an ACO achieves savings (ie, savings against the

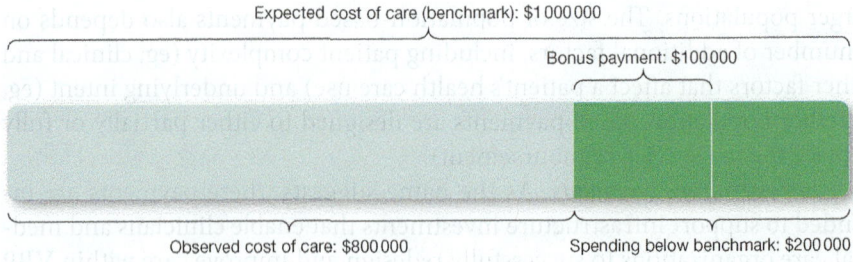

Figure 8.3 Reconciliation Payment, Bonus Payment Example. (Source: Data from Centers for Medicare and Medicaid Services. Shared savings program participation options for performance year 2024. Accessed December 18, 2023. https://www .cms.gov/Medicare/Medicare-Fee-for-Service-Payment/sharedsavingsprogram/ Downloads/ssp-aco-participation-options.pdf)

expected spending amount). If the ACO also has acceptable quality performance, it may be eligible to receive a bonus payment that is a portion of the spending below the benchmark (Figure 8.3).

Conversely, if the observed spending across the ACO's population exceeds the benchmark (ie, it is more than expected), the ACO fails to achieve savings. In some cases, it may then be required to pay a penalty that is a portion of the spending above the benchmark (Figure 8.4).

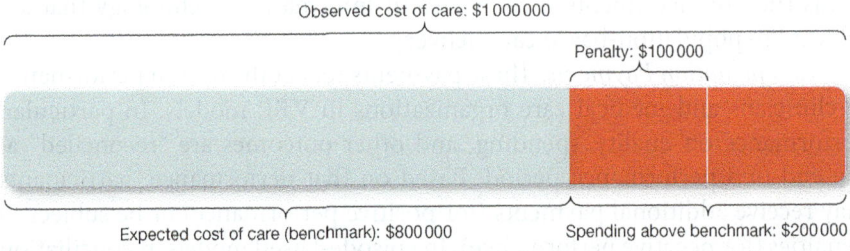

Figure 8.4 Reconciliation Payment, Penalty Example. (Source: Data from Centers for Medicare and Medicaid Services. Shared savings program participation options for performance year 2024. Accessed December 18, 2023. https://www.cms.gov/ Medicare/Medicare-Fee-for-Service-Payment/sharedsavingsprogram/Downloads/ ssp-aco-participation-options.pdf)

Performance-based payment. These payments represent incentives in VBP models intended to reward participants for actions or performance on specific measures or in specific areas. The focus on specific measures or focus areas distinguishes performance-based payments from reconciliation and other types of payments.

Performance-based payments can target clinical, quality, utilization, and/or cost performance, and can adopt several forms within VBP models. In "pay-for-reporting" approaches, medical care organizations or clinicians are eligible for performance-based payments for reporting their performance on quality measures. Because payments are made to participants on the sole basis of reporting, this approach is often used in early phases of VBP arrangements but phased out or evolved to other approaches over time. An alternative approach, "pay-for-performance," connects payment to results, either in the form of rewards for positive results, penalties for negative results, or both.

Back to the Clinical Case

In this case, the patient is facing a number of medical and nonmedical barriers to achieving desired diabetes-related health outcomes. Although not directly tied to medical decisions such as medication choice or doses, these barriers can have a large influence on the patient's health. Declining memory and forgetfulness can result in large negative consequences (eg, high blood sugar due to incomplete medication adherence) and put her at risk for end-stage complications and more ER or hospital utilization.

Under non-VBP models, such as fee-for-service, clinicians receive payment for any care delivered, no matter its quality or cost-efficiency. There are also few incentives and payments to encourage clinicians and their medical care organizations to meaningfully invest resources that could overcome barriers and help the patient manage her care in community settings. Conversely, VBP models can include incentives that shift clinicians' and medical care organizations' focus beyond health care facilities and visits, encouraging them to connect patients with or provide community-based resources.

TAKEAWAYS

- US health care has shifted toward VBP models, specific arrangements between a payer and medical care organizations governed by discrete rules that involve incentives for quality and cost performance.
- Two prominent types of VBP models are episode-based models (where participating medical care organizations agree to assume accountability for the quality and costs of care for a defined episode of care) and population-based models (where participating medical care organizations agree to assume accountability for the quality and costs of care for a defined patient population).
- Under VBP, quality of care is assessed through specific quality measures, which can be conceptualized as reflecting structure, process, outcomes, or utilization.

- VBP models are defined by a number of different types of payments, including population-based, infrastructure, reconciliation, and performance-based payments.

Clinical Case Continued

After hearing about Jessica and her husband's challenges with navigating health in the community, including difficulties in finding and cooking nutritious foods, her primary care clinician decides to introduce the couple to Melissa, a community health worker (CHW) who was hired after the primary care clinician's office decided to participate in VBP models.

The primary care clinician shares that the CHW will join Jessica and her husband in food shopping, help them identify healthy foods and recipes to cook for diabetes, and assist them in navigating any additional health-related needs. The CHW will also join for their future visits with the primary care clinician to help make sure the couple's needs are met and recommendations are communicated effectively. Jessica and her husband ask the CHW what other activities she performs as part of her job duties.

In this circumstance, the patient and her husband describe finding and cooking healthy foods as a health-related challenge. These concerns—those that occur in patients' everyday lives and community settings—are common and relevant to health. However, these concerns may be difficult for patients and clinicians to resolve in a visit. Like many others, the patient exhibits a pattern of receiving care from health care professionals during specific visits (eg, ambulatory care visit, urgent care visit, hospital stay) that punctuate periods of independent responsibility in the community during which she must implement medical advice.

As described in prior chapters, drivers of this pattern include prevalent reimbursement methods (eg, fee-for-service for ambulatory care) that financially compensate clinicians for services provided in the context of a visit, but infrequently for services provided in-between visits. However, with the emergence of VBP as well as other historical and contemporary drivers, medical care organizations are increasingly responsible for the cost and/or quality of care delivered to patients. In turn, a growing number of clinicians and medical care organizations increasingly possess stronger financial incentives to engage patients in managing their medical conditions in between visits during their daily lives in the community.

Part of this effort can involve strategies for helping patients navigate their care in the community, and a workforce for doing so. Individuals such as CHWs play a growing role in these efforts and represent a systems factor influencing community care.

SYSTEMS FACTOR: COMMUNITY HEALTH WORKERS

CHWs have existed in the United States since at least the 1950s. However, they have become increasingly prevalent and integrated into the US health care system over time. For instance, in 2010, there were 38 000 CHWs in the United States, a figure that grew to 67 000 by 2022 across a period when the ACA was passed and VBP models were implemented nationally. Further, according to the US Bureau of Labor Statistics, the 10-year anticipated annual job growth rate for CHWs in 2022 was 14%, compared to the national average of 3% for jobs in the United States overall.

The role for CHWs in health care settings will likely grow as VBP and other forces shape how health care is delivered in the United States. Therefore, understanding this growing workforce is critical to developing a complete understanding of community care.

Definition and History of Community Health Workers

Compared to other health care team members (eg, physicians, nurses), CHWs do not have a nationally required or standardized education process. Instead, CHWs are defined more by the relationships they have with, and the services they provide to, patients and communities. In turn, many formal definitions of CHWs exist. One of the most accepted definitions, created in 2009 by the American Public Health Association (APHA), is as follows:

> "A community health worker is a frontline public health worker who is a trusted member of and/or has an unusually close understanding of the community served. This trusting relationship enables the community health worker to serve as a liaison/link/intermediary between health/social services and the community to facilitate access to services and improve the quality and cultural competence of service delivery. A community health worker also builds individual and community capacity by increasing health knowledge and self-sufficiency through a range of activities such as outreach, community education, informal counseling, social support, and advocacy."

As this definition reflects, core components of what defines CHWs is their status as trusted members of a community, their service as a trusted intermediary between a particular community with medical or social services professionals, and their responsibility to assist individuals and communities by increasing health knowledge. Since the APHA definition was created, some states have made their own definitions of CHWs for purposes of scaling and tailoring the position within their state. Most definitions have roots in the APHA definition.

Importantly, CHWs have a rich international history. CHWs are believed to have their origins in Ding Xian, China in the 1920s. These first CHWs received 3 months of health-related training and were taught to provide vaccinations for smallpox and other diseases, provide first aid, teach communities about health-related topics, help maintain the cleanliness of community wells, and provide some basic medical care. These CHWs worked part time in their health-related role and part time as agricultural workers, embedded in their communities. Since this initial emergence, CHWs have grown in numbers in countries around the world. As of 2014, it was estimated that there were at least 5 million CHWs globally.

1950s to 1980s: Early Examples of Community Health Workers in the United States

Since their first emergence in the United States, CHWs have had a rich foundation in serving the health needs of communities through public health and grassroots efforts, rather than explicitly through the formal US health care system. CHWs are first believed to have emerged in the 1950s via grassroots efforts by indigenous workers to provide health outreach and education initiatives, with additional examples occurring in the mid-1960s to early 1970s. In these examples, CHWs were included in several anti-poverty-focused programs, where health was often a contributing focus of a broader program.

These programs also often focused on indigenous or impoverished populations, and the health focus of CHWs usually was centered on a specific condition. Some instances included the use of CHW as "neighborhood health aides" in a tuberculosis reduction program in New York City, as individuals improving adherence to clinician recommendations for pediatric respiratory infection treatment, and as team members in the Community Health Representative Program that was a part of a broader overall antipoverty initiative through a federal agency called the Office of Economic Opportunity. Despite these examples, over this period CHWs existed as part of specific programs, rather than as integrated parts of the broader health care system. For instance, despite Medicare and Medicaid being implemented in the mid-1960s, there was no documented effort in this time period to integrate CHWs.

From the mid-1970s to late 1980s, the use of CHWs continued to grow, mostly as a part of short-term projects or grants and linked to research efforts. In turn, although CHWs were still not a mainstream component of the health care workforce in the United States over this period, more examples of their use grew with a body of curricular training and literature supporting their effectiveness. One notable example from this time period was "Resource Mothers," a curriculum for CHWs developed in Virginia in the 1980s and implemented subsequently in many areas throughout the United States to train CHWs to support maternal and child health. Another example of a notable CHW program was the Health Education Training Centers program, which emerged in 1989 and was designed to helped train and promote the use of CHWs in public health projects serving immigrant communities near the US-Mexico border.

1990s: Increasing National Recognition for Community Health Workers

After this implementation of smaller prior programs, CHWs received more recognition in the 1990s. For example, in 1993, the Centers for Disease Control and Prevention (CDC) funded one of the first national conferences on CHW programs. In 1995, an *American Journal of Public Health* study framed CHWs as critical members of the health care workforce. In 1998, the Health Resources and Services Administration's Bureau of Primary Health Care organized a national conference that included a focus on discussing strategies for incorporating CHWs into larger nationally funded programs. During this time, several federal and state bills were introduced to scale and expand CHWs at either the state or the national levels.

1999 to Early 2000s: Increasing Adoption Into State and National Health Care Programs

During this time period, there was an increase in adoption of CHWs into broader health care programs and some efforts at standardizing credentialing and training. For instance, in 1999, Texas passed training and certification legislation and mandated CHW pilot projects in Medicaid-managed care programs. In 2003, Ohio passed formal credentialing legislation for CHWs, the University of Arizona began to develop a standardized CHW education program, and the Institute of Medicine published a report recommending incorporation of CHWs for the purpose of reducing health disparities. Medicare launched six different demonstration programs that incorporated CHW services for Medicare patients from minority communities living with cancer.

2010 to Present: The Affordable Care Act and Value-Based Payment Supporting Growth of Community Health Workers

The ACA, passed in 2010, was landmark legislation responsible for much of the recent growth and adoption of CHWs into US health care more broadly. The ACA supported the growth of CHWs both directly and indirectly. Directly, the ACA supported the growth of CHWs in pursuit of its goal to improve access to and delivery of care particularly for underserved, previously uninsured, and/or historically marginalized communities. Specifically, the ACA provided grant funding for projects that used CHWs to do the following:

- Conduct outreach for common health problems in underserved populations
- Promote healthy behavior
- Conduct outreach for the purpose of facilitating enrollment in insurance
- Identifying and referring people from underserved communities to health care and other community resources
- Provide home visiting services for pregnant women and prenatal care

While these initiatives provided direct opportunities to scale the use of CHWs, the indirect influence of the ACA might have had an even bigger impact. Embedded in the ACA were several programs that catalyzed the wide-scale adoption of VBP, including Medicare's ACO and patient-centered medical home programs, and statewide initiatives funded through the Centers for Medicare and Medicaid Services Innovation Center aimed at improving value in health care. These programs, and their emphasis on improving health outcomes, made community-based care a priority, which CHWs were equipped to address. It was under this context that CHWs became more broadly incorporated into US health care. Indeed, the year the ACA was passed (2010) was the first year the US Census listed "community health worker" as an occupation.

Studies have shown that CHWs have been used in various VBP models and value-based care initiatives, such as ACOs and patient-centered medical home programs. Appreciating the value of CHWs, policy efforts after the ACA have continued to support the growth of CHWs into US health care. As of 2022, at least 29 states allowed their Medicaid programs to directly reimburse CHW services. Further, in 2022, the American Rescue Plan provided $225 million in funding to train over 13 000 CHWs, representing the largest direct investment in CHWs from the federal government.

The Community Health Worker Workforce: Composition, Roles, and Qualification Expectations

Throughout their history, CHW initiatives have largely focused on serving underserved and historically marginalized groups. Since a core component of the definition of a CHW is that they be a "trusted member of and/or has an unusually close understanding of the community served," the CHW workforce is overall more diverse than other health workforce professions.

CHWs take on a variety of roles in assisting their communities' health needs, which can vary depending on identified health goals, nature of the CHWs' employers, or communities being served. However, in recent years, efforts have been undertaken to create a standardized understanding of what a CHW's core roles, or functions that CHWs take in the health care system. One of the more notable efforts to create this standardized understanding was the Community Health Worker Core Consensus Project in 2016. This project's overall aim was to create consensus surrounding what it means to be a CHW and facilitate greater understanding of CHWs. In creating the list of roles and competencies, the project was influenced by prior efforts, and directly solicited feedback from CHWs and CHW organizations spanning several practice settings. The project identified 10 roles. Each of these roles is explained in Table 8.2.

To fulfill these roles, CHWs use an understanding of their community and on-the-job training, as formal CHW training programs remain limited. However, as CHWs have become more widespread in US healthcare, some states have started to incorporate certification criteria for CHWs. As of 2022, 13 states operated their own certification program. New Jersey, for instance, includes 144 hours of required classroom training and between 1000 to 2000 hours of on-the-job training before individuals can be certified as a CHW. The classroom training is virtual and focuses on many of the same competencies outlined by the 2016 Community Health Worker Core Consensus Project, as well as other training topics such as COVID-19 education, safety, health equity and disparities, and adverse childhood experiences.

Still, most states do not include a formal certification program, and some have argued that there is a risk of overstandardizing the role in ways that may diminish what makes CHWs unique—roles as trusted members of the community they serve or individuals with shared life experience with community members—and enables them to gain trust in ways that clinicians and other individuals of traditional health care teams might not be able.

In lieu of formal certification and universal training requirements, one way to understand the CHW education and training expectations would be through the hiring practices of organizations that employ them. In a 2017 study, researchers performed a literature review, developed a database of known programs that hire CHWs, interviewed key informants, and cross-examined lists of competencies produced as expectations by states (eg, Texas) or major cities (eg, Boston). The study ultimately assessed the CHW hiring practices of 76 programs, 58% of which were led by medical care organizations (eg, hospitals, federally qualified health centers) and health insurance plans, 38% were

Table 8.2 Core Roles of CHWs

Role	Explanation
Cultural mediation among individuals, communities, and health and social service systems	Educating medical care organizations about the cultural practices of patients and educating patients on how to interact with the health care system to facilitate cross cultural communication
Providing culturally appropriate health education and information	Providing patients with information about health to prevent illness and about chronic illnesses to help with disease management in a language-concordant manner that respects cultural differences and norms
Care coordination, case management, and system navigation	Helping with follow-up on referrals, helping with transportation to visits, and informing clinicians about challenges patients and communities face
Providing coaching and social support	Providing one-on-one support for individual behavior change and disease self-management, facilitating support groups, and helping people obtain needed health services
Advocating for individuals and communities	Advocating for broader health system and policy changes, connecting individuals with community resources such as nutrition support, advocating for the perspective of patients within health care systems
Building individual and community capacity	Helping build community and individual self-sufficiency through the other nine roles and helping support other CHW groups in building their abilities
Providing direct service	Administering basic direct medical services, such as blood pressure measurement, diabetes foot checks, or administering first aid services
Implementing individual and community assessments	Helping to design and implement individual assessments (eg, home health assessments) and community-level assessments (eg, neighborhood safety initiatives)
Conducting outreach	Recruiting individuals, community leaders, and organizations to help support patients and the community, recruiting patients for needed services
Participating in evaluation and research	Evaluating the effectiveness of CHW interventions and engaging with career researchers on identifying community priorities for research and incorporating community perspectives

CHW, community health worker.

Source: Adapted from Rosenthal L. The community health worker core consensus (C3) a report of the C3 project: phase 1 and 2. Texas Tech University Health Sciences Center El Paso. Published December 2018. Accessed December 18, 2023. https://www.c3project.org/_files/ugd/7ec423_2b0893bcc93a422 396c744be8c1d54d1.pdf

led by community-oriented organizations and nonprofits, and 9% were led by local health departments or other health or social agencies.

Of these programs, half required that the CHW candidate live in the community served or have considerable prior experience with the community served. Only about 10% explicitly required a particular formal education attainment, most of which were for a high school diploma or GED (General Education Development). Instead, more than a third of the programs required some other type of training, such as achieving an asthma educator certification, and more than 20% of programs had requirements surrounding language proficiency. A minority of programs also required applicants to have what's referred to as peer status, meaning that the CHW share the same condition or life experience as the community served (eg, a CHW in a diabetes program would have peer status if they had diabetes themselves). Twenty percent of programs had no specific criteria listed.

Approaches for Integration of Community Health Workers

As CHWs have grown in number and scope in the US health care system, approaches have emerged for how they've integrated into the health care system. The four most common approaches of CHW integration into the health care system are shown in Figure 8.5.

In the first approach, CHWs can embed within community-oriented organizations to facilitate connection to resources through linkages. CHWs are employed by community-oriented organizations and collaborate via informal relationships with medical care organizations, government agencies, or payers to facilitate connection with community resources. Community-oriented organizations can be small community-based organizations that are located in and stem directly from local communities served, or broader, national, or international organizations that serve individual communities.

In this approach, CHWs receive referrals from linked organizations for patients who need support for social needs or health coaching. CHWs can work with community members directly, connect community members to medical care as one part of the several services they may offer, or receive referrals from clinicians for patients who need support for social needs or for health coaching. One example of this is City Health Works, an NYC-based organization that hires and trains CHWs to help peers in the community to manage their health and navigate the health care system. In this way, CHWs work with medical care organizations and serve as a bridge between the community and medical care organizations but are not directly employed by them.

A second approach for integrating CHWs is to embed them within medical care organizations. Here, CHWs are employed by such organizations and focus on interprofessional communication, increasing "trust in clinicians, and

Embed within community-oriented organizations to facilitate connection to community resources through linkages
- CHWs are employed by community-oriented organizations and collaborate via informal relationships with medical care organizations, government agencies, or payers to facilitate connection with community resources.
- CHWs receive referrals from linked organizations for patients who need support for social needs or health coaching.

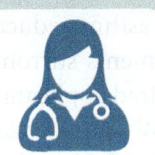
Embed within medical care organizations
- CHWs are employed by medical care organizations and focus on interprofessional communication, increasing trust in clinicians, and enhance patients' experience of care.
- CHWs provide support as part of care teams, participate in care during and between visits, help during high-risk periods such as after hospital discharge, and serve in overall outreach roles.

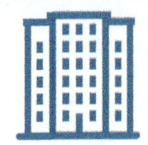
Embed within government agencies to provide coordination
- CHWs are employed by government agencies, such as departments of health or social services agencies, and provide services to the community at large, rather than from a community-oriented organization, medical care organization, or payer.

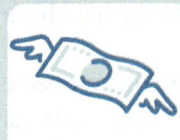
Embed within payers
- CHWs are employed by public or private payers to work with insured beneficiaries across multiple medical care organizations.
  or
- Payers provide funding specifically for medical care organizations to hire CHWs as part of their care teams.

Figure 8.5 Common Approaches for Integration of CHWs in US Health Care. CHWs, community health workers. (Source: Data from Centers for Medicare and Medicaid Services. Accountable health communities model overview and track 1 requirements. Accessed December 18, 2023. https://innovation.cms.gov/files/slides/ahcm-track1 overview-appreq.pdf)

enhance patients" experience of care. CHWs can support care as part of care teams, participate in care during and between visits, help during high-risk periods such as after hospital discharge and serve in overall outreach roles. One example of this model is Iora Health, which was founded as a primary care organization that used CHWs and participated in VBP models. One of the models used by Iora Health involved pairing clinicians with social workers, administrative staff, and employed CHWs, whose role was to serve as an advocate for patients during visits and help patients navigate health needs in between visits.

Another way to integrate CHWs is to provide care coordination by embedding them within government agencies, rather than community-oriented organizations, medical care organizations, or payers. In this third approach, CHWs are employed by entities such as departments of health or social services agencies and provide services to the community at large. One example of this is the role of some CHWs during the COVID-19 pandemic. In this instance, the CDC provided funding for state and local health departments to hire CHWs, where they worked in contact tracing to manage the spread of the virus, provided education about COVID-19, and helped facilitate access to the COVID-19 vaccine.

A fourth approach for CHW integration is to embed them within payers. In this approach, CHWs are employed by public or private payers to work with insured beneficiaries across multiple medical care organizations, or payers provide funding specifically for medical care organizations to hire CHWs as part of their care teams. One example of a payer directly hiring CHWs is Pennsylvania Medicaid's Community-Based Care Management program. This program included partnerships between Medicaid Managed Care Organizations (private payers that are paid to administer Medicaid benefits) and medical care organizations, where the Managed Care Organization allotted funding for or sometimes directly hired CHWs to provide services such as care coordination, medication management, social needs screening, and referral to community resources for patients.

These four approaches for CHW integration are not mutually exclusive. Rather, individuals can receive care from or be exposed to CHWs via multiple approaches simultaneously. For example, an individual could receive assistance from a CHW at the local health department to learn where they can access a COVID-19 vaccine; another CHW who is directly embedded in their medical care organization and coaches patients on healthy diet and exercise habits for diabetes; and another CHW who is embedded within their payer and helps facilitate connections to resources for health-related social needs such as transportation.

Back to the Clinical Case

In this case, the patient is connected by her physician to a CHW after describing difficulty navigating health in the community. In this role, the CHW is meant to help the patient navigate difficult tasks such as grocery shopping, healthy meal preparation, and may be present at future visits to help advocate for the patient. Some of the responsibilities the CHW may have include providing coaching and social support, advocating for individuals, building individual capacity, and providing direct service. It can be beneficial for the CHW to reside in the same community as the patient or have meaningful knowledge and experience of her community; an even stronger connection may result if the CHW is a "peer CHW"—for instance, someone living with the same condition as the patient (eg, diabetes). In this circumstance, it is likely that the CHW is operating under the CHW integration model of direct employment by medical care organizations, where she's employed and embedded in the patient's primary care team.

TAKEAWAYS

- CHWs have been a part of health care globally since the 1920s and in the United States since the 1950s, growing in prevalence over time and amid emphasis on community-based care driven by VBP and other systems factors.
- Throughout their history, CHWs have emphasized care and advocacy for historically underserved, impoverished, and indigenous populations.
- There are no national standardized accreditation or training requirements for CHWs, but there is some consensus about their core roles.
- Four common approaches for integrating CHWs into the US health care system include embedding them within community-oriented organizations, medical care organizations, government agencies, and payers.

Clinical Case Continued

The CHW helps Jessica and her husband identify recipes with affordable ingredients and teaches them how to prepare these meals. The CHW also helps Jessica and her husband create a system to make sure Jessica reliably takes her diabetes medication in between visits.

With these measures, her husband notices that Jessica's blood sugar improves. However, Jessica's memory continues to decline, and at her next visit, the CHW attends and advocates that the primary care clinician evaluate Jessica's memory changes further and consider referral to a neurologist. The primary care clinician performs a Montreal Cognitive Assessment, a screening test to detect early signs of cognitive impairment related to different etiologies of dementia.

Jessica's score is consistent with a likely diagnosis of dementia. The primary care clinician refers Jessica to a neurologist, who conducts additional testing and confirms the diagnosis of Alzheimer disease.

Jessica's ability to care for herself continues to diminish as a result of her disease. Unable to afford 24-hour home care, her husband decides to further reduce his work hours so that he can take a larger role in managing Jessica's care throughout the day. Her husband starts to experience depression, loneliness, and fatigue, and even misses his own medical visits, as a result of his caregiver responsibilities. Compounding these challenges, he has not been able to afford extra help at home or groceries for nutritious meals due to reduced income from time off work. Her husband mentions all of this to Jessica's CHW, who shares this information with the primary care clinician.

In this circumstance, the patient and her husband are facing several barriers to optimal care for the patient's medical conditions. Some of those barriers are clinical in nature. For instance, even though the clinicians explained Alzheimer disease treatment options and its disease course, the patient's husband still needs education to fully prepare him to care for the patient's every day clinical needs and understand how the disease will impact their daily life in the community. Other barriers are nonmedical, such as more limited ability to afford groceries in light of the patient's husband reducing his employment (and, in turn, income) to care for her. Each of these nonmedical barriers, if unaddressed, can have a serious and detrimental impact on the patient's health.

Medical care organizations that assume accountability for patient outcomes such as those participating in VBP models or already engaging CHWs, might still benefit from outside resources that can help address patients' nonmedical needs, such as health education, peer support, or direct provision of health-related services between visits. These are needs that can potentially be filled by organizations oriented to community needs—both local community-based organizations and broader organizations targeting individual communities. Such community-oriented organizations, and the supports they can provide, represent a health systems factor that can complement patients' medical care to address overall health.

SYSTEMS FACTOR: COMMUNITY-ORIENTED ORGANIZATIONS

Community-oriented organizations can represent broader, national or international organizations with a local community focus, as well as smaller community-based organizations that are located in and stem directly from local communities served. Community-oriented organizations offer a variety of resources that can help patients address both medical and nonmedical drivers of health in community settings.

Although community-oriented organizations have an important history serving communities, more recent trends toward VBP—and clinicians and medical care organizations assuming accountability for health outcomes— may prompt these groups to increase their focus and efforts on working with community-oriented organizations to address patients' health needs in community settings in ways that complement medical care. Community-oriented organizations can achieve this through many different services, including health education, peer support, direct provision of health-related services, and programs addressing health-related nonmedical needs.

Health Education

As community-oriented organizations, disease-specific nonprofits can offer services that complement health education provided by clinicians. For example, consider the patient in this clinical case and her diagnosis of Alzheimer disease—a progressive and terminal disease that influences individuals' cognition and ability to care for activities of daily living and instrumental activities of daily living. Patients living with Alzheimer disease can increasingly rely on informal (eg, family members, friends) or formal (eg, home health aides, personal care aides) to care for their medical, legal, and personal needs, which can be challenging to navigate.

The Alzheimer's Association, a national nonprofit with local chapters throughout the country, complements the health education provided by clinicians through free online and in-person classes for people living with dementia and loved ones who often act as caregivers. Topics include navigating financial and legal planning for someone with dementia, using communication strategies to connect with and better understand loved ones with the disease, and preparing participants on how to be a caregiver as well as what to expect in early, middle, and late stages of the disease. Such health education resources are not unique to Alzheimer disease, as national and local disease-specific organizations offer education programs for many medical conditions.

Health education can be embedded in community settings rather than dedicated educational locations. For instance, consider hypertension—a major risk factor for heart attacks, strokes, kidney disease, and a number of other medical conditions—and the dangers it poses in particular for Black men (Black men experience hypertension at higher rates, have a higher risk of developing organ damage from hypertension at younger ages, and, on average, have less access to medical care than White men).

Given the familiarity and comfort that men can have with barbershops, there have been efforts to incorporate hypertension-related health education within barbershop settings. In one study of 52 barbershops serving a high proportion of Black men, barbers were trained as hypertension educators. When customers came to the barbershop, they had their blood pressure measured and barbers educated them about the disease, its risks, lifestyle strategies to reduce blood pressure, and benefits of seeing their primary care clinician. For one group in the study, barbers also connected customers with hypertension with pharmacists, who were able to prescribe blood pressure medication, if indicated.

Six months after this intervention, the mean systolic blood pressure for the group who received education from barbers and were connected with a pharmacist fell by 27 mm Hg. The mean systolic blood pressure for the group who received education but were not connected with pharmacists also fell, by 9.3 mm Hg. Hypertension education delivered in barbershops represents one example of the broader potential to deliver health education to individuals in familiar community settings.

One community-oriented organization that coordinates barbershop-based health initiatives such as the hypertension-related intervention is the Black Barbershop Health Outreach Program, a Los Angeles organization founded in 2006 whose mission is to address health disparities in Black men. After their success in screening for hypertension in barbershops in Los Angeles and coordinating similar efforts nationally, the Black Barbershop Health Outreach Program expanded its model to also focus on addressing other medical conditions that disproportionately impact Black men, including diabetes and COVID-19.

Peer Support

When used in health care, peer support—which involves direct interaction and support between people who share similar experiences of being diagnosed with a particular medical, mental health, or substance use condition—can improve health outcomes and people's attitudes about their illness. However, despite these benefits, such supports remain broadly underutilized in many parts of the health care system. Community-oriented organizations can be positioned to address this gap and be facilitators of peer support, especially in areas of mental health and substance use.

One notable example is Alcoholics Anonymous (AA). An international nonprofit organization with local chapters, AA incorporates a 12-step sobriety program with peer support/mentorship for people recovering from an alcohol use disorder at no financial cost to the individual. Peer support comes through anonymous group meetings where people share their experiences with their illness and recovery, and through direct mentor-mentee dyad relationships. Groups meetings are offered every day, and people can look up groups occurring near them online (in 2015, there were more than 60 000 AA groups across the United States).

Peer mentorship also occurs through relationships between AA participants and their sponsors—more experienced members of AA further in their recovery who offer mentorship to newer members in guiding them through the 12-steps of the AA program. AA describes itself as a fellowship, where individual groups share their loose affiliation, but individuals can find a group most in line with their values and preferences. Similar community-oriented organizations have created similar peer support environments for individuals with other substance use disorders, as well as for family members of people with similar illnesses.

Peer supports provided through community-oriented organizations can not only promote particular goals such as sobriety but also create a sense of connection and community as important goals themselves. One notable example is Fountain House, a national nonprofit community-oriented organization focused on creating supportive community environments for people with serious mental illness as a group that can have smaller and less satisfactory social networks. Fountain House and other organizations throughout the United States achieve this goal through what is sometimes referred to as a clubhouse model, in which intended groups (individuals with serious mental illness, in Fountain House's case) have membership and access to a community-oriented physical space at no cost.

In the Fountain House clubhouse, members can receive a number of services, including crisis intervention, support with employment, housing, education, and meals. Members work alongside staff to carry out all daily operations to maintain the space and community, with every member assigning themselves a job from predetermined options, including meal prep, cleaning, gardening, clerical work, or research. This approach is intended to facilitate a sense of ownership over the clubhouse for all members, dignity, agency, independence, and relationships with other clubhouse members.

One community-based organization that follows the clubhouse model is Hero House Northwest, which operates three clubhouses in the greater Seattle area. Beyond direct services, Hero House Northwest creates a sense of community for members through shared social events and wellness activities, such as trips to baseball games, the local zoo, museums, game nights, and community walks.

Direct Provision of Health-Related Services

Community-oriented organizations can complement clinicians and medical care organizations by directly providing health-related services. For example, consider exercise as one of the most effective nonmedication treatments for a range of conditions including osteoarthritis. Despite this recognition, individuals with osteoarthritis may need more help to plan and execute exercise plans than traditional medical care organizations can provide. Community-oriented organizations such as the Young Men's Christian Association can fill this gap by promoting balance and range of motion via aerobic and tai chi classes.

Additionally, people who are responsible for caring for loved ones with a serious illness (eg, dementia, amyotrophic lateral sclerosis, cancer) can sometimes suffer from caregiver fatigue, which is an overall state of physical or emotional exhaustion arising from efforts to meet another person's care needs. As many as 75% of caregivers experience symptoms of anxiety and depression, and caregivers who are older in age and experience emotional distress have higher mortality rates than people who aren't caregivers.

Community-oriented organizations can provide relief through respite care programs, where a trained person comes to the home to provide temporary caregiving duties while the primary caregiver takes a break to tend to their own needs. Respite care can be expensive, but several community-oriented organizations offer affordable or free respite care services, including faith-based organizations and non-faith-based organizations. One example, Elder Helpers, offers a national online service that prescreens and shares a list of local volunteers who can help with a few hours of respite care and basic chores, at no cost to the recipient.

Programs Addressing Health-Related Nonmedical Needs

Health-related nonmedical needs are issues arising from an individual's environment that can have a large impact on health outcomes. Examples include, but are not limited to, housing instability, food insecurity, challenges with transportation to visits or in general, having difficulty meeting electricity or utility bills, unemployment, and intimate partner violence. Because these needs are generally difficult to address directly in the context of a visit, community-oriented organizations exist to address many of these needs.

The Rhode Island Community Food Bank, for instance, is a community-based organization that provides food to more than 75 000 Rhode Islanders annually through a network of more than 140 local groups that provide food directly to Rhode Islanders in need of food assistance. Other community-oriented organizations work to assist people experiencing housing instability, providing shelter to more than 300 000 people experiencing homelessness in a given night, and also working to provide safe housing for people in particularly sensitive or traumatic situations. Yet other community-oriented organizations are designed to help individuals with transportation barriers, providing free rides to food banks, medical visits, or for critical errands such as grocery shopping.

Given the different potential resources offered through community-oriented organizations, connecting patients to community-based resources can be a challenge in itself. Organizations have emerged to address this need. For instance, an organization called Aunt Bertha offers a free directory, searchable by zip code, where people can learn about the resources and organizations in their community that help with a number of health-related social needs (eg, food, housing, transit, legal assistance, employment). An additional free resource is the 2-1-1, which people can use—either via a website, or by dialing 2-1-1 on the telephone—to find similar information by zip code in all 50 states and Puerto Rico, and in 180 languages.

Still, connection to and use of community-based resources could be further aided by better identification of patients' health-related needs (eg, resources that would be most beneficial for a given patient) and existing community resources (eg, resources that currently do or do not exist through community-oriented organizations in a given community).

Payment and Care Models Addressing Health-Related Nonmedical Needs

By virtue of holding clinicians accountable for health outcomes, VBP and care models have the potential to prompt medical care organizations to design and implement care innovations that involve community-oriented organizations and provide patients with supports in community settings. While most payment and care models have yet to do this at scale, early pilots exist.

In particular, the Medicare Accountable Health Communities Model was specifically designed and funded to support medical care organizations in efforts to build relationships with community-oriented organizations to help address patients' health-related social needs. Implemented between 2017 and 2022, the model required participating organizations to create processes to identify Medicare patients with health-related social needs—with emphasis on five core types of need, which are utilities, food security, transportation, interpersonal violence, and housing instability—and connect individuals with identified needs with "community service providers" that could address those needs (Figure 8.6).

At the center of the Accountable Health Communities Model were bridge organizations, groups tasked with coordinating with medical care organizations (eg, hospitals, clinician offices) and community service providers, state Medicaid agencies, and other stakeholders to ensure that individuals receiving care under the model were receiving needed community resources. Notably, the model was not prescriptive about eligibility as a bridge organization. In turn, approximately half of the groups participating as bridge organizations were medical care organizations that provided patients with direct clinical care, as opposed to community-oriented or other types of organizations.

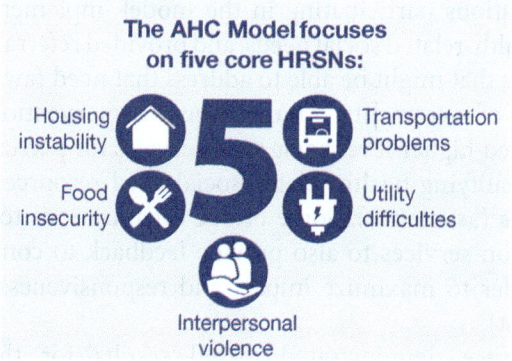

Figure 8.6 HRSNs in the AHC Model. AHC, Accountable Health Communities; HRSNs, health-related social needs. (Source: Adapted from Centers for Medicare and Medicaid Services. Accountable health communities model 2018-2021. Accessed December 18, 2023. https://innovation.cms.gov/data-and-reports/2023/ahc-second-eval-rpt-fg)

    The model sought to test the impact of three types of interventions with different and increasing intensity levels (Figure 8.7). Specifically, the model sought to understand the impacts of increasing awareness about patients' needs through screening, education, and referral; providing assistance via navigation resources to help patients access community service providers; and promoting alignment between medical care organizations and community service providers.

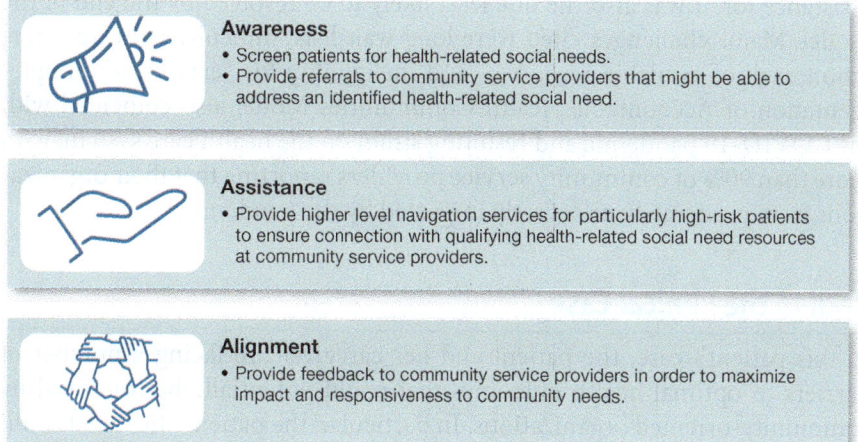

Figure 8.7 Interventions Tested in the Accountable Health Communities Model. (Source: Adapted from Centers for Medicare and Medicaid Services. Accountable health communities model overview and track 1 requirements. Accessed December 18, 2023. https://innovation.cms.gov/files/slides/ahcm-track1overview-appreq.pdf)

All organizations participating in the model implemented a universal screening for health-related social needs, and provided referrals to community service providers that might be able to address that need (awareness). To test the effectiveness of incrementally more intensive interventions, bridge organizations provided higher level navigation services for particularly high-risk patients with qualifying health-related social need resources at community service providers (assistance). Some bridge organizations took extra efforts beyond navigation services to also provide feedback to community service providers in order to maximize impact and responsiveness to community needs (alignment).

Early evidence demonstrated mixed results for the Accountable Health Communities Model. On one hand, evaluations reported that the model reduced emergency room (ER) visits, and more than 75% of eligible patients accepted navigation assistance. Most community service providers reported being able to address more than one health-related social need for referred patients, and most organizations reported an increased capacity to address health-related social needs at the end of the model compared to at the beginning.

On the other hand, more than half of the patients receiving care through the model and who agreed to receive patient navigation services for identified health-related social needs had none of their health-related social needs resolved and were not connected to a community service provider that addressed their need. Although food insecurity was the most commonly identified need and the one that individuals said they were most likely to accept assistance for, it was also the one least likely to be resolved by the end of the model. Major challenges cited were long wait lists, difficulty with transportation, lack of available resources, and ineligibility for services. The implementation of Accountable Health Communities Model also coincided with the COVID-19 pandemic and resulting strain on the health care system, with more than 90% of community service providers reporting that their organizations were moderately or severely impacted by the pandemic.

Back to the Clinical Case

In this patient's case, the patient and her caregiver are facing a number of barriers to optimal health outcomes that could potentially be improved by community-oriented organizations. In particular, the patient's husband could attend classes through organizations such as a local chapter of the Alzheimer's Association to better equip himself to care for the patient's needs, and access respite care resources so that he can better tend to his own needs as a longer term caregiver. Both the patient and her husband could benefit from the resources of a local food bank, helping to supplement their groceries so that the patient's husband does not need to prepare and purchase ingredients for all meals. Although not necessarily applicable in this case, expansion of programs such as the Accountable Health Communities Model could increase the ability and incentives for the patient's clinicians to screen patients such as the one in this case, and for identified needs, connect individuals to community-oriented organizations.

TAKEAWAYS

- Community-oriented organizations can serve as a complement to clinical care, helping individuals navigate their health in the community through health education, peer support, direct provision of health-related services, and programs that address health-related nonmedical needs.
- Programs that address health-related nonmedical needs focus on issues arising from an individual's environment that can have a large impact on health outcomes (eg, housing instability, food insecurity, challenges with transportation) that are generally difficult to address directly in the context of a visit.
- The Accountable Health Communities Model is an early example of a payment and care model focused on meeting patients' health-related nonmedical needs through engaging medical care organizations to create greater awareness, assistance, and alignment with community service providers.

Clinical Case Continued

The CHW identifies food assistance as a health-related social need for Jessica and her husband. This information is conveyed to the primary care clinician, who is participating in the Accountable Health Communities Model. The primary care clinician's office refers Jessica to the local chapter of the Alzheimer's Association (which enrolls her husband in their course on caring for loved ones with dementia and a respite care program) as well as the local food bank. The primary care clinician, CHW, and Jessica decide to have another visit in 3 months.

Two weeks later, the patient's husband goes to his first Alzheimer's Association course. During the session, one of the other attendees shares that before becoming a caregiver for a loved one experiencing Alzheimer disease, he used to love going to the gym. He adds that although he now has less time to do so since taking on caregiver duties, his health insurance company recently started including a free gym membership as part of its benefits. This piques the husband's interest, as he is unfamiliar with health insurance plans paying for a gym membership.

This situation highlights the potential variation and nature of health insurance plan benefits. Many plans, including Traditional Medicare (TM), only cover a set of health care services provided through clinicians and medical care organizations. However, some insurance plans cover additional health-related benefits focused on wellness and community-based care, such as gym memberships.

In particular, certain insurance companies enable flexibilities that allow gym memberships, and other services such as transportation or meal supports, to be included as covered benefits. To the extent that some of these services exist in community rather than health care settings, health insurance benefit design represents a systems factor potentially affecting community-based care.

SYSTEMS FACTOR: HEALTH INSURANCE BENEFIT DESIGN FOR COMMUNITY-BASED CARE

Clinicians, particularly those engaged in VBP models that create reinforcing incentives, can incorporate community-based care into care delivery processes. Analogously, payers—and in particular those adopting value-based approaches—can incorporate plan benefits that involve community-based services to support better quality and cost outcomes. Notable examples include Medicare Advantage (MA) plans and Medicaid waivers.

Medicare Advantage

Individuals who are eligible for Medicare choose to receive coverage through either MA or TM. A major difference is that while MA is privately administered via managed care (Medicare pays commercial insurance companies to administer and manage plans), TM is publicly administered via indemnity insurance (Medicare pays directly for covered services). So long as they cover all inpatient and outpatient benefits provided through TM, MA plans can incorporate additional plan design features. Many apply managed care principles to benefit design, create provider networks, and implement patient cost sharing and prior authorization measures.

MA plans possess this flexibility because, in essence, they operate under VBP incentives. In particular, Medicare pays MA plans using a risk-adjusted per-beneficiary ("per capita") lump sum. MA plans then endeavor to achieve high-quality, cost-efficient care within the confines of this fixed lump sum payment—that is, under value-based accountability for quality and cost outcomes. One way that plans seek to achieve these goals is by structuring plans to incorporate supplemental benefits not covered under TM.

Initially, allowable supplemental benefits were narrowly defined and limited to medical benefits such as vision or dental coverage. However, Medicare loosened this restriction in 2019 and began permitting MA plans to incorporate nonmedical supplemental health benefits as well. Under those changes, MA plans could institute a new benefit so long as it was intended to address one of several requirements as specifically defined in Medicare regulation:

- Diagnose, prevent, or treat an illness or injury
- Compensate for physical impairments
- Ameliorate the functional/psychological impact of injuries or health conditions
- Reduce avoidable emergency and health care utilization to all beneficiaries

In addition, in 2020, Congress passed the Creating High-Quality Results and Outcomes Necessary to Improve Chronic Care Act, which permitted MA plans to offer benefits tailored specifically to beneficiaries with certain chronic conditions, so long as such benefits might improve the overall health and functioning of people with that condition.

As a collective result of these changes, many MA plans have incorporated a number of community-based care benefits (Figure 8.8). Setting aside unique circumstances for plans covering special needs populations, covered community-based care benefits include the following:

Fitness. Nearly every MA plan includes a fitness benefit, such as a free gym membership.

Meal support. Approximately half of all beneficiaries enrolled in an MA plan include a home-delivered meal benefit. In most cases, the home-delivered meal benefit is focused on assisting beneficiaries with meals after a hospitalization or other major health event, and is usually limited to a certain amount of time or number of meals rather than long-term support. The meal benefit is a maximum of 30 days in more than 90% of MA plans that include it, and includes a maximum of 60 meals in more than 70% of the plans that include a meal benefit. In some cases, MA plans will include longer term home-delivered meal support.

Medical and nonmedical transportation. A little more than one-third of MA plans include a transportation benefit. In most cases, the transportation benefit is limited to transportation to and from visits, but in some circumstances includes transportation assistance to grocery shopping, the bank, or other essential errands. MA plans vary in whether they cover dedicated medical transportation vehicles, public transportation, taxi or ride shares, or other transportation modalities.

Structural home modifications. People with disabilities, for example those who use a wheelchair for ambulation, may require structural home modifications in order to live safely in their home and community. In 2020, 10% of MA plans included coverage for home modifications in their benefit design, such as building permanent ramps or widening halls or doorways.

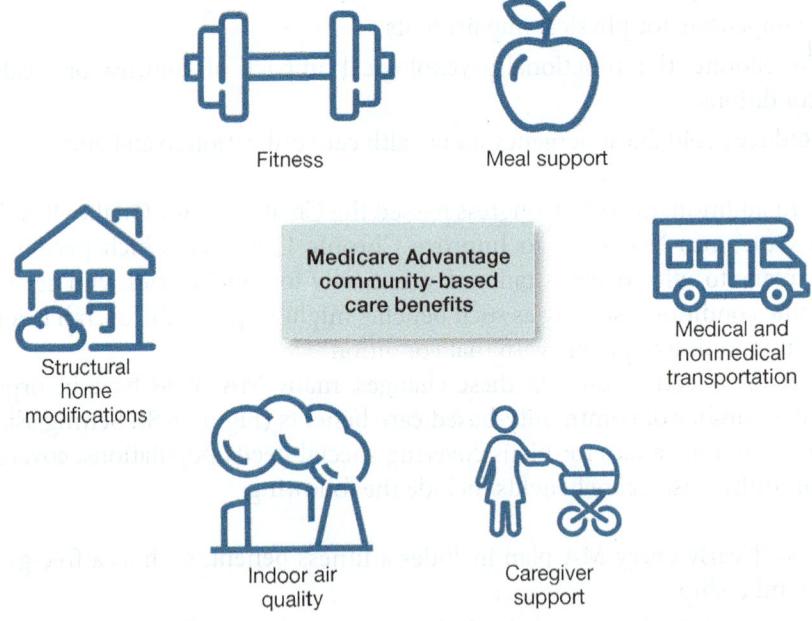

Figure 8.8 Examples of Medicare Advantage (MA) Benefits That Relate to Community-Based Care. (Source: Data from Centers for Medicare and Medicaid Services. Implementing supplemental benefits for chronically ill enrollees. Updated April 24, 2019. Accessed December 18, 2023. https://www.cms.gov/Medicare/Health-Plans/HealthPlansGenInfo/Downloads/Supplemental_Benefits_Chronically_Ill_HPMS_042419.pdf; Kornfield T, Kazan M, Frieder M, et al. Medicare advantage plans offering expanded supplemental benefits: a look at availability and enrollment. Commonwealth Fund. Updated February 10, 2021. Accessed from December 18, 2023. https://www.commonwealthfund.org/publications/issue-briefs/2021/feb/medicare-advantage-plans-supplemental-benefits#4)

Caregiver support. Approximately 4% of MA beneficiaries are enrolled in a plan that includes caregiver supports, such as basic training on how to care for people with particular health conditions, or respite care assistance.

Indoor air quality. A small proportion of MA plans also include supplemental benefits that focus on indoor air quality. Indoor air quality is important for health overall, but particularly impactful to health for people with chronic lung conditions such as asthma or chronic obstructive pulmonary disease (COPD). Some MA plans (1% in 2020) cover equipment to help with indoor air quality, such as through putting in air conditioning units, dehumidifiers, air filters, and carpet cleaning.

Medicaid Waivers

Over time, Medicaid programs—health insurance programs jointly funded by state and federal governments and operated by states for the benefit of eligible low-income adults, children, pregnant women, and people with disabilities—have incorporated benefits related to community-based care. This can occur when a Medicaid program pursues particular "waivers," which permit state Medicaid programs to deviate from federal requirements under certain circumstances, which would otherwise generally restrict Medicaid benefits to health care services. States have used two particular types of waivers, the 1915(c) waiver and the 1115 waiver, to pursue community-based care benefits.

The 1915(c) waiver allows states to develop new home- and community-based services that are intended to meet the needs of people who prefer to receive long-term services and support needs at home, rather than in an institution such as a skilled nursing facility. Eligibility for waivers is determined in part by clinical appropriateness and cost considerations—specifically, that the new benefit would not cost more than services provided in an institution; and that the new benefit meets the needs of the intended population and follows an individualized and person-centered plan of care.

One example is Washington state, which has obtained and used a 1915(c) waiver to create a new community-based care benefit through its Community Options Program Entry System and Family Caregiver Support Program. These waiver-authorized programs encompass a set of benefits that enable individuals who would otherwise require nursing home–level care to remain and access care supports in the community. Some benefits mirror those observed in MA plans, such as home modifications and meal support. Additional community-based care-related benefits under the Washington 1915(c) waiver include the following:

Adult day care. Medicaid will provide certain community-residing older adults (those needing daytime supervision for safety or additional social interaction) access to nonresidential facilities during regular business hours for meals, activities, time with peers, and some medical services.

Alternative housing. Medicaid will pay a portion of the fee for a person to live in an assisted living facility or adult family home instead of a skilled nursing facility.

Caregiver support. If a beneficiary's spouse is serving as their unpaid caregiver, Medicaid will help pay for respite care, counseling for the caregiver, and for training classes. If the caregiver is not the spouse of the beneficiary and meets requirements to become a certified caregiver, then a person that the beneficiary chooses (eg, stranger, friend, non-spouse relative) can be paid by Medicaid to provide caregiving services.

Whereas a 1915(c) waiver can create benefits for a specific subpopulation, a Medicaid 1115 waiver allows for broader changes and expanded benefits in a Medicaid program, so long as they are aligned with overall program mission and considered budget neutral. State Medicaid programs receive an initial 5-year authorization for a 1115 waiver and can be renewed for an additional 3 to 5 years.

One of the approaches taken by states under 1115 waivers has been to expand benefits that relate to community-based care. In addition to support with housing, nutrition, and respite care for caregivers, some of the benefits incorporated by different states through state 1115 waiver programs include the following:

Peer support services. In California, patients experiencing a mental illness or substance use disorder can be connected with a peer specialist. In this circumstance, peer specialists are members of the community who have direct lived experience or are close family members with someone with experience recovering from serious mental illness or a substance use disorder, are committed to recovery, and achieve a certification requirement as a peer specialist. Through this benefit, peer specialists coach patients to try to prevent a return to substance use or worsening of a mental illness, educate patients about a range of topics, and link patients to community resources.

Disease prevention programs. In North Carolina, patients who are at risk for diabetes participate in a 1-year education program that is delivered by a lifestyle coach and offered online and in the community. The program follows CDC guidelines and focuses on healthy eating and physical activity.

Back to the Clinical Case

In this case, the patient is dually eligible for Medicare and Medicaid and could therefore potentially benefit from additional community-based care-related resources available through MA plans or Medicaid waivers. For instance, home meal delivery could help alleviate some of the financial and time pressures of cooking. Respite care, adult day care, and caregiver training can assist the patient's husband in his caregiver responsibilities.

> ### TAKEAWAYS
>
> - Flexibility in insurance benefit design can enable payers to create new benefits, including those that relate to or impact community-based care.
> - Notable examples of such flexibilities include MA and Medicaid waivers.
> - Some benefits related to community-based care include gym memberships, home-delivered meals, transportation benefits, chronic disease prevention classes, peer supports, respite care, and home modifications.

Implications

The systems factors in this chapter have implications for patients' access to care. For instance, CHWs directly facilitate access to new types of care (eg, coaching, advocacy, capacity building). Overall, the majority of research suggests that CHW programs improve access to clinicians and help ensure follow-up through regular visits. It is critical to evaluate access holistically, particularly because expanded access to certain services (such as observed under MA plans) does not guarantee expanded, or even stable, access to other services.

A 2022 study comparing access to care for low-income Medicare beneficiaries found no differences in most measures of access to care between those insured through MA compared to TM. For example, there were no differences between the two groups with respect to their likelihood of receiving diabetes screening, hypertension screening, or flu vaccination.

The systems factors pose implications for quality of care. On one hand, most VBP models have neither substantially worsened nor improved quality of care. For example, Medicare population-based VBP models have not been associated with differences in quality of care or patient experience. Similarly, episode-based VBP models have not been associated with differences in measured quality outcomes for surgical procedures or common medical conditions.

On the other hand, VBP models are still poised to affect quality generally through an increased focus on patients' nonmedical needs and community supports. As this occurs, there is a potential for VBP to encompass and capture the benefits observed in community-based programs like those discussed in this chapter, such as improved blood pressure among individuals receiving education in barbershops, and reduced mental health symptoms among individuals experiencing serious mental illness who engage with a clubhouse model of community place–based resources. To the extent that VBP encourages organizations to emphasize community-based care and coordination with community-oriented organizations, such models are poised to affect health care quality.

Although not a VBP model per se, MA encompasses value-based incentives in a way that can impact quality of care. In particular, the ability to provide supplemental benefits that advance community-based care could lead to greater quality for insured individuals. Robust peer-reviewed literature detailing the impact of MA community-based supplemental benefits remains scant. Nonetheless, many MA beneficiaries are very satisfied overall with their insurance benefits. In a June 2022 survey, 88% of beneficiaries expressed satisfaction with their plan, 86% would recommend MA to a family member or friend, and only 6% were dissatisfied with their plan. In the same survey, 61% of respondents who previously had other forms of Medicare insurance said they were more satisfied with MA.

The systems factors also have implications for health care costs. In contrast to limited effects on quality, population- and episode-based VBP models have been demonstrated to achieve cost savings. For instance, studies of national Medicare episode-based VBP models have found that participation was associated with lower 90-day spending for both surgical and medical episodes. Large population-based VBP models have also yielded cost savings. MA plans can also have cost implications. In particular, some analyses have estimated that Medicare spends more per individual for those insured through MA, compared to what it spends per individual insured through TM.

Lastly, systems factors discussed in this chapter have important equity implications. Some factors can directly target disparities. CHWs, for example, have a rich history and ongoing track record of serving historically underserved populations. Due to their history of working to address health inequity and the evidence supporting their role in promoting quality of care, the Institute of Medicine specifically urged "programs to support the use of CHWs." Further, community-oriented organizations, and programs that seek to increase connection between traditional medical care and community-oriented organizations, can potentially affect health equity. For instance, programs such as the Accountable Health Communities Model can directly target health disparities by addressing nonmedical needs that drive them (eg, food insecurity, transportation barriers). Despite mixed overall results, Black individuals who receive care through the model were more likely to report using community resources and have their food needs addressed than Black individuals not receiving care under the model.

However, the broader movement to VBP has been accompanied by health equity concerns. Since they include clinician accountability to cost of care, VBP models could unintentionally discourage clinicians from caring for historically underserved groups that could have high overall health care spending, and for whom quality improvements and cost savings could be particularly difficult to achieve. Early physician participation in population-based VBP models was higher in high-income communities than in communities with a high percentage of the population identifying as Black, being uninsured, having lower overall education levels, or living with disabilities. In some recent primary care VBP models, very few participating groups were located in rural communities or areas with a high percentage of the population being low income or identifying as Hispanic.

Medicare has started to address these concerns through VBP models designed to address health disparities. For instance, launched in 2023, the ACO Realizing Equity, Access, and Community Health model required participating medical care organizations to establish plans for addressing health equity and collect data on nonmedical drivers of health. As another example, Medicare announced Making Care Primary in 2023, seeking to focus on health equity through the program via financial payments and incentives to improve community-based care (eg, quality measures related to screening and referral for nonmedical needs).

Multiple-Choice Questions

1. Dr Ali is a surgeon participating in a VBP model where she receives an episode-based payment for patients receiving coronary artery bypass graft. In the model, episode-based payments will increase if she performs in the 90th percentile on predefined quality measures. Under the structure-process-outcomes-utilization quality measure types, which of the following would be considered an outcomes quality measure?

   A. Percentage of patients prescribed a high-intensity statin medication

   B. Percentage of patients who visit an ER for any reason within 30 days of surgery

   C. Use of a certified electronic health record that patients can use to see their test results and ask questions

   D. Percentage of patients who experience an acute myocardial infarction within 3 months of surgery

2. Louise is a CHW. She works for an organization located in a local community and focused on supporting people in that community who are living with HIV. She has a list of long-term patients for whom she attends visits and facilitates connection to other community resources. Which approach for integration of CHW does this represent?

   A. Embed within community-oriented organizations

   B. Embed within medical care organizations

   C. Embed within government agencies

   D. Embed within payers

3. Bill, a 64-year-old man experiencing homelessness, is diagnosed with pneumonia and admitted to a hospital participating in the Accountable Health Communities Model as a bridge organization. While hospitalized, the patient is screened for health-related social needs, and identified needs include assistance with food and housing. The hospital makes referrals to community service providers and assigns a care navigator to the patient. The hospital does not provide feedback to community service providers to improve impact on or responsiveness to the patient's needs. Which of the Accountable Health Community interventions did the hospital implement?

   A. Awareness

   B. Assistance

   C. Alignment

   D. Awareness and assistance

4. Through 1115 waivers, state Medicaid programs can create new community-based care benefits if:

   A. Changes are budget neutral

   B. New benefits align with the overall mission of the Medicaid program

   C. New benefits last 3 years before they are reevaluated for continuation

   D. A and B

Answers

1. The correct answer is D. An acute myocardial infarction is a clinical outcome that could be related to the quality of a coronary artery bypass graft surgery.

2. The correct answer is A. The CHW is employed by a community-oriented organization that has informal relationships with medical care organizations.

3. The correct answer is D. The hospital acted to address awareness by screening the patient for health-related social needs, making referrals, and making the patient aware of those referrals. The hospital also provided assistance by providing the patient with navigation services.

4. The correct answer is D. The Medicaid 1115 waiver allows for broader changes and expanded benefits in a Medicaid program, so long as they are aligned with overall program mission and considered budget neutral. State Medicaid programs receive an initial 5-year authorization for a 1115 waiver and can be renewed for an additional 3 to 5 years.

Bibliography

AARP. Respite care: how to give yourself the caregiving break you need. Published September 22, 2010. Accessed December 18, 2023. https://www.aarp.org/caregiving/life-balance/info-2017/respite-care-plan.html

Agency for Healthcare Research and Quality. Identifying and addressing social needs in primary care. Accessed December 18, 2023. https://www.ahrq.gov/sites/default/files/wysiwyg/evidencenow/tools-and-materials/social-needs-tool.pdf

Agency for Healthcare Research and Quality. Six domains of healthcare quality. Accessed December 18, 2023. https://www.ahrq.gov/talkingquality/measures/six-domains.html

Aggarwal R, Gondi S, Wadhera RK. Comparison of Medicare advantage vs traditional Medicare for health care access, affordability, and use of preventive services among adults with low income. *JAMA Netw Open.* 2022;5(6):e2215227.

Alcoholics Anonymous. Find A.A. near you. Accessed December 18, 2023. https://www.aa.org/find-aa

Alzheimer's Association. Education Center. Accessed December 18, 2023. https://training.alz.org/?5=page/1/page-size/10

American Diabetes Association. Find a diabetes education program. Accessed December 18, 2023. https://diabetes.org/tools-support/diabetes-education-program

American Public Health Association. Support for community health workers to increase health access and to reduce inequities. Published November 10, 2009. Accessed December 18, 2023. https://www.apha.org/policies-and-advocacy/public-health-policy-statements/policy-database/2014/07/09/14/19/support-for-community-health-workers-to-increase-health-access-and-to-reduce-health-inequities

Arthritis Foundation. Benefits of exercise for osteoarthritis. Accessed December 18, 2023. https://www.arthritis.org/health-wellness/healthy-living/physical-activity/getting-started/benefits-of-exercise-for-osteoarthritis

Association of State and Territorial Health Officials. Ever-changing picture: state approaches to CHW certification. Updated May 2022. Accessed December 18, 2023. https://www.astho.org/topic/brief/state-approaches-to-community-health-worker-certification/

Asthma and Allergy Foundation of America. Asthma and allergy education programs. Accessed December 18, 2023. https://aafa.org/programs/education-programs/

ATI Advisory. A deep dive on in-home, caregiver, and social supports in Medicare advantage: can these benefits meaningfully meet member needs and support independence?

Published March 2023. Accessed December 18, 2023. https://www.ltqa.org/wp-content/themes/ltqaMain/custom/images/ATI-TSF_Report-032323.pdf

BBC. The many groups that have copied Alcoholics Anonymous. Published June 9, 2015. Accessed December 18 2023. https://www.bbc.com/news/magazine-33049093

Biniek JF, Cubanski J, Neuman T. Higher and faster growing spending per Medicare advantage enrollee adds to Medicare's solvency and affordability challenges. Kaiser Family Foundation. Published August 17, 2021. Accessed December 18, 2023. https://www.kff.org/medicare/issue-brief/higher-and-faster-growing-spending-per-medicare-advantage-enrollee-adds-to-medicares-solvency-and-affordability-challenges/

Biniek JF, Sroczynski N, Freed M, Neuman T. Extra benefits offered by Medicare advantage firms vary. Kaiser Family Foundation. Published November 16, 2022. Accessed December 18, 2023. https://www.kff.org/medicare/issue-brief/extra-benefits-offered-by-medicare-advantage-firms-varies/

Black Barbershop. About. The Black Barbershop Health Outreach Program. Accessed December 18, 2023. https://www.blackbarbershop.org/about

Blyler CA, Rader F. Sustainability of blood pressure reduction in black barbershops. *Curr Opin Cardiol*. 2019;34(6):693-699.

Cacal SL, Spock N, Quensell ML, Sentell TL, Stupplebeen DA. Legislative definitions of community health workers: examples from other states to inform Hawai'i. *Hawaii J Med Public Health*. 2019;78(6 suppl 1):23-29.

California Department of Health Care Services. California Advancing and Innovating Medi-Cal. Published December 2021. Accessed December 18, 2023. https://www.dhcs.ca.gov/CalAIM/Documents/CalAIM-Waiver-Announcement-Issue-Brief-a11y.pdf

California Department of Health Care Services. Medi-Cal Peer Support Services Specialist Program—frequently asked questions. Accessed December 18, 2023. https://www.dhcs.ca.gov/Pages/Medi-Cal-Peer-Support-Services-Specialist-Program-Frequently-Asked-Questions.aspx#:~:text=The%20law%20does%20not%20make,family%20member%20of%20the%20consumer.%22

Carter J, Hassan S, Walton A, Yu L, Donelan K, Thorndike AN. Effect of community health workers on 30-day hospital readmissions in an accountable care organization population: a randomized clinical trial. *JAMA Netw Open*. 2021;4(5):e2110936.

Cella D, Hahn EA, Jensen SE, et al. *Patient Reported Outcomes in Performance Measurement*. RTI Press; 2015.

Centers for Medicare and Medicaid Services. Comprehensive primary care plus 2018 payer and practice solicitation. Published December 15, 2016. https://www.cms.gov/newsroom/fact-sheets/comprehensive-primary-care-plus-cpc-2018-payer-and-practice-solicitation

Centers for Medicare and Medicaid Services. Implementing supplemental benefits for chronically ill enrollees. Published April 24, 2019. Accessed December 18, 2023. https://www.cms.gov/Medicare/Health-Plans/HealthPlansGenInfo/Downloads/Supplemental_Benefits_Chronically_Ill_HPMS_042419.pdf

Centers for Medicare and Medicaid Services. Kidney Care First and Comprehensive Kidney Care Contract models. Published July 10, 2019. https://www.cms.gov/newsroom/fact-sheets/kidney-care-first-kcf-and-comprehensive-kidney-care-contracting-ckcc-models

Centers for Medicare and Medicaid Services. 2021 national impact assessment of the Centers for Medicare & Medicaid Services quality measures report. Published June 2021. https://www.cms.gov/files/document/2021-national-impact-assessment-report.pdf

Centers for Medicare and Medicaid Services. 2023 MIPS improvement activities user guide. Published March 14, 2023. https://qpp.cms.gov/resources/document/b57b97f7-23d0-495a-a170-beaebbee37d5

Centers for Medicare and Medicaid Services. Medicare shared savings program saved more than $1.8 billion in 2022 and continues to deliver high-quality care. Published August 24, 2023. Accessed December 18, 2023. https://www.hhs.gov/about/news/2023/08/24/medicare-shared-savings-program-saves-medicare-more-1-8-billion-2022-continues-deliver-high-quality-care.html

Centers for Medicare and Medicaid Services. About section 1115 waivers. Accessed December 18, 2023. https://www.medicaid.gov/medicaid/section-1115-demonstrations/about-section-1115-demonstrations/index.html

Centers for Medicare and Medicaid Services. Accountable Health Communities model 2018-2021. Accessed December 18, 2023. https://innovation.cms.gov/data-and-reports/2023/ahc-second-eval-rpt-fg

Centers for Medicare and Medicaid Services. Accountable Health Communities model overview and track 1 requirements. Accessed December 18, 2023. https://innovation.cms.gov/files/slides/ahcm-track1overview-appreq.pdf

Centers for Medicare and Medicaid Services. Announcement of calendar year (CY) 2019 Medicare advantage capitation rates and Medicare advantage and part D payment policies and final call letter. Published April 2, 2018. Accessed December 18, 2023. https://www.cms.gov/MEDICARE/HEALTH-PLANS/MEDICAREADVTGSPECRATESTATS/DOWNLOADS/ANNOUNCEMENT2019.PDF

Centers for Medicare and Medicaid Services. Bundled payments for care improvement initiative: general information. Accessed December 18, 2023. https://www.cms.gov/priorities/innovation/innovation-models/Bundled-Payments

Centers for Medicare and Medicaid Services. Comprehensive primary care initiative: primary care practice solicitation. Accessed December 18, 2023. https://www.cms.gov/priorities/innovation/files/x/cpc_practicesolicitation.pdf

Centers for Medicare and Medicaid Services. Gym memberships and fitness programs. Accessed December 18, 2023. https://www.medicare.gov/coverage/gym-memberships-fitness-programs

Centers for Medicare and Medicaid Services. Home & Community-Based Services 1915 (c). Accessed December 18, 2023. https://www.medicaid.gov/medicaid/home-community-based-services/home-community-based-services-authorities/home-community-based-services-1915c/index.html

Centers for Medicare and Medicaid Services. Making care primary request for applications. Accessed December 18, 2023. https://www.cms.gov/files/document/mcp-rfa.pdf

Centers for Medicare and Medicaid Services. Measures management system. Accessed December 18, 2023. https://www.cms.gov/Medicare/Quality-Initiatives-Patient-Assessment-Instruments/MMS/Downloads/Structural-Measures.pdf

Centers for Medicare and Medicaid Services. Medicaid. Accessed December 18, 2023. https://www.medicaid.gov/medicaid/index.html

Centers for Medicare and Medicaid Services. Medicare shared savings program advance investment payments. Accessed December 18, 2023. https://www.cms.gov/files/document/mssp-aip-glance.pdf

Centers for Medicare and Medicaid Services. Primary care first request for applications cohort 2 version: 3. Last Modified April 12, 2023. https://www.cms.gov/priorities/innovation/media/document/pcf-cohort2-rfa

Centers for Medicare and Medicaid Services. Quality measure FAQs. Accessed December 18, 2023. https://mmshub.cms.gov/about-quality/new-to-measures/what-is-a-measure

Centers for Medicare and Medicaid Services. Quality measures. Accessed December 18, 2023. https://www.cms.gov/Medicare/Quality-Initiatives-Patient-Assessment-Instruments/QualityMeasures

Centers for Medicare and Medicaid Services. Shared savings program participation options for performance year 2024. Accessed December 18, 2023. https://www.cms.gov/Medicare/Medicare-Fee-for-Service-Payment/sharedsavingsprogram/Downloads/ssp-aco-participation-options.pdf

Centers for Medicare and Medicaid Services. The hospital value-based purchasing program. Accessed December 18, 2023. https://www.cms.gov/medicare/quality/value-based-programs/hospital-purchasing

Centers for Medicare and Medicaid Services Innovation Center. Oncology care model overview. Accessed December 18, 2023. https://www.cms.gov/priorities/innovation/files/slides/ocm-overview-slides.pdf

Cigna Healthcare. What is managed care? Accessed December 18, 2023. https://www.cigna.com/knowledge-center/what-is-managed-care

Cleveland Clinic. Caregiver burnout. Accessed December 18, 2023. https://my.clevelandclinic.org/health/diseases/9225-caregiver-burnout

Commonwealth Fund. Putting health coaches front and center: Q&A with Rushika Fernandopulle of Iora Health. Published December 17, 2014. https://www.commonwealthfund.org/publications/2015/dec/putting-health-coaches-front-and-center-qa-rushika-fernandopulle-iora-health

Congress.gov. H.R. 3590 Patient Protection and Affordable Care Act. 111th Congress of the United States. 2009-2010. Accessed November 1, 2023. https://www.congress.gov/bill/111th-congress/house-bill/3590/text

Crook HL, Saunders RS, Roiland R, Higgins A, McClellan MB. A decade of value-based payment: lessons learned and implications for the Center for Medicare and Medicaid Innovation, part 1. *Health Affairs Blog*. 2021. https://www.healthaffairs.org/do/10.1377/forefront.20210607.656313/

Cunningham SD, Sutherland RA, Yee CW, et al. Group medical care: a systematic review of health service performance. *Int J Environ Res Public Health*. 2021;18(23):12726.

Dale SB, Ghosh A, Peikes DN, et al. Two-year costs and quality in the comprehensive primary care initiative. *N Engl J Med*. 2016;374:2345-2356.

Damberg CL, Sorbero ME, Lovejoy SL, Martsolf GR, Raaen L, Mandel D. Measuring success in health care value-based purchasing programs: findings from an environmental scan, literature review, and expert panel discussions. *Rand Health Q*. 2014;4(3):9.

Donabedian A. Evaluating the quality of medical care. 1966. *Milbank Q*. 2005;83(4):691-729.

Draper Richards Kaplan. City Health Works. Accessed December 18, 2023. https://www.drkfoundation.org/organization/city-health-works/

Dummit LA, Kahvecioglu D, Marrufo G, et al. Association between hospital participation in a Medicare bundled payment initiative and payments and quality outcomes for lower extremity joint replacement episodes. *JAMA*. 2016;316:1267-1278.

eHealth. Spotlight on Medicare advantage: an eHealth survey. Published June 2022. Accessed December 18, 2023. https://news.ehealthinsurance.com/_ir/68/20225/Spotlight_On_Medicare_Advantage_eHealth_Survey_June2022.pdf

Findhelp. Find help. Accessed December 18, 2023. https://www.findhelp.org/

Fountain House. Our services. Accessed December 18, 2023. https://www.fountainhouse.org/services

George R, Gunn R, Wiggins N, et al. Early lessons and strategies from statewide efforts to integrate community health workers into Medicaid. *J Health Care Poor Underserved.* 2020;31(2):845-858.

Haldar S, Hinton E. State policies for expanding Medicaid coverage of community health worker services. Kaiser Family Foundation. Published January 23, 2023. https://www.kff.org/medicaid/issue-brief/state-policies-for-expanding-medicaid-coverage-of-community-health-worker-chw-services/

Halpern DJ, Clark-Randall A, Woodall J, Anderson J, Shah K. Reducing imaging utilization in primary care through implementation of a peer comparison dashboard. *J Gen Intern Med.* 2021;36(1):108-113.

Health Care Payment Learning and Action Network. Measuring progress: adoption of alternative payment models in commercial, Medicare advantage, and state Medicaid programs. 2016. https://hcp-lan.org/workproducts/apm-measurement-final.pdf

Health Care Payment Learning and Action Network. APM measurement progress of alternative payment models: 2022 methodology and results report. 2022. http://hcp-lan.org/workproducts/apm-methodology-2022.pdf

Health Resources and Services Administration. Community Health Worker National Workforce Study. Published March 2007. Accessed December 18, 2023. https://bhw.hrsa.gov/sites/default/files/bureau-health-workforce/data-research/community-health-workforce.pdf

Healthinsurance.org. What is an indemnity health plan? Accessed December 18, 2023. https://www.healthinsurance.org/glossary/indemnity-health-plan/

Hinton E. A look at recent Medicaid guidance to address social determinants of health and health-related social needs. *Kaiser Family Foundation.* Published February 22, 2023. Accessed December 18, 2023. https://www.kff.org/policy-watch/a-look-at-recent-medicaid-guidance-to-address-social-determinants-of-health-and-health-related-social-needs

Horstman C, Lewis C. Engaging primary care in value-based payment: new findings from the 2022 Commonwealth Fund survey of primary care physicians. *Commonwealth Fund.* Published April 13, 2023. https://www.commonwealthfund.org/blog/2023/engaging-primary-care-value-based-payment-new-findings-2022-commonwealth-fund-survey#

Hughes DL. CMS innovation center launches new initiative to advance health equity. *Health Affairs Forefront.* 2022. https://www.healthaffairs.org/content/forefront/cms-innovation-center-launches-new-initiative-advance-health-equity

Ingram M, Reinschmidt KM, Schachter KA, et al. Establishing a professional profile of community health workers: results from a national study of roles, activities and training. *J Community Health.* 2012;37(2):529-537.

Institute of Medicine. *Crossing the Quality Chasm: A New Health System for the 21st Century.* National Academy Press; 2001.

Islam N, Nadkarni SK, Zahn D, Skillman M, Kwon SC, Trinh-Shevrin C. Integrating community health workers within Patient Protection and Affordable Care Act implementation. *J Public Health Manag Pract.* 2015;21(1):42-50.

James PA, Oparil S, Carter BL, et al. 2014 evidence-based guideline for the management of high blood pressure in adults: report from the panel members appointed to the eighth Joint National Committee (JNC 8). *JAMA*. 2014;311(5):507-520.

Joynt Maddox KE, Orav JE, Zheng J, Epstein AM. Evaluation of Medicare's bundled payments initiative for medical conditions. *N Engl J Med*. 2018;379:260-269.

Kaiser Family Foundation. Medicaid waiver tracker: approved and pending section 1115 waivers by state. Published December 14, 2023. Accessed December 18, 2023. https://www.kff.org/medicaid/issue-brief/medicaid-waiver-tracker-approved-and-pending-section-1115-waivers-by-state/

Knowles M, Crowley AP, Vasan A, Kangovi S. Community Health worker integration with and effectiveness in health care and public health in the United States. *Annu Rev Public Health*. 2023;44:363-381.

Kornfield T, Kazan M, Frieder M, Duddy-Tenbrunsel R, Donthi S, Fix A. Medicare advantage plans offering expanded supplemental benefits: a look at availability and enrollment. Commonwealth Fund. Published February 10, 2021. Accessed from December 18, 2023. https://www.commonwealthfund.org/publications/issue-briefs/2021/feb/medicare-advantage-plans-supplemental-benefits#4

L&M Policy Research. Evaluation of CMMI accountable care organization initiatives Advanced Payment ACO final report. Published November 25, 2016. Available from: https://innovation.cms.gov/files/reports/advpayaco-fnevalrpt.pdf

Liao JM, Navathe AS. What comes next in prioritizing equity in payment? The ACO REACH Model. *Health Affairs Forefront*. 2022. https://www.healthaffairs.org/content/forefront/comes-next-prioritizing-equity-payment-aco-reach-model

Liao JM, Navathe AS. Using advanced payments in population-based models to address equity. *Health Affairs Forefront*. 2023. https://www.healthaffairs.org/content/forefront/using-advanced-payments-population-based-models-address-equity

Liao JM, Huang Q, Wang E, et al. Performance of physician groups and hospitals participating in bundled payments among Medicare beneficiaries. *JAMA Health Forum*. 2022;3(12):e224889.

Liao JM, Navathe AS, Werner RM. The impact of Medicare's alternative payment models on the value of care. *Annu Rev Public Health*. 2020;41:551-565.

Malcarney MB, Pittman P, Quigley L, Horton K, Seiler N. The changing roles of community health workers. *Health Serv Res*. 2017;52(suppl 1):360-382.

Matiz LA, Peretz PJ, Jacotin PG, Cruz C, Ramirez-Diaz E, Nieto AR. The impact of integrating community health workers into the patient-centered medical home. *J Prim Care Community Health*. 2014;5(4):271-274.

Maung TZ, Bishop JE, Holt E, Turner AM, Pfrang C. Indoor air pollution and the health of vulnerable groups: a systematic review focused on particulate matter (PM), volatile organic compounds (VOCs) and their effects on children and people with pre-existing lung disease. *Int J Environ Res Public Health*. 2022;19(14):8752.

McCarthy-Alfano M. Care management for Medicaid patients. Penn Leonard Davis Institute. Published August 27, 2020. Accessed December 18, 2023. https://ldi.upenn.edu/our-work/research-updates/care-management-for-medicaid-patients/

Mistry SK, Harris E, Harris M. Community health workers as healthcare navigators in primary care chronic disease management: a systematic review. *J Gen Intern Med*. 2021;36:2755-2771.

MoCA Cognition. Montreal cognitive assessment. Accessed December 18, 2023. https://mocacognition.com/

Mutschler C, Junaid S, McShane K; Canadian Clubhouse Research Group. Clubhouses response to COVID-19: member challenges and clubhouse adaptations. *Community Ment Health J.* 2021;57(3):424-437.

Narcotics Anonymous World Services. Welcome to www.na.org. Accessed December 18, 2023. https://na.org/

National Academy for State Health Policy. State community health worker models. Accessed December 18, 2023. https://nashp.org/state-community-health-worker-models/

National Alliance to End Homelessness. State of homelessness: 2023 edition. Accessed December 18, 2023. https://endhomelessness.org/homelessness-in-america/homelessness-statistics/state-of-homelessness/

National Association of Community Health Workers. Community health worker: advancing diversity in community health. https://nachw.org/wp-content/uploads/2022/08/chw_diversity_2.pdf

Navathe AS, Liao JM. Aligning value-based payments with health equity: a framework for reforming payment reforms. *JAMA.* 2022;328(10):925-926.

NC Department of Health and Human Services. NC Medicaid managed care healthy opportunities pilot fee schedule and service definitions. Published March 2023. Accessed December 18, 2023. https://www.ncdhhs.gov/healthy-opportunities-pilot-fee-schedule-and-service-definitions/open

New Jersey Department of Health. Family Health Services. Accessed December 18, 2023. https://www.nj.gov/health/fhs/clgi/training/

Ogunniyi M, Commodore-Mensah Y, Ferdinand K, et al. Race, ethnicity, hypertension, and heart disease. *J Am Coll Cardiol.* 2021;78(24):2460-2470.

Paying For Senior Care. Washington COPES Medicaid Waiver Program. Published February 24, 2023. Accessed December 18, 2023. https://www.payingforseniorcare.com/washington/medicaid-waivers/copes-waiver

Perry HB, Zullinger R, Rogers MM. Community health workers in low-, middle-, and high-income countries: an overview of their history, recent evolution, and current effectiveness. *Annu Rev Public Health.* 2014;35:399-421.

Porter ME. A strategy for health care reform—toward a value-based system. *N Engl J Med.* 2009;361(2):109-112.

Ramchand R, Ahluwalia SC, Xenakis L, Apaydin E, Raaen L, Grimm G. A systematic review of peer-supported interventions for health promotion and disease prevention. *Prev Med.* 2017;101:156-170.

Rosenthal L. The Community Health Worker Core Consensus (C3) a report of the C3 project: phase 1 and 2. Texas Tech University Health Sciences Center El Paso. Published December 2018. Accessed December 18, 2023. https://www.c3project.org/_files/ugd/7ec423_2b0893bcc93a422396c744be8c1d54d1.pdf

RTI International. Accountable Health Communities model evaluation second evaluation report. Published May 2023. Accessed December 18, 2023. https://www.cms.gov/priorities/innovation/data-and-reports/2023/ahc-second-eval-rpt

Rural Health Information Hub. Accountable Health Communities model. Accessed December 18, 2023. https://www.ruralhealthinfo.org/new-approaches#:~:text=Accountable%20Health%20Communities%20Model,costs%20and%20reduce%20healthcare%20utilization

Seattle Clubhouse: A Program of Hero House NW. A bit about us. Accessed December 18, 2023. seattleclubhouse.org/about

Singh P, Chokshi DA. Community health workers—a local solution to a global problem. *N Engl J Med*. 2013;369(10):894-896.

Smedley BD, Stith AY, Nelson AR, eds. *Unequal Treatment: Confronting Racial and Ethnic Disparities in Health Care*. Institute of Medicine; 2002:17-18.

Sound Generations. Transportation. Accessed December 18, 2023. https://soundgenerations. org/our-programs/transportation/

Staloff J, Morenz AM. Making equity primary in the making care primary model. *Health Affairs Forefront*. 2023. https://www.healthaffairs.org/content/forefront/making-equity-primary-making-care-primary-model

Staloff J, Diop M, Matuk R, Riese A, White J. Caring for caregivers: burnout and resources for caregivers in Rhode Island. *R I Med J (2013)*. 2018;101(9):10-11.

Substance Abuse and Mental Health Services Administration. Peer support. Accessed December 18, 2023. https://www.samhsa.gov/sites/default/files/programs_campaigns/brss_ tacs/peer-support-2017.pdf

The Salvation Army. The Salvation Army domestic violence programs in Seattle. Accessed December 18, 2023. https://seattle.salvationarmy.org/seattle_services/domestic-violence-programs-and-shelters/

US Bureau of Labor Statistics. Implementing the 2010 Standard Occupational Classification in the Occupational Employment Statistics. Published May 2013. Accessed December 18, 2023. https://www.bls.gov/opub/mlr/2013/article/implementing-the-2010-standard-occupational-classification-in-the-occupational-employment-statistics-program.htm

US Bureau of Labor Statistics. Community health workers. Accessed December 18, 2023. https://www.bls.gov/ooh/community-and-social-service/community-health-workers.htm

US Department of Health and Human Services. Social determinants of health. Accessed December 18, 2023. https://health.gov/healthypeople/priority-areas/social-determinants-health

Valeriani G, Sarajlic Vukovic I, Bersani FS, Sadeghzadeh Diman A, Ghorbani A, Mollica R. Tackling ethnic health disparities through community health worker programs: a scoping review on their utilization during the COVID-19 outbreak. *Popul Health Manag*. 2022;25:517-526.

Victor RG, Lynch K, Li N, et al. A cluster-randomized trial of blood-pressure reduction in Black Barbershops. *N Engl J Med*. 2018;378(14):1291-1301.

Washington State Department of Social and Health Services. Agencies that help. Accessed December 18, 2023. https://www.dshs.wa.gov/altsa/home-and-community-services/agencies-help#FCSP

Washington State Department of Social and Health Services. Becoming a paid caregiver. Accessed December 18, 2023. https://www.dshs.wa.gov/altsa/home-and-community-services/becoming-paid-caregiver

Yasaitis LC, Pajerowski W, Polsky D, Werner RM. Physicians' participation in ACOs is lower in places with vulnerable populations than in more affluent communities. *Health Aff (Millwood)*. 2016;35(8):1382-1390.

Young Men Christian's Association. Aqua fitness. Accessed December 18, 2023. https://www .seattleymca.org/programs/fitness/water-fitness/water-fitness/aqua-fitness

Young Men Christian's Association. Tai Chi. Accessed December 18, 2023. https://www .ymca.org/what-we-do/healthy-living/fitness/older-adults

Part II

Solutions to Change Health Care

9

Approaching the Problem

Clinical Case

Dr Jackson reviews utilization data for her patient panel and notices that one of her new patients, Jessica, has had three total recent visits to the emergency room and urgent care. After reviewing Jessica's medical record, Dr Jackson concludes that some of those visits could have potentially been prevented if Jessica had received care in the clinic. While Dr Jackson recognizes potentially preventable emergency room and urgent care visits as a problem requiring action, she is unsure how to approach the problem.

This situation, where a clinician recognizes a potential problem in their practice, is common. While it may be tempting to immediately begin problem-solving or implementing solutions, clinicians and their teams should instead systematically approach the problem. While they can do so in a number of ways, four approaches—Lean, Six Sigma, Kotter's Eight-Step Change Model, and Design Thinking—have been used widely in health care and represent health systems solutions with the potential to improve patient care.

SYSTEMS SOLUTION: LEAN

As a precursor to Lean, the Toyota Production System (TPS) was developed throughout the 1950s to 1960s to provide best quality products or services at the lowest cost and shortest lead time through the elimination of waste. TPS was founded on two pillars, just-in-time and Jidoka—a production system that only made products based on demand and a process in which any worker who spots a problem in a process had the authority to stop the production, respectively.

In 1990, recognition of TPS as the model production system grew rapidly with the publication of *The Machine That Changed the World*. A new paradigm at the time, TPS later evolved into Lean production. The Lean concept focuses on waste reduction in a number of areas, as originally defined by Taii-chi Ohno, the chief engineer at Toyota:

■ Waste of overproduction (considered the largest waste)
■ Waste of waiting
■ Waste of transportation
■ Waste of overprocessing
■ Waste of inventory
■ Waste of motion
■ Waste of defect

Although not originally included in the TPS, waste of talent was later added as a focus area to Lean production.

Principles Used in Lean

Lean incorporates five principles: value, value stream, flow, pull, and perfection. They can be summarized as follows:

Value. Value is defined as what the customer is willing to pay for. Teams should have a firm understanding of the customers' expectations with respect to a product or service. Through interviews, surveys, and demographic information, teams can discover what customers want in a product or service, how they want it to be delivered, and how much they can afford to pay for it.

Value stream. Using customer value as the reference point, teams should undergo a process to identify all steps and components that contribute toward increasing value—collectively known as mapping the value stream. Any steps and components outside of the value stream, which by definition do not add value, can be target areas for waste reduction. Waste can be categorized into two general types: no value added but necessary and no value added and unnecessary. The first type of waste should be minimized, while the second type should be eliminated.

Flow. After removing waste from the value stream, teams should ensure that the remaining steps and components run smoothly. Teams can aim to reconfigure production steps and level out the workload to minimize interruptions, delays, or bottlenecks.

Pull. Teams should reduce waste via actions to create products or deliver services based on customer demand. This goal is supported by systems in which production or processes are "pulled" by demand. Pull systems can reduce waste when compared to "push" systems that deliver services or create products partially or wholly uncoupled from demand. Establishing a pull system enables manufacturing that occurs just-in-time, where products and services are created at the appropriate time and in needed quantities.

Perfection. Teams should repeat the first four steps (value, value stream, flow, and pull) iteratively toward an aspirational state of perfection that is defined by perfect value creation and no waste.

Concepts and Tools Used in Lean

- *Value stream mapping:* A tool for teams to identify all steps and components that contribute toward value offered by a product or service
- *Plan-Do-Study-Act (PDSA) cycle:* A tool that teams can use for the iterative development of a process, product, or service
- *Single-minute exchange or die:* A concept that teams can use to reduce changeover time—the time required to replace a piece of malfunctioning manufacturing equipment
- *The 5 S's (sort, set in order, shine, standardize, and sustain):* A tool for teams to address physical space and create a well-organized and orderly workplace
- *Kaizen:* A concept of continuous improvement based on the belief that team members' commitment and constant pursuit of excellence have a greater impact on a team's development than significant but sporadic improvements
- *Error proofing (also referred to as poka-yoke):* A tool that helps teams avoid mistakes by preventing, correcting, or drawing attention to human errors as they occur
- *Gemba walk:* A tool that refers to teams walking through the workplace, observing processes, and engaging with employees to gain insights for improvements
- *Root cause analysis*: A concept for teams to identify the underlying reason for a problem; there are several tools that can support root cause analysis, including using the Five Whys and Ishikawa diagrams.
- *Five Whys:* A tool for teams to ask repeatedly (usually at least 5 times) "why" a problem occurs in order to uncover the root causes
- *Ishikawa diagram (also referred to as the fishbone or the cause-and-effect diagram):* A tool that aims to identify all potential underlying primary and other causes of a problem
- *Andon cord:* A tool that reflects the principles of Jidoka and consists of the ability for any team member of the production process to "pull the cord" to stop production and correct the problem

Applying Lean: Hospital Lean Production System

In 2002, Virginia Mason Hospital created the Virginia Mason Production System (VMPS) as an institutional approach for focusing on high quality, zero defects, exceptional service, innovation, and respect for patients. The VMPS was built on the belief that by eliminating waste, Virginia Mason Hospital could improve quality and safety and reduce costs for patients.

VMPS embodies a number of principles, concepts, and tools used in Lean. VMPS defines value and maps the value stream to patients using the motto that the patient is always first. VMPS also seeks to empower all clinicians and staff to "stop the line" (ie, pull the Andon cord) in order to address any problems that may put patients at risk.

VMPS has used PDSA cycles to drive change in a number of areas, including better early identification and treatment of patients with sepsis via a nurse-driven protocol. The protocol has been used to promote timely administration of evidence-based sepsis therapies within an hour of identifying patients with sepsis, a period of time termed "Sepsis Power Hour." In 2017, the Sepsis Power Hour protocol was associated with a 54% reduction in the time to completion of sepsis therapies and a 45% reduction in sepsis mortality rates.

SYSTEMS SOLUTION: SIX SIGMA

Six Sigma was developed under the leadership of Bob Galvin and Bill Smith at Motorola in the late 1980s as a method for managing quality. Motorola began to use statistical approaches to reduce process variation, limit defects, and ensure that products or services only went into design when certain specifications were met. Motorola coined the term Six Sigma to mean that if a product operates within six sigmas or standard deviations to the mean, the defect rate is nearly zero and represents a very high proportion of products or services within certain specifications (Figure 9.1).

In 1988, Motorola was recognized with the Malcolm Baldrige National Quality Award for its achievement in quality improvement and in turn many

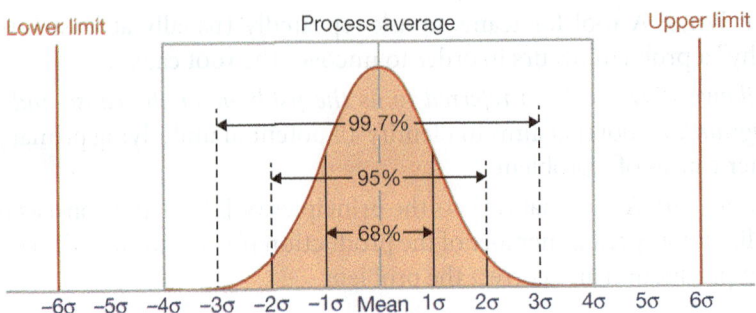

Figure 9.1 Six Sigma Quality. (Source: Reproduced with permission from John Clarkson, University of Cambridge. Improving improvement. https://www.iitoolkit .com/improvement/sigma.html)

organizations began to adopt the Six Sigma approach. By the late 1990s, companies such as General Electric, Samsung, Ford, Microsoft, and Amazon had begun to use Six Sigma to improve their products and services.

Principles Used in Six Sigma

Six Sigma involves a number of principles, which can be summarized as follows:

Focus on the customers. Teams should aim to maximize benefits for customers. By keeping the customers' benefits at the forefront, teams can ensure that their strategy is designed to meet the customers' needs.

Identify the root cause. Teams should outline all the steps and components of a process to identify potential root causes to a problem.

Reduce variation. After identifying root causes, teams should eliminate any steps or components that will cause variation in product or service development, predicated on the idea that eliminating variation will reduce defects.

Involve stakeholders. Teams should collaborate with all stakeholders to find solutions to complex issues. Such efforts should involve diverse stakeholders for a product or service, such as those from management, engineering, and sales.

Create a flexible system. Teams should be flexible and adapt processes as needed. The process required for change should not be so complex that team members would rather work within a broken process than fix it.

Concepts and Tools Used in Six Sigma

- *Defects per million opportunities (DPMO):* A tool that teams can use to measure chances of defects and track process performance for a product or service
- *Pareto chart:* A tool that teams can use to identify areas of priority for improvement; a Pareto chart is based on "80/20 rule" that states that approximately 80% of problems are the result of 20% of causes.
- *Control chart:* A tool to display characteristic measures (eg, weight, length, temperature) and their variation over time
- *Define, measure, analyze, improve, control (DMAIC):* A concept that teams can use to focus on incrementally improving an existing process, product, or service through defect reduction
- *Define, measure, analyze, design, verify (DMADV):* A concept that teams can use for the development of a new process, product, or service

- *Problem statement:* A tool for teams to define and address the problem at hand; the problem statement identifies the gap between identified problems and goals.

The Six Sigma and Lean approaches also share a number of concepts and tools:

- *Value stream mapping:* A tool for teams to identify all steps and components that contribute toward value offered by a product or service
- *PDSA cycle:* A tool that teams can use for the iterative development of a process, product, or service
- *Root cause analysis:* A concept for teams to identify the underlying reason for a problem; there are several tools that can support root cause analysis, including using the Five Whys and Ishikawa diagrams.
- *Five Whys:* A tool for teams to ask repeatedly (usually at least 5 times) "why" a problem occurs in order to uncover the root causes
- *Ishikawa diagram (also referred to as the fishbone or the cause-and-effect diagram):* A tool that aims to identify all potential underlying primary and other causes of a problem

Applying Six Sigma: Operating Room Turnaround

A hospital used the Six Sigma approach to reduce variation in turnaround time between surgical cases and increase operating room capacity. The hospital used the DPMO tool to measure operating room "defects" (in this case, delays in turnaround time) and record DPMO for three operating room categories: time to "patient out to patient in," time to "patient in to surgeon in," and time to "surgeon out to surgeon in."

Using the DMAIC concept, the hospital found that the defects in turnaround time were largely from variations in nurse/anesthesia communication, patient preparation process, and surgeon availability. Using control charts, the hospital was able to track the following measures over time:

- A 15% improvement in average operating room turnaround time
- A 32% improvement in DPMO
- Increased operating room capacity, translating into the potential for 1106 additional cases per year
- Potential annual benefit of $1 355 282 in revenue from additional cases

Integration of Lean and Six Sigma

During the early 2000s, a trend emerged to combine Lean, which focuses on waste reduction and high process efficiency, and Six Sigma, which focuses on defect reduction and low process variation, into a "Lean Six Sigma" approach. A number of organizations have adopted this integrated approach—which leverages the fact that Lean and Six Sigma can share certain concepts and tools—in their improvement efforts.

SYSTEMS SOLUTION: KOTTER'S EIGHT-STEP CHANGE MODEL

Kotter's Eight-Step Change Model is heavily influenced by Lewin's Three-Step Model of Change, the first notable approach in the field of change management—which focuses on the process of successfully guiding an organization to make lasting change. Kurt Lewin, a psychologist considered by many to be the father of change management, first described his Model in the 1940s after decades of research on individual-level change and group dynamics. Lewin's research found several key lessons that informed his model and subsequently Kotter's Eight-Step Change Model.

The first lesson was that change cannot be successful unless one considers the personalities of individuals in the group, the structure of the group, and the group's ideology and culture. The second lesson was that all members of a group need to be active participants in decisions related to a change for it to be effective. The third lesson was that groups often have relatively stable dynamics or productivity, which in turn may create a particular frozenness or resistance to change. Lewin used these three lessons to design his Three-Step Model of Change, which can be summarized as follows (Figure 9.2):

Unfreeze. This step acknowledges that initial effort is needed to overcome an organization's initial frozenness or resistance to change and create motivation to engage in change. Lewin believed that unfreezing—considered by some to be the most important step of the model—could be accomplished by directing behavior away from the equilibrium, removing forces that oppose change, or both.

Change. Sometimes called the movement step, this step involves actual change making. Work in this step focuses on altering an organization's structures, systems, processes, and behaviors to align with the intended change.

Refreeze. This step recognizes that once a change has been made, efforts should be made to ensure that the change endures (or "refreezes") so that the organization does not regress to its prior state, which would render the change process irrelevant.

While several change management models emerged in the decades after Lewin's Three-Step Model of Change, Kotter's Eight-Step Change Model has become one of the most prominent and studied in health care contexts.

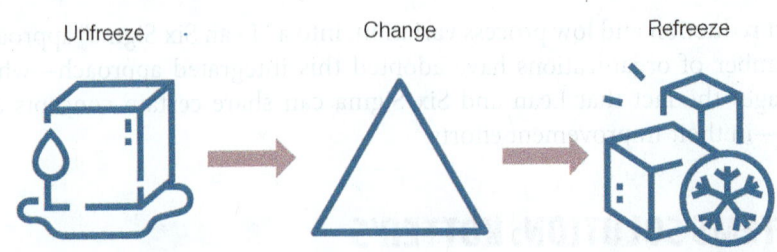

Unfreeze   Change   Refreeze

Figure 9.2 Lewin's Three-Step Model of Change.

A professor at Harvard Business School, John Kotter first described concepts underlying his Eight-Step Change Model in an article entitled "Leading Change: Why Transformation Efforts Fail" as well as in a subsequent book *Leading Change*. In his article, Kotter explained that over the course of 10 years, he observed more than 100 companies attempt to make transformational changes in how business was conducted to cope with new, more challenging market environments. He observed that some were successful at making an organization-wide change, but most were not.

In his study of the successful organizations, Kotter observed that change required a series of overlapping steps requiring a significant amount of time, and that skipping steps resulted in the illusion of a speedy change without yielding lasting results. In addition, Kotter noted that critical errors made in any of the steps usually had a devastating impact on the change effort, either by significantly slowing progress or damaging previous progress.

These observations informed a set of eight errors that Kotter believed organizations made when attempting transformational change. In turn, he identified eight corresponding steps that organizations could take to position themselves to successfully make transformational change (Figure 9.3).

The first phase of the Kotter's Eight-Step Change Model, collectively referred to as "creating a climate for change," involves three steps that can be summarized as follows:

Step one: Establishing a sense of urgency. This step acknowledges that successful change requires the active participation of people throughout an organization. Organizations and leaders desiring transformational change first need to create a sense of urgency to inspire people's intrinsic motivation to participate in change. Failure to achieve this step—or not establishing a great enough sense of urgency—could make getting any change off the ground unlikely.

Step two: Creating a powerful guiding coalition. In this step, Kotter acknowledged that while transformational change efforts may start with just one or two people, a critical mass of people who buy into the notion of change is needed for any change efforts to move forward. Failure to achieve this step—or not creating a powerful enough guiding coalition—might not

Eight Errors

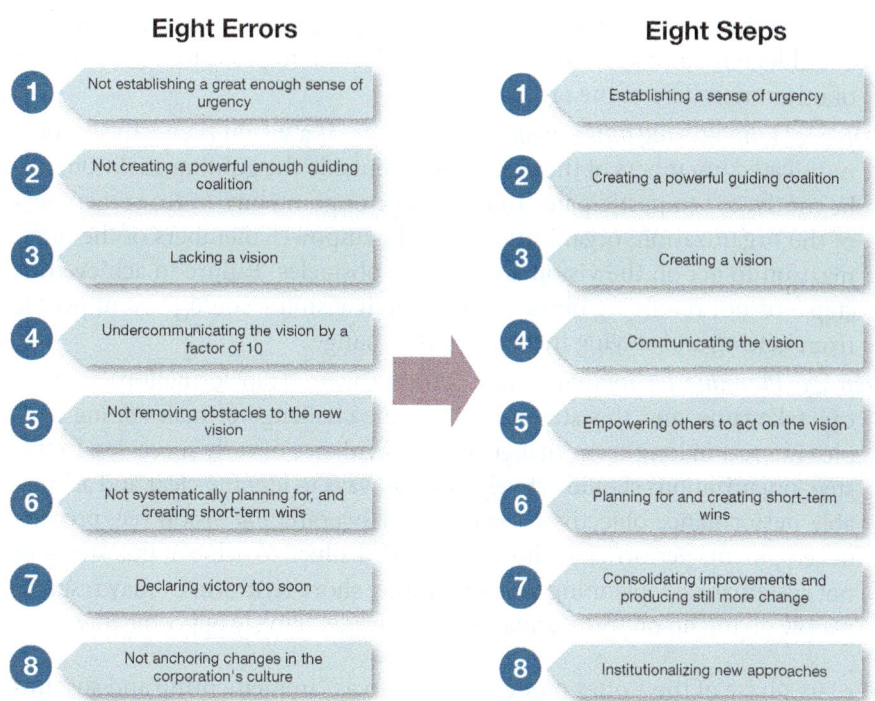

1	Not establishing a great enough sense of urgency
2	Not creating a powerful enough guiding coalition
3	Lacking a vision
4	Undercommunicating the vision by a factor of 10
5	Not removing obstacles to the new vision
6	Not systematically planning for, and creating short-term wins
7	Declaring victory too soon
8	Not anchoring changes in the corporation's culture

Eight Steps

1	Establishing a sense of urgency
2	Creating a powerful guiding coalition
3	Creating a vision
4	Communicating the vision
5	Empowering others to act on the vision
6	Planning for and creating short-term wins
7	Consolidating improvements and producing still more change
8	Institutionalizing new approaches

Figure 9.3 Kotter's Eight Errors and Corresponding Eight-Step Change Model. (Source: Data from Kotter JP. Leading change: why transformation efforts fail. *Harvard Business Review*. Published May-June 1995. https://hbr.org/1995/05/leading-change-why-transformation-efforts-fail-2)

hinder an organization's ability to make initial change. However, it could make overcoming any inevitable opposition to change more challenging.

Step three: Creating a vision. Once built, the guiding coalition must develop a vision of what the future would be like once transformational change is implemented and the overall direction in which the organization should move. Failure to achieve this step—or lacking a vision—could result in a transformational change effort devolving into disparate projects without a clear direction, projects heading in a different direction than originally intended, or members of the organization becoming confused and uninspired.

The second phase of the Kotter's Eight-Step Change Model, referred to as "engaging and enabling the whole organization," can be summarized in the form of three steps:

Step four: Communicating the vision. Once a vision is created, the next step is appropriate quantity and quality communication of that vision. Failure to achieve this step—or undercommunicating the vision by a factor of 10—could lead to an organizational change effort failing to capture the buy-in of other members of the organization.

Step five: Empowering others to act on the vision. If a vision is effectively communicated, members of the organization outside the guiding coalition may be motivated to participate. To encourage ongoing buy-in from members of the organization, organizations should empower members of the organization to act on the vision and remove obstacles. Failure to achieve this step—or not removing obstacles to the new vision—could prevent people from getting and staying involved in the change.

Step six: Planning for and creating short-term wins. Transformational change can take time, and this step recognizes the challenge of maintaining people's interest in long-term change without evidence of early successes. In this step, organizations should actively look for ways to identify clear and achievable performance objectives related to the overarching vision (eg, product development, performance improvement). Failure to achieve this step—or not systematically planning for and creating short-term wins—may result in people giving up on transformational change or actively opposing it.

The last phase of the Kotter model, referred to as "implementing and sustaining change," includes these final two steps:

Step seven: Consolidating improvements and producing still more change. This step acknowledges that in some cases, organizations may be inclined to claim success for the whole vision after achieving just a first small win. Instead of indulging this inclination, organizations should build on the credibility gained by a short-term win to focus on addressing an even bigger challenge related to the overall vision. Failure to achieve this step—or declaring victory too soon—could result in the progress of a short-term win fizzling out or lead to change opponents claiming that the change cycle is over.

Step eight: Institutionalizing new approaches. This step focuses on engraining transformational change in the overall organizational structure. Failure to achieve this step—or not anchoring changes in the corporation's culture—can result in the breakdown of some or all the progress made by the change efforts.

Since its introduction, Kotter's Eight-Step Change Model has been utilized by numerous organizations aiming to make transformational change. Indeed, the model and other change management principles described by Kotter have been used domestically and internationally across sectors (eg, government, private corporations) and industries (eg, energy, health care, manufacturing, education).

SYSTEMS SOLUTION: DESIGN THINKING

Design Thinking became mainstream during the 1980s and 1990s. In 1988, Don Norman wrote the book *The Design of Everyday Things* and explained how human-centered design methods, broadly referred to as Design Thinking, could improve products and services. He described Design Thinking as "an approach that puts human needs, capabilities, and behaviors first, then designs to accommodate those needs, capabilities, and ways of behaving."

As a design and innovation company founded in the 1990s, IDEO was one of the first organizations to apply and practice Design Thinking on a large scale. In particular, the company introduced customer friendly terminology, steps, and toolkits to make Design Thinking methodologies more accessible to customers.

In 2004, Stanford University established the Hasso Plattner Institute of Design to focus on Design Thinking development, education, and implementation. The Institute incorporated fields of business, law, medicine, social sciences, humanities, engineering, and product design into its curriculum. Through IDEO and the Hasso Plattner Institute of Design, Design Thinking began to gain momentum and spread across companies such as Google, Apple, and General Electric.

Principles Used in Design Thinking

IDEO encourages teams to start with the lens of what is desirable from a user point of view followed by what is technologically feasible and financially viable. IDEO's three lenses of Design Thinking can be summarized as follows (Figure 9.4):

Desirability. Teams start by looking at the needs and behaviors of the end users. Teams listen with empathy to understand what the end users desire. Teams then brainstorm interventions to satisfy needs from the end user's point of view.

Feasibility. Having identified potential interventions, teams determine whether implementation is feasible. Given finite resources and time constraints, teams evaluate if potential interventions are worth pursuing. Such considerations may require teams to iterate on interventions to make them more technologically feasible.

Viability. Interventions must be financially practical. Using Design Thinking, teams consider viability after desirability and feasibility.

Concepts and Tools Used in Design Thinking

- Journey map: A tool that teams can use to visually showcase the series of actions, mindsets, and emotions of users to accomplish a goal

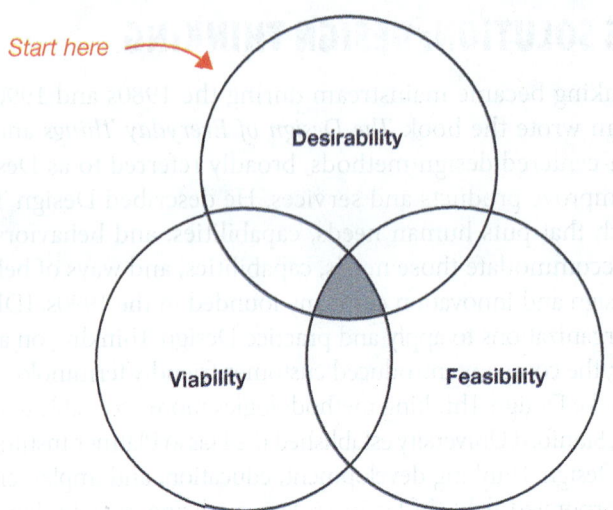

Figure 9.4   IDEO's Three Lenses of Design Thinking. (Source: Reproduced with permission from IDEO U. What is design thinking? Accessed April 29, 2024. https://www.ideou.com/blogs/inspiration/what-is-design-thinking/)

- Persona: A tool that teams can use to create fictional characters to represent different users of a product or service
- Affinity diagram (also known as an affinity map or affinity chart): A tool that helps teams organize a large amount of information into themes, according to the affinity or similarity between different pieces of information
- How Might We question: A tool that helps teams frame ideation for brainstorming sessions
- Brainstorming: A concept that helps teams generate ideas to solve clearly defined problems
- Rapid prototyping: A concept that teams can use to quickly test and validate interventions early in the design process
- Field research: A tool that teams can use to gather qualitative data regarding the problem through observation of and interaction with users in their natural environment
- Pain/gain map: A tool that teams can use to evaluate the user's motivations and decisions by understanding the pains and gains of a situation
- Powerful questions: A concept that helps teams ask open-ended questions to elicit deeper understanding and gain new insights
- User experience surveys: A tool that helps teams gather both qualitative and quantitative data about user experiences
- User shadowing: A concept that teams can use to test new interventions and observe user interaction with the interventions in their natural environment

◼ Five stages of Design Thinking: A concept developed by the Hasso Plattner Institute of Design. The stages include empathize, define, ideate, prototype, and test, which are not always meant to be completed linearly. Teams can conduct them out of order, in reverse order, or on a repeated basis as needed (Figure 9.5).

  ◼ *Empathize.* Crucial to Design Thinking, empathy allows teams to set aside assumptions and gain insight into users. Teams aim to understand the problem by conducting interviews or observations with those affected by the problem and reviewing existing knowledge of the issue. This stage allows teams to also understand what users are currently doing to solve or work around the problem.

  ◼ *Define.* Teams analyze all information and synthesize them to define the problem (ie, problem statement). Based on the problem statement, teams can develop a plan for learning more about their users through tools such as journey maps, personas, affinity diagrams, and How Might We questions.

  ◼ *Ideate.* During this stage, teams ideate or think outside the box, using information gathered from prior stages to brainstorm ideas for interventions to defined problems. Teams come up with as many interventions as possible, even if they are at first impractical or naive. Afterward, teams narrow and choose the most viable and feasible interventions.

  ◼ *Prototype.* In this stage, teams turn interventions into inexpensive, scaled-down products or services—prototypes. The prototypes should be low-fidelity, digital, or even paper prototypes. Teams should design multiple versions of prototypes that are intuitive to use.

  ◼ *Test.* Teams test prototypes with end users and evaluate whether the prototypes solve the problem. Based on user feedback, teams may refine

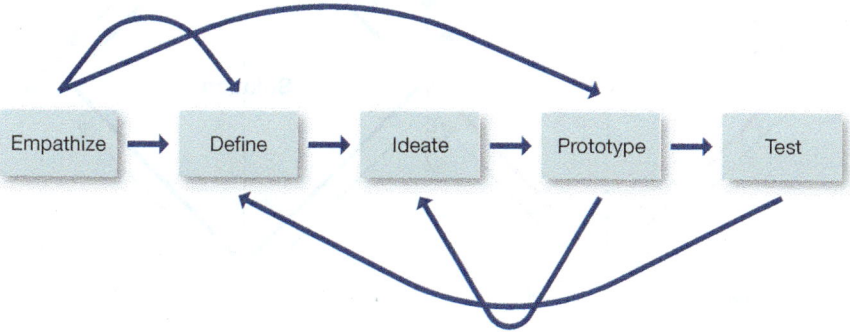

Figure 9.5 Five Stages of Design Thinking. (Source: Data from An introduction to design thinking process guide. Hasso Plattner Institute of Design at Stanford University; 2010. https://web.stanford.edu/~mshanks/MichaelShanks/files/509554.pdf)

the prototypes or go back to the Define stage. The prototypes become increasingly refined with cycles of testing on the path to a final design.

■ Double Diamond (DD) model: A concept adopted from a preceding divergence-convergence model, the DD model was popularized by the British Design Council. As the name suggests, the model consists of two diamonds—one in the problem space and then in the solution space (Figure 9.6) that represent alternating diverging (widening perspective, considering all possibilities) and converging (narrowing perspective, focusing in) activities.

The four steps of the DD Model—Discover, Define, Develop, and Deliver—can be summarized as the following:

■ *Discover.* In this step, teams work to better understand the problem. The Discover step is considered divergent in the sense that teams widen their perspective and aim to examine all possible ideas and information. Potential tools include field research, journey maps, and personas.

■ *Define.* Using insights gathered from the Discover step, teams work to define the problem. This step is considered convergent insomuch as teams aim to focus in and organize ideas to reach a clear definition (eg, problem statement). Potential tools include How Might We questions, pain/gain maps, and affinity diagrams.

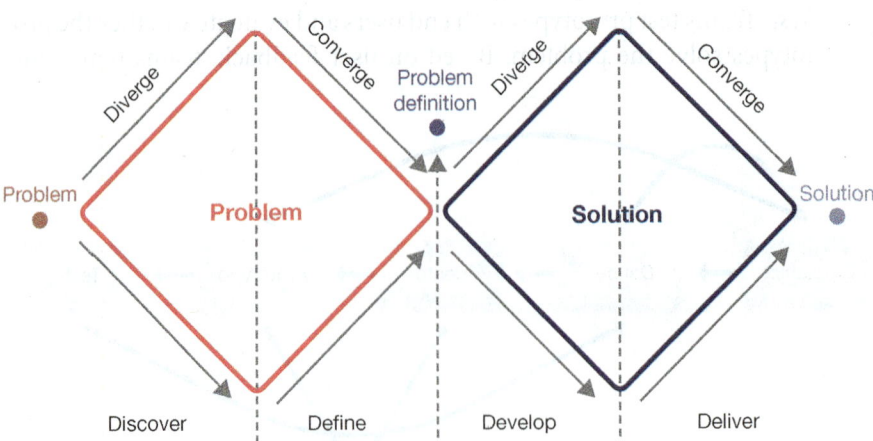

Figure 9.6 The DD Model. (Source: Reproduced with permission from Sobrinho R. UX process: the double diamond. Hi Interactive. July 13, 2023. Accessed May 7, 2024. https://www.hi-interactive.com/blog/ux-process-the-double-diamond/)

- *Develop.* In this step, teams ideate, create, and test prototypes with end users—divergent activities given the desire to generate multiple ideas and prototypes that could solve the problem. Tools that can be used in this step include brainstorming, rapid prototyping, and journey maps.
- *Deliver.* Teams focus on refining and validating prototypes through testing and user feedback. This step is considered convergent because teams use feedback to iteratively improve and narrow toward specific versions of the intervention. Relevant tools encompass powerful questions, user experience surveys, and user shadowing.

Applying Design Thinking: Managing Medications

PillPack, an online pharmacy and a former start-up company at IDEO, used the Design Thinking approach to support older adults who need to manage their medications. Through field research and pain/gain maps, PillPack was able to better understand the challenges and constraints of older adults trying to keep track of their medications. These insights allowed the company to create journey maps and personas of individuals who might use their services.

Through How Might We questions and subsequent rapid prototyping sessions, PillPack designed a prescription home delivery system that organizes medications into presorted, easy-to-open packets. These packets are labeled by date and time and sent directly to patients through mail. Instead of having numerous prescriptions in separate bottles, patients receive all medications combined into packets with clearly marked time stamps (Figure 9.7).

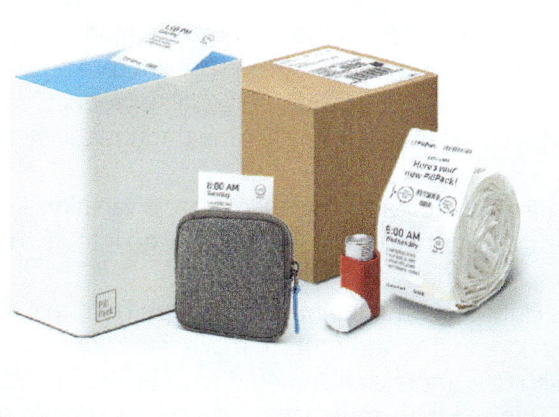

Figure 9.7 PillPack Prescription Packets. (Source: Reproduced with permission from IDEO. This startup revolutionized an industry through design. Accessed April 29, 2024. https://www.ideo.com/works/this-startup-revolutionized-an-industry-through-design/)

Back to the Clinical Case

In this case, the clinician and their team can adopt any of the four health systems solutions in efforts to reduce potentially preventable patient visits to the emergency room or urgent care. Using Lean, the team can define value and map value streams to the patients in order to reduce inefficient processes and non-value-added steps that could be considered waste.

Using Six Sigma, the team can use DPMO to measure the rate of defects—in this case, the rate of potentially avoidable emergency room or urgent care visits. Through the DMAIC concept, the team can work toward identifying and reducing variation in clinic process.

Using Kotter's Eight-Step Change Model, the team can motivate, guide, and manage change. Change management can be essential given the multiple factors that must change to reduce potentially preventable emergency room and urgent care visits.

Lastly, the team can use Design Thinking to approach problems via empathy—in this case, by first understanding why patients are choosing to go to the emergency room or urgent care. Then the team can focus on potential interventions that the patients would find desirable and interventions that would have long-term feasibility and viability for the clinic.

Importantly, these approaches are not mutually exclusive; clinicians and their teams can use them alone or together, in different combinations or sequences, to approach a problem.

TAKEAWAYS

- Lean, Six Sigma, Kotter's Eight-Step Change Model, and Design Thinking represent ways to approach health care problems.
- Lean is an approach to provide best quality products or services at the lowest cost and shortest lead time through the elimination of waste.
- Six Sigma is an approach to reduce process variation, limit defects, and ensure that products or services only go into design when certain specifications are met.
- Kotter's Eight-Step Change Model is an approach that aims to guide organizations in their attempts to make transformational changes to cope with new, more challenging market environments.
- Design Thinking is an approach predicated on what is desirable from users' point of view followed by what is technologically feasible and financially viable.

Multiple-Choice Questions

1. A hospital administrator sets the goal to decrease the spread of in-hospital infections. Which of the following Lean concepts or tools can the administrator use to empower all clinicians and staff members to speak up and correct the problem?

    A. Gemba walk

    B. Ishikawa diagram

    C. Kaizen

    D. Andon cord

2. The director of the surgery department would like to decrease the rate of postoperative complications from preventable errors. Which of the following Six Sigma concepts or tools can the director use to first measure chances of defects per million cases and track performances?

    A. DMAIC

    B. DMADV

    C. DPMO

    D. VMPS

3. Which of the following is not a stage of Kotter's Eight-Step Change Model?

    A. Creating a climate for change

    B. Engaging and enabling the whole organization

    C. Implementing and sustaining change

    D. Unfreeze

4. A primary care clinician is notified that only half of the patients on his panel are receiving age-appropriate colon cancer screening. To better understand patient actions, mindset, and emotions required to receive appropriate screening, the primary care clinician should use which of the following Design Thinking concepts or tools?

    A. Affinity diagrams

    B. How Might We questions

    C. Journey maps

    D. Rapid prototyping

Answers

1. The correct answer is D. Andon cord is a tool that reflects the principles of Jidoka and consists of the ability for any team member of the production process to "pull the cord" to stop the production and correct the problem.

2. The correct answer is C. DPMO is a tool that teams can use to measure chances of defects and track process performance for a product or service.

3. The correct answer is D. Unfreeze is a stage of Lewin's Three-Step Model of Change, not Kotter's Eight-Step Model of Change.

4. The correct answer is C. Journey maps are a Design Thinking tool that teams can use to visually showcase the actions, mindset, and emotions involved in individuals accomplishing a goal.

Bibliography

Adams R, Warner P, Hubbard B, Goulding T. Decreasing turnaround time between general surgery cases: a six sigma initiative. *J Nurs Adm.* 2004;34(3):140-148.

American Society for Quality. DMAIC process: define, measure, analyze, improve, control. https://asq.org/quality-resources/dmaic

American Society for Quality. Six Sigma definition—what is Lean Six Sigma? https://asq.org/quality-resources/six-sigma

American Society for Quality. Six Sigma tools: DMAIC, Lean & other techniques. https://asq.org/quality-resources/six-sigma/tools

Association for Supply Chain Management. Principles of lean manufacturing. https://www.ascm.org/lp/principles-of-lean-manufacturing/

Burnes B. The origins of Lewin's three-step model of change. *J Appl Behav Sci.* 2020;56(1): 32-59.

Co-Active Training Institute. Powerful questions. 2019. https://inclusion.uoregon.edu/sites/inclusion2.uoregon.edu/files/co-active-coaching-toolkit-powerful_questions.pdf

Coates E, Villarreal A, Gordanier C, Pomernacki L. Sepsis power hour: a nursing driven protocol improves timeliness of sepsis care. *J Hosp Med.* 2015;10(suppl 2). https://shmabstracts.org/abstract/sepsis-power-hour-a-nursing-driven-protocol-improves-timeliness-of-sepsis-care/

Corporation Finance Institute. Six Sigma—definition, principles, methods, explain. https://corporatefinanceinstitute.com/resources/management/six-sigma/

Design Council. Framework for innovation. https://www.designcouncil.org.uk/our-resources/framework-for-innovation/

Do D. The five principles of lean. The Lean Way. https://theleanway.net/The-Five-Principles-of-Lean

Ewenstein B, Smith W, Sologar A. Changing change management. McKinsey. Published July 1, 2015. https://www.mckinsey.com/featured-insights/leadership/changing-change-management

Fatemi F. Why design thinking is the future of sales. Forbes. https://www.forbes.com/sites/falonfatemi/2019/01/15/why-design-thinking-is-the-future-of-sales/

Feldman K. Driving quality improvement with DPMO: a roadmap to process excellence. ISIXSIGMA. https://www.isixsigma.com/dictionary/defects-per-million-opportunities-dpmo/

Feldman K. What is Six Sigma? *ISIXSIGMA.* https://www.isixsigma.com/getting-started/what-six-sigma/

Gökce K. Successful organizational transformation—Kotter's 8-steps change model. Evolutionizer. Published February 12, 2014. https://www.evolutionizer.com/en-blog/kotter-change-management-8-steps-model

Griffiths B. Top 25 lean manufacturing tools. Lean Transition Solutions. https://www.leantransitionsolutions.com/Lean-Technology/Top-25-Lean-Manufacturing-Tools

Harrison R, Fischer S, Walpola RL, et al. Where do models for change management, improvement and implementation meet? A systematic review of the applications of change management models in healthcare. *J Healthc Leadersh*. 2021;13:85-108.

Harvard Business School. A 3-step change management framework for businesses. Published November 2, 2017. https://online.hbs.edu/blog/post/a-3-step-framework-for-managing-organizational-change

Hasso Plattner Institute of Design at Stanford University. An introduction to design thinking: process guide. https://web.stanford.edu/~mshanks/MichaelShanks/files/509554.pdf

IDEO. Design thinking defined. https://designthinking.ideo.com/

IDEO. This startup revolutionized an industry through design. https://www.ideo.com/works/this-startup-revolutionized-an-industry-through-design

IDEO U. What is design thinking? https://www.ideou.com/blogs/inspiration/what-is-design-thinking

Interaction Design Foundation. What is design thinking? Updated 2024. https://www.interaction-design.org/literature/topics/design-thinking

Kotter. What we do. https://www.kotterinc.com/what-we-do/

Kotter JP. Leading change: why transformation efforts fail. Harvard Business Review. Published May-June 1995. https://hbr.org/1995/05/leading-change-why-transformation-efforts-fail-2

Kotter JP. *Leading Change*. Harvard Business School Press; 1996.

Kritsonis A. Comparison of change theories. *Int J Sch Acad Intellect Divers*. 2004-2005; 8(1):1-7. https://globalioc.com/wp-content/uploads/2018/09/Kritsonis-Alicia-Comparison-of-Change-Theories.pdf

Lean Enterprise Institute. Lean thinking and practice. https://www.lean.org/lexicon-terms/lean-thinking-and-practice/

Lean Enterprise Institute. Toyota production system. https://www.lean.org/lexicon-terms/toyota-production-system/

Lean Six Sigma Institute. Lean Six Sigma certification and implementation. https://leansixsigmainstitute.org/

Lewin K. Frontiers in group dynamics: concept, method and reality in social science; social equilibria and social change. *Hum Relations*. 1947;1(1):5-41.

Liedtka J, Ogilvie T. 10 design thinking tools: turn creativity and data into growth. UVA Darden Ideas to Action. https://ideas.darden.virginia.edu/10-design-thinking-tools-turn-creativity-and-data-into-growthLin M. *Beating the Clock to Stop Sepsis in One Hour*. Virginia Mason Institute; 2017.

McKinsey & Company. Enduring ideas: the 7S framework. McKinsey quarterly. Published March 1, 2008. https://www.mckinsey.com/capabilities/strategy-and-corporate-finance/our-insights/enduring-ideas-the-7-s-framework

Norman DA. *The Design of Everyday Things*. Basic Books; 2013.

Purdue University. Lean tools and their applications. https://www.purdue.edu/leansixsigmaonline/blog/lean-tools/

Purdue University. What are the Lean Six Sigma principles? LSS certification. https://www
.purdue.edu/leansixsigmaonline/blog/lean-six-sigma-principles/

Raza M. Lewin's 3 stage model of change explained. The Business of IT Blog. Published November 5, 2019. https://www.bmc.com/blogs/lewin-three-stage-model-change/

Six Sigma. Lean Six Sigma certification. 6 Sigma training. https://www.6sigma.us/

Six Sigma. What are the different Lean Six Sigma Tools? https://www.6sigma.us/lean-six-sigma-articles/what-are-the-different-lean-six-sigma-tools/

Sobrinho R. UX process: the double diamond. Hi Interactive. https://www.hi-interactive.com/blog/ux-process-the-double-diamond

Stanford University. About—Stanford d.school. https://dschool.stanford.edu/about

Stobierski T. Organizational change management: what it is & why it's important. Harvard Business School. Published January 21, 2020. https://online.hbs.edu/blog/post/organizational-change-management

Terra J. Six Sigma tools: here's top powerful tools you should know in 2024. UMass Amherst. https://bootcamp.umass.edu/blog/quality-management/six-sigma-tools

Toyota. Toyota production system: vision & philosophy. Toyota Motor Corporation official global website. https://global.toyota/en/company/vision-and-philosophy/production-system/

Toyota Europe. Toyota production system. https://www.toyota-europe.com/about-us/toyota-vision-and-philosophy/toyota-production-system

UMass Amherst. Six Sigma principles: a comprehensive guide to implementing and optimizing your processes. https://bootcamp.umass.edu/blog/quality-management/six-sigma-principles

University of Cambridge. Six Sigma: improving improvement. https://www.iitoolkit.com/improvement/sigma.html

University of Exeter. The change curve. https://www.exeter.ac.uk/media/universityofexeter/humanresources/documents/learningdevelopment/the_change_curve.pdf

UX Planet. The design thinking toolkit: 100+ method cards to create innovative products. https://uxplanet.org/the-design-thinking-toolbox-100-tools-to-create-innovative-products-50ede1f5e3c1

Villanova University. 6 effective Lean Six Sigma tools & techniques. https://www.villanovau.com/articles/six-sigma/practical-lean-six-sigma-tools/

Virginia Mason Franciscan Health. VMPS success stories. https://www.vmfh.org/about-vmfh/research-care-quality/virginia-mason-production-system/vmps-success-stories

Virginia Mason Institute. Improve sepsis bundle & training protocols. https://www.virginiamasoninstitute.org/empowering-teams-to-identify-and-address-sepsis-in-under-one-hour/

Vorne. Lean manufacturing tools and techniques: lean production. https://www.leanproduction.com/top-25-lean-tools/

Womack JP, Jones DT, Roos D; Massachusetts Institute of Technology. *The Machine That Changed the World: Based on the Massachusetts Institute of Technology 5-Million Dollar 5-Year Study on the Future of the Automobile.* Rawson Associates; 1990.

10

Identifying the Problem and Solutions

Case

This pattern of preventable emergency room and urgent care visits for Dr Jackson's patients has been ongoing for years. She would like to better understand the scope of the problem and the root cause for its occurrence.

This case reflects a common situation, in which clinicians and their teams must identify the nature of a problem as an early step in pursuing change and improvement. Because health care is complex and involves interplay between medical care organizations, clinicians, and patients, there may be differing conceptions of the scope and drivers of problems. Several health systems solutions—Problem Statements, Five Whys, and Ishikawa diagrams—can support efforts to identify health care problems.

SYSTEMS SOLUTION: PROBLEM STATEMENTS

Developing problem statements—one- or two-sentence summary statements that define problems that teams plan to address—can be useful in a number of different situations. There is no universal method for creating such statements; teams can use a number of different approaches to do so. Two notable examples to crafting problem statements include the Six Sigma approach and Design Thinking approach, each of which offers a distinct lens to teams working to conceptualize a problem.

Six Sigma Approach to Problem Statements

Six Sigma is an overarching method for reducing process variation based on the premise that defects in a product or service can be minimized by identifying and eliminating variations that impact performance. The Six Sigma approach is predicated on the assumption that most variation from the mean exists within six sigmas or standard deviations to the mean. In turn, performance outside the bounds of these six sigmas reflects potential problems.

One useful Six Sigma concept to identify problems is DMAIC—Define, Measure, Analyze, Improve, Control. The development of a problem statement is integrated in the Define stage where a team identifies a process of interest that is not occurring optimally and a particular issue (termed a "pain point") in that process. In particular, to facilitate the development of the problem statement, the team asks themselves the following:

- What is the pain?
- Where is it hurting?
- When—is it current? How long has it been?
- What is the extent of the pain?

In answering these questions, teams seek not to assign blame to an individual, identify a root cause of the problem, or propose an intervention. Instead, the problem statement is intended to recognize a gap between how a process should be operating and how it is actually operating. Structurally, the problem statement should be concise, specific, fact- or data based, and focused on a single issue. When used in business contexts, problem statements can also include information on the financial impact of the problem.

In a Six Sigma approach, problem statements can be developed alongside goal statements, which are informed by problem statements in order to define what teams plan to achieve through their work. The goal statement is an action-oriented sentence that names specific, measurable, attainable, relevant, and time-bound goals; the aims statement does not detail root causes or particular interventions.

Applying the Six Sigma Approach to a Problem Statement: Patient Satisfaction in the Hospital

The Six Sigma approach was used by a medical telemetry unit in an acute care hospital to develop a problem statement focused on performance in patient satisfaction surveys. A team from the unit recognized that the existing processes for promoting patient satisfaction (as measured by a tool called the Hospital Consumer Assessment of Healthcare Providers and Systems [HCAHPS]) were suboptimal and needing change. In particular, the team identified two pain points: low "overall unit rating" and low patient responses to a question about whether they would "recommend this hospital."

This process yielded a problem statement that could be summarized as follows:

A medical telemetry unit in a medium-sized hospital reported HCAHPS percent ratings below the competition for "Overall Unit Rating" and "Would you Recommend this Hospital." The baseline scores of nine of ten responses were 56 percent, and 61 percent of respondents stated "Definitely Yes" to "Would You Recommend this Hospital."

This problem statement included elements such as what is the pain (scores on HCAHPS patient satisfaction surveys), and where is it hurting (the medical telemetry unit in a medium-sized hospital). Notably, the statement did not include information about how long the pain has existed (months, years), the extent of the pain (how far below the competition the unit performed), or the consequences of the pain (reduced reimbursement, fewer patients).

Design Thinking Approach to Problem Statements

Design Thinking is an approach to innovation anchored around human-centered design. The approach emphasizes interventions to a problem instead of the problem itself, as well as the person behind the problem and intervention. Design Thinking has five stages: Empathize, Define, Ideate, Prototype, and Test.

Design Thinking incorporates empathy as a core element of problem statements. First, in the Empathize stage, teams perform an analysis intended to gain insight into users and their needs, for instance, by conducting interviews with people affected by an issue. Then, in the Define stage, teams create a problem statement with the intent of synthesizing lessons learned from empathy analysis and defining the problem in a way that centers end user needs.

Often called a point-of-view problem statement, this type of Design Thinking-based problem statement combines knowledge about issues with knowledge about users, their needs, and reasons for identified needs. Teams are also encouraged to consider the following Design Thinking concepts when making a point-of-view problem statement:

Make it human centered. Problem statements should be framed with end users in mind, integrating insights gained from the Empathize stage and focusing on humans affected rather products or technologies.

Make it broad enough to allow for creativity. Problem statements should not overly focus on an individual process or include specific technical requirements. Instead, teams should be encouraged to think in ways that might bring unexpected value and fail to emerge from a more technical or narrowly focused problem statement.

Make it narrow enough to be achievable. Problem statements should not be so broad that they seem unachievable or possess scope that will overwhelm teams. Achieving this point while maintaining enough breadth to enable creativity is a key task for teams seeking to create a Design Thinking–informed problem statement.

Applying a Design Thinking Approach to Developing a Problem Statement: Patient Care Handoffs

A team consisting of individuals in an internal medicine residency program, medical informaticists, architects, and designers used a Design Thinking approach to develop a problem statement to address patient care handoffs in hospitals using the electronic medical record. An inherent aspect of hospital care, patient care handoffs create potential safety and quality risks—in particular, when a patient's care is passed from one clinician to another, there are risks of miscommunicating information that can lead to errors or low-quality care. While electronic medical records can improve health care delivery, clinicians must use technology effectively while avoiding risks such as transcription errors.

In this context, the impetus for creating a problem statement was several fold: suboptimal use of standardized approaches to patient care handoffs by internal medicine residents, despite training on how to do so and frequent need to lead handoffs; and usability issues in the electronic medical record for handoffs.

After completing the Empathize stage through end user interviews, directly observed handoffs, and other empathy-focused analysis methods, the team developed a series of point-of-view problem statements, including the following:

> "A medicine resident needs a way to import patient data from the [electronic medical record] so that he/she never makes a transcription error when updating the list."

In this example, the team developed a problem statement that was broad enough to allow for creativity (did not assign how data from the electronic medical record needed to be visualized or what specific data needed to be included in the handoff tool) and narrow enough to be manageable (focused on existing data that internal medicine residents had access to) while being human centered and focused on users (medical residents), their needs (access to and transfer of patient data into a useful form for patient care handoffs), and insight about reasons for those needs (so no transcription errors in the electronic medical record take place).

SYSTEMS SOLUTION: FIVE WHYS

The Five Whys is a root cause analysis tool first developed by Sakichi Toyoda, a Japanese inventor who founded Toyoda Automatic Loom Works, Ltd (now known as Toyota Industries) in 1926. As a young man, Toyoda became interested in handlooms used on farms, which at the time required two peo-ple to operate. Hoping to make handlooms more efficient and easy to use, Toyoda began building and taking them apart.

Even after earning his first patent for a single-person-operated wooden han-dloom in 1891, Toyoda continued to spend decades iteratively inventing more advanced looms. His work culminated in the invention of the automatic loom in 1924, the Type G, which at the time produced the world's highest quality textiles at the greatest efficiency. In his work, Toyoda used the Five Whys to identify root causes for problems he encountered, having been attributed to saying "by repeat-ing why five times, the nature of the problem as well as its solution becomes clear."

Subsequently, the Five Whys became widely known due to its incorpora-tion in the Toyota Production System, a multifaceted production system that was developed in the 1950s and 1960s by Taiichi Ohno, Toyota's chief of pro-duction after World War II, and focused on providing high-quality, low-cost, and efficient production of automobiles through waste elimination.

Ohno described the Five Whys as the "basis of Toyota's scientific ap-proach." The tool has since been adopted into root cause analysis efforts across industries as well as in other approaches to addressing problems, such as Six Sigma and Lean.

The Five Whys can be used by teams seeking to uncover root causes of an already identified problem. The tool is best used by teams with expertise in the problem(s) at hand who have articulated a clear problem statement.

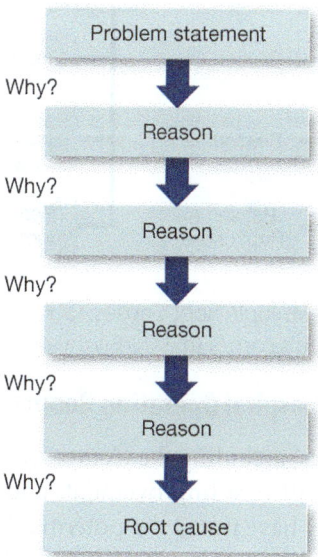

Figure 10.1 The Five Whys, One Root Cause. (Source: Data from Businessmap. Unlock the power of 5 whys: root cause analysis made easy. https://businessmap.io/lean-management/improvement/5-whys-analysis-tool)

To begin, a team facilitator asks "why" the issue targeted in the problem statement occurred. Members of the team are then encouraged to present data-supported reasons as to why the problem occurred, with a focus on systems or process errors. The facilitator then asks "why" in response to those reasons, and again in iterative cycles (generally, at least 5 times; hence the name of the tool) until root causes are identified. In response to each "why," team members can present a single cause (Figure 10.1) or multiple root causes (Figure 10.2). In the latter case, each branching reason that emerges can be further interrogated in parallel to ultimately illuminate multiple root causes.

Once the team has asked "why?" iteratively and identified what it believes to be root causes, the facilitator can help validate these findings by asking whether the problem could be prevented if identified causes were fixed. The ability to answer affirmatively supports the idea that a true root cause has been identified. Despite the name of the tool, it is possible that fewer or more than five iterations of "why?" will be needed to identify root causes.

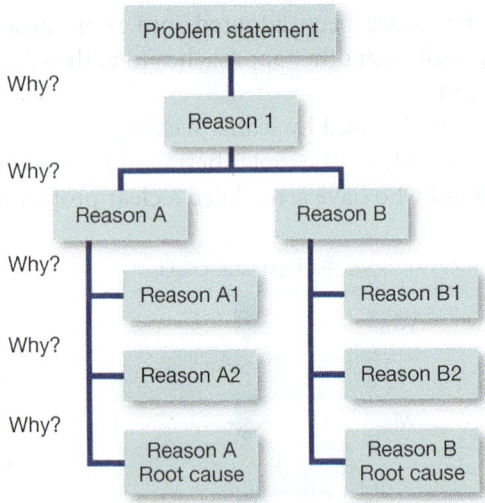

Figure 10.2 The Five Whys, Multiple Root Causes. (Source: Data from MindTools. 5 whys. https://www.mindtools.com/a3mi00v/5-whys)

Applying the Five Whys: Hospital Operating Room Delays

A number of organizations, including the Centers for Medicare and Medicaid Services, Institute for Healthcare Improvement, and the Agency for Healthcare Research and Quality have noted the potential benefit of the Five Whys. One application, as noted by England's National Health Service, relates to hospital operating room delays.

In this case, the problem at hand is that surgeries are delayed in a hospital operating room. After asking why a first time, the team working through the problem may learn that a patient who was scheduled early in the day's schedule

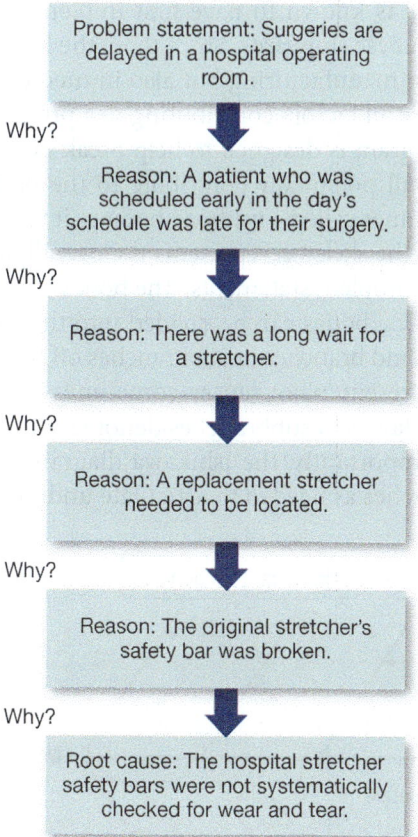

Figure 10.3 Using the Five Whys to Identify the Root Cause of Hospital Operating Room Delays.

was late for their surgery, thereby creating a cascade of delay throughout the rest of the schedule. Asking why a second time, the team may learn that the patient was late because there was a long wait for a stretcher. Asking why the third and fourth times might yield insight that a replacement had to be located due to a broken safety bar on the original stretcher. A fifth time of asking may identify the root cause: that safety bars had not been systematically checked for wear and tear (Figure 10.3).

SYSTEMS SOLUTION: ISHIKAWA DIAGRAMS

The Ishikawa diagram, also referred to as the fishbone or the cause-and-effect diagram, is a tool that aims to identify all potential causes for a problem. The Ishikawa diagram was popularized in the 1960s by Kaoru Ishikawa. A professor of engineering at the University of Tokyo and a student of W. Edwards Deming, Ishikawa was a pioneer in developing processes to manage quality in manufacturing. He is known to have first implemented the use of Ishikawa diagrams in Japanese shipyards. Since then, the Ishikawa diagrams have been used not only in manufacturing but also in medical care organizations to identify and analyze all factors contributing to a problem.

The Ishikawa diagram is designed to help break down, in successive layers, root causes that all potentially contribute to the problem. The diagram (Figure 10.4) is sometimes called a fishbone because it visually resembles a fish skeleton. The head of the skeleton represents the overall problem as identified through tools such as problem statements. The bones of the skeleton represent the potential causes. The bones can be divided into the backbone (horizontal line toward the head) and branches or subbranches off the backbone.

The branches represent major causes, sometimes termed primary causes, while the subsequent layers of subbranches denote root causes (ie, secondary, or tertiary causes). Importantly, the Ishikawa diagram is flexible enough to include as many branches as needed to articulate underlying causes.

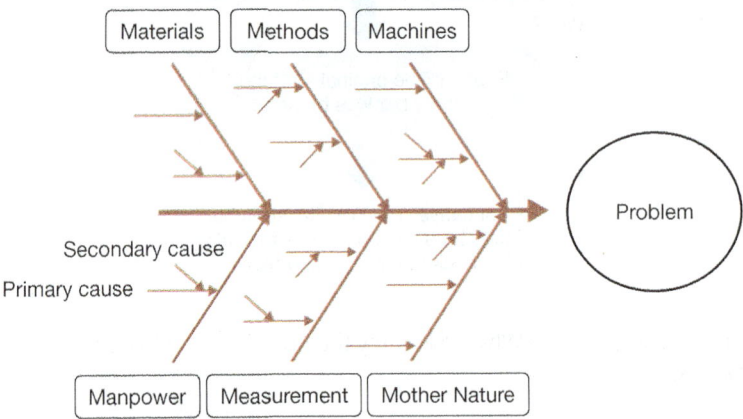

Figure 10.4 Example of an Ishikawa Diagram. (Source: Data from Gartlehner G, Schultes MT, Titscher V, et al. User testing of an adaptation of fishbone diagrams to depict results of systematic reviews. *BMC Med Res Methodol.* 2017;17(1):169.)

Ishikawa diagrams are versatile for use in different situations. A number of commonly applicable types of Ishikawa diagrams have been established across health care and other industries. While clinicians, teams, and medical care organizations must tailor diagrams to their specific uses and situations, they can benefit from familiarity with common diagram types:

3Ms diagram. This type of diagram organizes major causes into three categories: manpower, machineries, and materials. It is commonly used in the manufacturing industry.

6Ms diagram. This type of diagram organizes major causes into six categories: materials, methods, machines, manpower, measurement, and mother nature. It is also commonly used in the manufacturing industry.

4Ss diagram. This type of diagram organizes major causes into four categories: suppliers, systems, surroundings, and skills. It is commonly used in the service industry.

8Ps diagram. This type of diagram organizes major causes into eight categories: procedures, policies, places, products, people, processes, prices, and promotions. It is commonly used in the marketing industry.

Each diagram type can apply to different settings or scenarios within health care. For instance, machines and materials can be relevant in the context of surgery, procedures, and medical devices. Systems, surroundings, and skills can be relevant to the process of delivering health care services. Causes such as policies and prices can be salient to the policy and payment environments in which patient care occurs. Ishikawa diagrams can be made via a series of steps:

Identify a problem statement. The problem statement must be specific about how and when the problem occurs. The problem statement is placed at one end of the diagram (ie, head of the fish) with a horizontal line (ie, backbone) drawn toward the head of the fish (Figure 10.5).

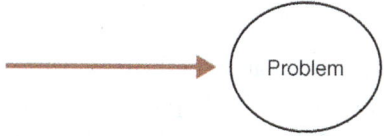

Figure 10.5 Identify a Problem Statement.

Identify major causes. In this step, teams must brainstorm and identify the major causes of the identified problem. Some teams may find it helpful to begin with, and adapt from, one of the commonly used types of Ishikawa diagrams (eg, 3Ms, 4Ss, 6Ms, or 8Ps), versus starting from scratch. Regardless, the output of this step is to generate main branches emanating from the backbone and reflecting major causes of the problem (Figure 10.6).

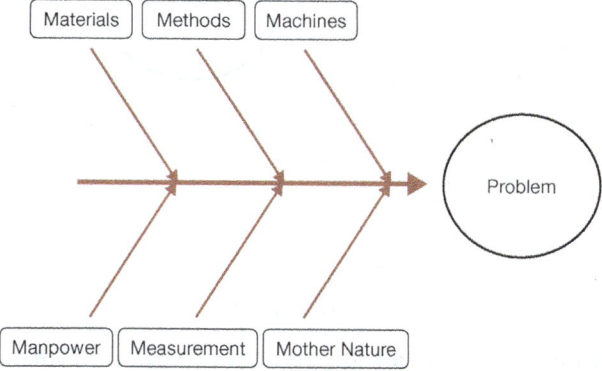

Figure 10.6 Identify Major Causes.

Identify root causes. With the major causes identified, the teams' next step is to brainstorm and identify deeper secondary and tertiary—that is, root—causes related to each major cause. During this step, tools such as the Five Whys may be helpful. While some root causes fit neatly underneath a single major cause, others may relate to and be most appropriately listed under multiple major causes (Figure 10.7).

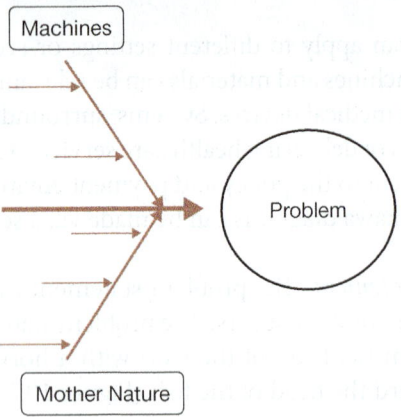

Figure 10.7 Identify Root Causes.

Analyze root causes. As a continuation of the prior step, teams should continue to use tools such as the Five Whys to pursue iteratively deeper understanding of the root causes contributing to the problem. Ultimately, this process may yield several layers of subbranches. Teams can prioritize the root causes based on the significance of their impact on the problem (Figure 10.8).

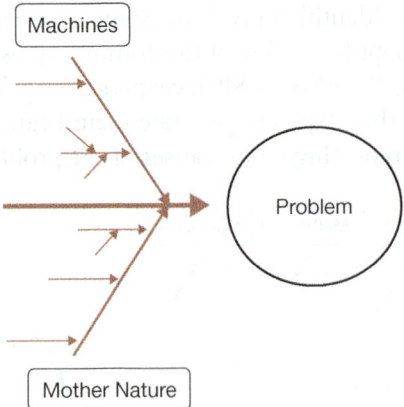

Figure 10.8 Analyze Root Causes.

Applying the Ishikawa Diagram: Delayed Test Results

A hospital team chooses to use the Ishikawa diagram to identify potential causes of delayed test results (ie, problem statement). Delayed test results, as the problem statement, is placed at the head of the diagram. The team identifies people, environment, materials, methods, and equipment as the major causes to be connected as ribs to the backbone. Physicians, laboratory technicians, dispatchers, secretaries, escorts, and phlebotomists are all identified as people involved. The Five Whys (or more) are asked to discuss each role and how they could cause delays in test results. Upon repeating the Five Whys and analyzing other potential root causes for deeper understanding (Figure 10.9), the team chooses to prioritize minimizing transcription errors (under environment) and pager malfunction (under equipment).

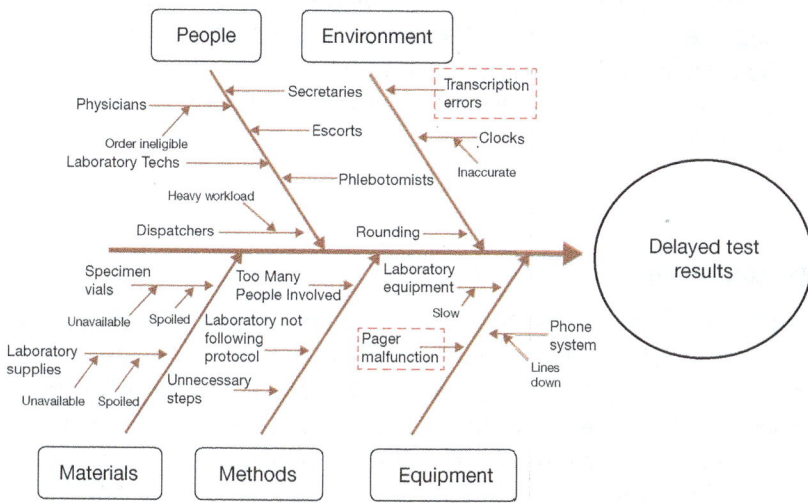

Figure 10.9 Ishikawa Diagram for Delayed Test Results. (Source: Data from Picarillo AP. Introduction to quality improvement tools for the clinician. *J Perinatol.* 2018;38[7]:929-935.)

Back to the Case

In this case, the clinician and the team can adopt any of the three health systems solutions. By developing a problem statement using a Six Sigma approach, the team can clearly define the "pain point" of potentially preventable emergency room and urgent care visits. Using a Design Thinking approach to developing a problem statement, the team can frame the problem by first empathizing with why patients may feel the need to use the emergency room or urgent care rather than the clinic. In using the Five Whys or an Ishikawa diagram, the team can further analyze the problem to identify its root causes that can potentially be intervened upon. The team can use one or a combination of these health systems solutions to identify the problem.

TAKEAWAYS

- Several health systems solutions—problem statements, Five Whys, and Ishikawa diagrams—can support efforts to identify health care problems.
- A problem statement is a one- or two-sentence summary statement that defines the problem teams plan to address.
- Different approaches—including Six Sigma and Design Thinking—offer different lenses for developing problem statements.
- The Five Whys can identify one or multiple root causes and is best used after articulation of a clear problem statement.
- The Ishikawa diagram is designed to help break down, in successive layers, root causes that all potentially contribute to the problem.

Case Continued

The team identifies limited hours of operation—in particular, the lack of evening or weekend hours—as a root cause for potentially preventable emergency room and urgent care visits. Dr Jackson and her colleagues suspect that the issue will likely continue in the absence of a change addressing this root cause, but they are unsure of how to design a potential solution.

Having identified the problem(s) at hand, clinicians and teams must then turn their attention to identifying solutions; affinity diagrams represent a particularly salient health systems solution that provides a structured way for teams to do so.

SYSTEMS SOLUTION: AFFINITY DIAGRAMS

An affinity diagram—sometimes known as an affinity map or affinity chart—is a visual tool that helps teams organize a large amount of information into themes, according to the affinity or similarity between different pieces of information. The process of creating an affinity diagram can be summarized in the following ways:

Record ideas. After a brainstorming session where teams generate ideas, the team should visualize ideas in collective format. In particular, team members should record all ideas—notes and observations related to a product, process, or service—on individual sticky notes, with the goal of generating as many sticky notes as relevant. Each team member is then encouraged to place sticky notes onto a board or wall (Figure 10.10). When done by all individuals, this step provides teams an overall perspective and a master set of ideas from which to start visualizing information.

Person One		Person Two		Person Three		Person Four		Person Five	
Idea	Idea	Idea	Idea	Idea	Idea	Idea	Idea	Idea	Idea
Idea	Idea	Idea	Idea	Idea	Idea	Idea	Idea	Idea	Idea
Idea	Idea	Idea	Idea	Idea	Idea	Idea	Idea	Idea	Idea
Idea	Idea	Idea	Idea	Idea	Idea	Idea	Idea	Idea	Idea

Figure 10.10 Record Ideas.

Categorize ideas. Once all ideas are visualized on the board or wall, teams can then engage in a systematic effort and discussion to identify patterns or themes across the sticky notes. Ideas that have similarities (ie, affinity) with others can be grouped together into groups. This should be an iterative, flexible process: in initial parts of this process, groups of two or three sticky notes can be grouped into clusters; subsequently, these clusters may be revisited, reorganized, or further aggregated into larger groups. To the extent possible, teams should attempt to categorize all sticky notes into groups (Figure 10.11).

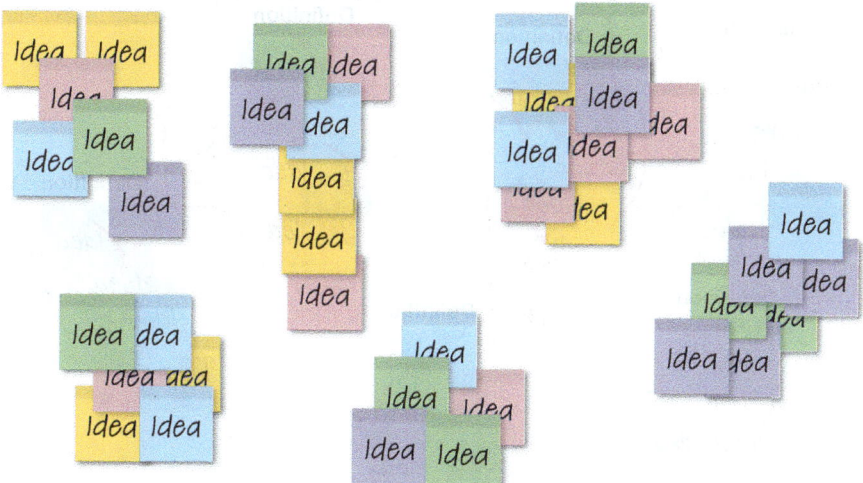

Figure 10.11 Categorize Ideas.

Define groups. Once sticky notes have been aggregated by groups, teams should discuss each group in detail to identify themes for each. Although different themes may apply to a given group, work in this step should result in short, three- to five-word consensus definitions for each group. These definitions can be placed at the head of each group (Figure 10.12).

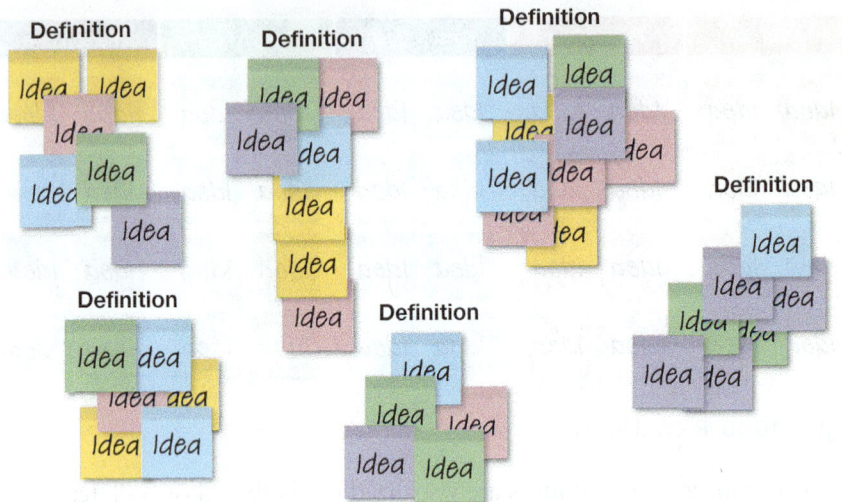

Figure 10.12 Define Groups.

Generate insights. With all information categorized, defined, and visualized for all individuals, teams can generate insights for each group of ideas, and, subsequently, translate insights into potential solutions. As a final step, teams can vote to prioritize insights (eg, red check marks and circles around groups) based on actionability and feasibility (Figure 10.13).

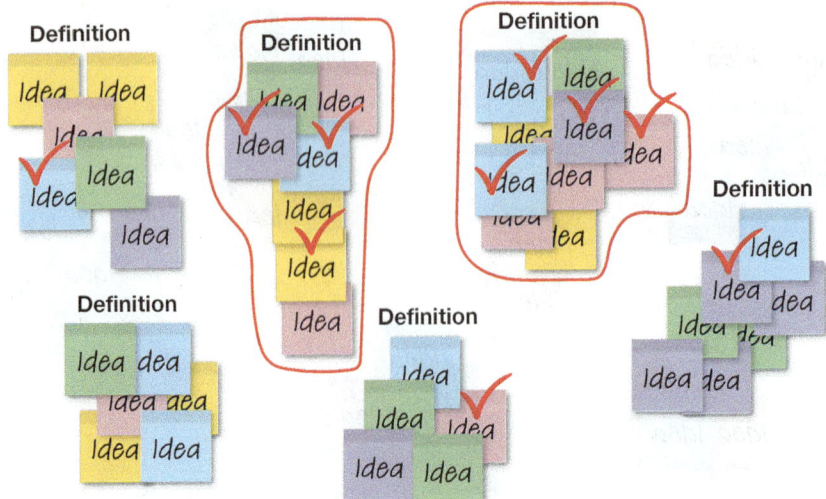

Figure 10.13 Generate Insights.

Ultimately, affinity diagrams are meant to help teams visualize, discuss, and collectively organize a large amount of information into useful themes that generate insights.

Applying the Affinity Diagram: Improving Radiology Workflow

A team of radiologists used affinity diagrams to improve how radiology images are processed and reported back to the ordering clinicians. The team interviewed nearly 50 clinicians (from the department of surgery, internal medicine, and emergency medicine) and recorded over 350 ideas onto individual sticky notes.

The team categorized the ideas into five clusters that were defined as follows: "we need you to know us better" (ie, clinicians believed radiologists left out findings pertinent to their respective specialties), "we need you to consider our workflow" (ie, clinicians wanted faster imaging reports), "we need more from your services" (ie, clinicians wanted more detail regarding certain anatomies and measurements), "we want to review your data in certain ways" (ie, clinicians wanted to customize how they review data), and "we want to do more with you" (ie, clinicians wanted to collaborate more with radiologists).

The team used these clusters to generate nine insights before prioritizing four in particular that deserved immediate action. These four insights—that referring clinicians are under the pressure of time, need key information, want imaging data reviewed over time as well as in specific ways—were applied toward identifying solutions in the radiology software. The other five insights were determined to be better suited as long-term initiatives (eg, teaching curriculum for trainees).

Back to the Case

In this case, the clinician can work with her team to use affinity diagrams and record, categorize, and define ideas for potential solutions to address limited hours of operation for the clinic. Affinity diagrams can help the clinician and her team to generate insights and vote on potential solutions based on their actionability and feasibility.

TAKEAWAYS

- An affinity diagram—sometimes known as an affinity map or affinity chart—is a visual tool that helps teams identify solutions.
- Affinity diagrams can help teams visualize, discuss, and collectively organize a large amount of information into useful themes.
- Steps for using affinity diagrams include recording ideas, categorizing ideas, defining groups, and generating insights.

Multiple-Choice Questions

1. After a hospital receives low consumer satisfaction scores, a nurse in a hospital ward leads a team focused on patient laboratory draw schedules. Before making a problem statement, the nurse interviews five patients about when they prefer to have laboratory tests drawn and imagines how laboratory draws in the middle of the night impact sleep. Afterward, the nurse drafts a problem statement focused on the patient and their need for a different laboratory draw schedule for improved rest. Which approach to drafting a problem statement did the nurse use?
   A. Design Thinking approach
   B. Six Sigma approach
   C. A and B
   D. None of the above

2. A medical team is trying to determine why an incorrect medication was given to the patient. After using the Five Whys, they determine an underlying reason for why the error occurred. What is another term for this underlying reason?
   A. Root cause
   B. Core issue
   C. Main mistake
   D. Person to blame

3. During which of the following steps in creating an affinity diagram do teams vote to prioritize potential solutions to a problem?
   A. Record each idea
   B. Categorize ideas
   C. Define each group
   D. Generate insights

Answers

1. The correct answer is A. After first conducting Empathize stage activities (eg, patient interviews), the nurse develops a problem statement focused on the user, the user's need, and insight from the user, which is in line with the Design Thinking approach to developing problem statements.

2. The correct answer is A. The Five Whys can be used to identify one or more root causes, which, if fixed, would have prevented the problem.

3. The correct answer is D. As a final step—generate insights—teams can vote to prioritize potential solutions based on actionability and feasibility.

Bibliography

6sigma. Types of fishbone diagrams aka "Ishikawa diagram." Published November 30, 2020. https://6sigma.com/types-of-fishbone-diagrams/

Agency for Healthcare Research and Quality. Job aid: 5 whys and fishbone diagram. https://www.ahrq.gov/sites/default/files/wysiwyg/ncepcr/resources/job-aid-5-whys.pdf

American Society for Quality. Five whys and five hows. https://asq.org/quality-resources/five-whys

American Society for Quality. What is an affinity diagram? 2009. https://asq.org/quality-resources/affinity

American Society for Quality. Kaoru Ishikawa. 2019. https://asq.org/about-asq/honorary-members/ishikawa

American Society for Quality. What is a fishbone diagram? Ishikawa cause & effect diagram. 2019. https://asq.org/quality-resources/fishbone

American Society for Quality. What is Six Sigma? https://asq.org/quality-resources/six-sigma

API. Five whys tool for root cause analysis. https://www.cms.gov/medicare/provider-enroll-ment-and-certification/qapi/downloads/fivewhys.pdf

Best M, Neuhauser D. Kaoru Ishikawa: from fishbones to world peace. *Qual Saf Health Care.* 2008;17(2):150-152.

Boll DT, Rubin GD, Heye T, Pierce LJ. Affinity chart analysis: a method for structured collection, aggregation, and response to customer needs in radiology. *AJR Am J Roentgenol.* 2017;208(4):W134-W145.

Businessmap. Unlock the power of 5 whys: root cause analysis made easy. https://businessmap.io/lean-management/improvement/5-whys-analysis-tool

Dam RF, Siang TY. Affinity diagrams: how to cluster your ideas and reveal insights. The Interaction Design Foundation. Published May 2, 2022. https://www.interaction-design.org/literature/article/affinity-diagrams-learn-how-to-cluster-and-bundle-ideas-and-facts?utm_source=linkedin&utm_medium=post

Dam RF, Siang TY. Stage 2 in the design thinking process: define the problem and interpret the results. Interactive Design Foundation. https://www.interaction-design.org/literature/article/stage-2-in-the-design-thinking-process-define-the-problem-and-interpret-the-results

Gartlehner G, Schultes MT, Titscher V, et al. User testing of an adaptation of fishbone diagrams to depict results of systematic reviews. *BMC Med Res Methodol.* 2017;17(1):169.

Institute for Healthcare Improvement. 5 whys: finding the root cause. https://www.ihi.org/resources/tools/5-whys-finding-root-cause

Juran. How to write a Six Sigma problem statement. Published December 19, 2019. https://www.juran.com/blog/how-to-write-a-six-sigma-problem-statement/

Juran. Improving patient satisfaction via Lean Six Sigma. https://www.juran.com/results/case-studies/patient-satisfaction-improve-patient-experience/

Lean Enterprise Institute. 5 whys. https://www.lean.org/lexicon-terms/5-whys

Lean Enterprise Institute. Toyota production system. https://www.lean.org/lexicon-terms/toyota-production-system/

Lesselroth BJ, Park H, Monkman H, Duncan A, Thompson G, Yarnall R. Designing Shift Hand-off Software: clinical learners and design students collaborate using the "design thinking" process. *Stud Health Technol Inform.* 2021;281:974-978.

MindManager. What is an Ishikawa diagram and how to use it? https://www.mindmanager.com/en/features/ishikawa-diagram/

MindTools. 5 whys. https://www.mindtools.com/a3mi00v/5-whys

MiroBlog. Affinity diagrams: a powerful way to organize ideas—and make them easier to act on. Published September 19, 2019. https://miro.com/blog/create-affinity-diagrams/

Muir I, Cano M, Terry A. A tool application model for root cause analysis. University of the West of Scotland. Published September 30, 2016. https://core.ac.uk/reader/287152370

National Health Service. Using five whys to review a simple problem. https://aqua.nhs.uk/wp-content/uploads/2023/07/qsir-using-five-whys-to-review-a-simple-problem.pdf

Picarillo AP. Introduction to quality improvement tools for the clinician. *J Perinatol.* 2018;38(7):929-935.

Six Sigma. The five whys: understanding the root cause of a problem. Published February 22, 2017. https://www.6sigma.us/it/five-whys-root-cause-analysis/

Six Sigma Institute. Six Sigma DMAIC problem statement & project charter. https://www.sixsigma-institute.org/Six_Sigma_DMAIC_Process_Define_Phase_Six_Sigma_Project_Charter.php

Toyota Industries Corporation. The story of Sakichi Toyoda. https://www.toyota-industries.com/company/history/toyoda_sakichi/

11

Planning and Implementing the Solutions

Clinical Case

After completing an affinity diagram exercise, Dr Jackson concludes that a potential intervention would be to expand hours of operation for the clinic. Dr Jackson has never been part of a clinic that offered expanded hours and does not know how to plan or implement this change. She also recognizes that expanded hours would be a transformative change requiring staff buy-in and patient engagement. Dr Jackson wonders how to begin planning and implementing this potential intervention.

This is a common circumstance: A clinician has identified a potential intervention to solve a problem but is uncertain of how to plan as an initial step and then implement an intervention. In the context of health care, planning and implementing involves multiple components to ensure candidate solutions are backed by organizational and team support while also being appealing and helpful to patients. A number of health systems solutions that can help teams in planning and implementing change include Plan-Do-Study-Act (PDSA) cycle and the Model for Improvement, Kotter's Eight-Step Change Model, and the Double Diamond (DD) model.

SYSTEMS SOLUTION: PLAN-DO-STUDY-ACT CYCLE AND THE MODEL FOR IMPROVEMENT

The PDSA cycle evolved over years of iterative development from multiple contributors. As a method for planning interventions with origins in industrial quality control, PDSA involves a cyclical method to improving and testing change.

Dr Walter Shewhart, an American engineer and statistician known by many as the father of modern quality control, aimed to bring the scientific method to his work as an engineer at the Hawthorne Plant of Western Electric, a telephone equipment manufacturing company in the 1920s. He initially developed a linear three-step process, "Specification, Production, and Inspection," which can be summarized as follows:

- Specification: naming the desired change to be made to an existing product
- Production: carrying out or executing the specified change to a product
- Inspection: evaluating whether the change to the product met expectations

Shewhart later reimagined Specification, Production, Inspection as cyclical in his 1939 book, *Statistical Method from the Viewpoint of Quality Control*. He changed the process from linear to cyclical to demonstrate product development and quality control as an iterative process rather than one that ends after a single cycle (Figure 11.1).

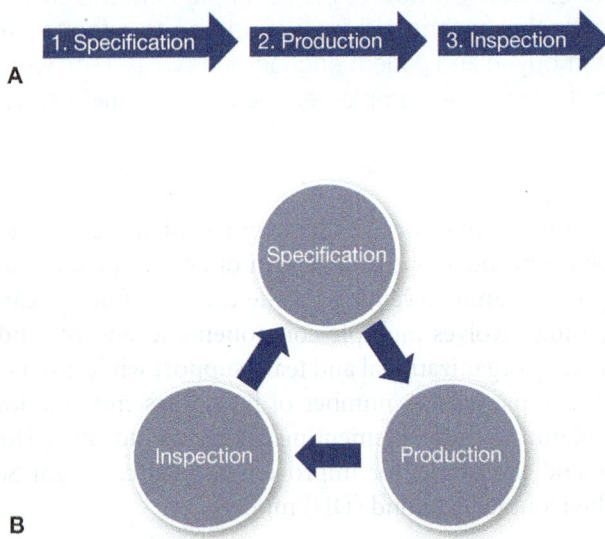

Figure 11.1 Evolution of Specification, Production, Inspection from (A) Linear to (B) Cyclical. (Source: Data from Shewhart WA. *Statistical Method from the Viewpoint of Quality Control*. United States Department of Agriculture; 1939.)

While at the Hawthorne Plant, Shewhart introduced the Specification, Production, Inspection cyclical quality control process to his colleague, Dr Edward Deming. In 1950, inspired by Shewhart's idea of cyclical improvement, Deming presented a new four-step cyclical process to product development at a seminar on quality control for executives at the Japanese Union of Scientists and Engineers. The cycle, later called the Deming Wheel, had four steps that can be summarized in the following way (Figure 11.2):

- Design: conceiving the product
- Produce: making and testing the product in laboratory
- Sell: bringing the product to market
- Redesign: learning through market research what works and does not work for the purposes of making iterative changes to the product

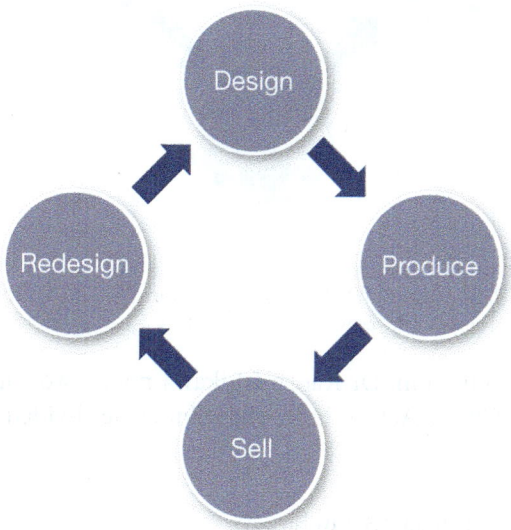

Figure 11.2 The Deming Wheel. (Source: Data from Moen RD. Foundation and history of the PDSA cycle. The W. Edwards Deming Institute. https://deming.org/wp-content/uploads/2020/06/PDSA_History_Ron_Moen.pdf)

After the presentation, Japanese executives adapted the Deming Wheel and repurposed it for problem-solving in general, rather than specifically for product development. This new process, created in 1951, followed a cycle of four steps, which can be summarized as follows (Figure 11.3):

- Plan: conceptualizing a problem, its possible root causes, and propose solutions
- Do: implementing the proposed solutions
- Check: assessing what worked and what did not work for the implemented solutions
- Act: deciding whether to return to the planning stage if the solutions did not work, or incorporating the solutions into standard processes if the solution did work

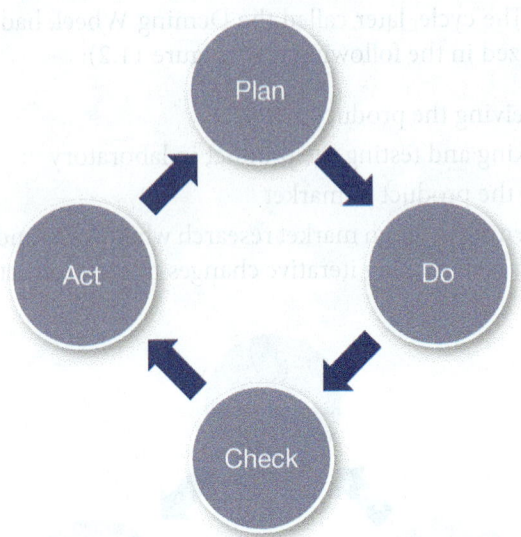

Figure 11.3 The Plan-Do-Check-Act Cycle. (Source: Data from Moen RD. Foundation and history of the PDSA cycle. The W. Edwards Deming Institute. https://deming.org/wp-content/uploads/2020/06/PDSA_History_Ron_Moen.pdf)

After its introduction, Dr Kaoru Ishikawa made two suggested changes to this Plan-Do-Check-Act cycle in 1985. First, he divided "Plan" into the following steps:

- Step one: Determine goals and targets.
- Step two: Determine methods of reaching goals.

Second, he divided "Do" into two component steps:

- Step one: Engage in education and training.
- Step two: Implement the work.

As the Plan-Do-Check-Act cycle gained prominence, Dr Deming objected to the notion that it had intellectual grounding in the initial Deming Wheel, stating that the two "bear no relation to each other." To contrast with Plan-Do-Check-Act, Deming made an adaptation to the Deming Wheel in 1986 that he called the Shewhart Cycle, a six-step cyclical process aimed at guiding teams through solving a problem that can be summarized in the following way (Figure 11.4):

- Step one: Teams ask what desirable changes can be made, what data can be utilized, and what additional observations are needed before making a

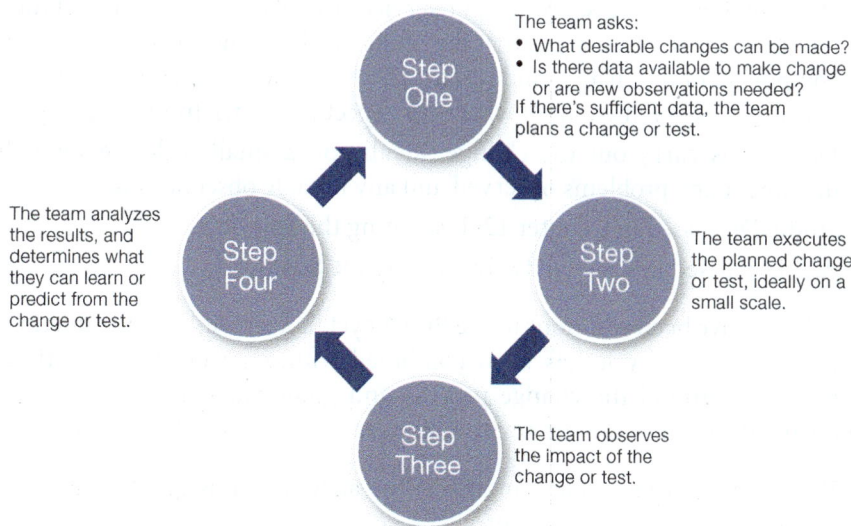

The team asks:
• What desirable changes can be made?
• Is there data available to make change or are new observations needed?
If there's sufficient data, the team plans a change or test.

Step One

The team analyzes the results, and determines what they can learn or predict from the change or test.

Step Four

Step Two

The team executes the planned change or test, ideally on a small scale.

Step Three

The team observes the impact of the change or test.

Step 5: The team repeats step one with the benefit of the insights gained.
Step 6: The team repeats steps two through four.

Figure 11.4 The Shewhart Cycle. (Source: Data from Moen RD, Norman CL. Circling back: clearing up methods about the deming cycle and seeing how it keeps evolving. Basic Quality. November 2010. https://deming.org/wp-content/uploads/2020/06/circling-back.pdf)

change. If there are sufficient data, teams will decide how to use the data to plan a change or test.

- Step two: Teams execute the planned change or test, ideally on a small scale.
- Step three: Teams observe the impact of the change or test.
- Step four: Teams analyze the results and determine what they can learn or predict from the implemented change or test.
- Step five: Teams repeat step one with the benefit of the insights gained.
- Step six: Teams repeat steps two through four.

Over time, Deming continued to iterate on the Shewhart cycle. In 1993, he revealed what he called the Shewhart Cycle for Learning and Improvement, which is now more commonly referred to as the PDSA cycle.

The PDSA cycle provides a systemic approach that teams can use for the iterative development of a process, product, or service. The four steps of the PDSA cycle can be summarized as follows:

- Plan: It is this step that can be used to help teams plan an intervention as part of an iterative change process. During this step, teams plan a change aimed at improving a process, product, or service. The Plan step includes defining the objective of the change, what the change will be, who will carry out each component of the change, and when and where it will be carried out. Teams will also make predictions of what they expect to happen from the change.

■ Do: Teams carry out the change, ideally on a small scale. Teams will document any problems observed and any notable observations.
■ Study: Discussed in Chapter 12: Evaluating the Solutions
■ Act: Discussed in Chapter 12: Evaluating the Solutions

There have been additions to the PDSA cycle since its initial introduction. Most notably, the cycle has been combined with a set of three questions intended to ground the change process and guide steps in the cycle. The following three questions are revisited for each iteration of the PDSA cycle:

■ What are we trying to accomplish? (The answer to this question is often referred to as an aim statement.)
■ How will we know that a change is an improvement?
■ What change can we make that will result in improvement?

These three questions, coupled with the PDSA cycle, are collectively known as the Model for Improvement. The Model has been used in and out of health care environments to guide iterative change (Figure 11.5).

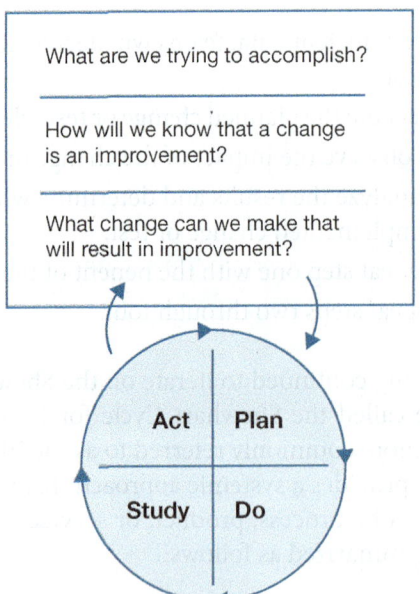

Figure 11.5 The Model for Improvement. (Source: Reproduced with permission from Langley GJ, Moen RD, Nolan KL, et al. *The Improvement Guide: A Practical Approach to Enhancing Organizational Performance.* 2nd ed. Wiley Books; 2009.)

Applying the Plan and Do Steps of the Plan-Do-Study-Act Cycle: Teach-Back Method in Primary Care

Communication can often create challenges between clinicians and patients. An estimated 50% of patients leave visits not understanding what their clinician told them, and 50% of patients do not understand how they were supposed to take a prescribed medication.

In the "teach-back" method, patients or caregivers are asked to explain medical information or instructions that have just been told to them using their own words. Then the clinician is able confirm that their understanding is accurate or correct any misunderstandings. The teach-back method has demonstrated potential benefit for improving patient understanding and self-efficacy.

The Plan and Do steps of the PDSA cycle in the Model for Improvement can be used to increase use of the teach-back method as a practice change.

Plan-Do-Study-Act Cycle

- What are we trying to accomplish?

  To increase clinician use of the teach-back method.

- How will we know that a change is an improvement?

  Clinicians who try the method will affirm its usefulness and plan to use it in the future without finding teach-back to be too time-consuming or onerous.

- What change can we make that will result in an improvement?

  Train clinicians who may not be aware of the teach-back method and ask them to utilize it.

- Plan: The clinic manager selects five clinicians in the practice as an initial sample. The manager shows them a video training on the use of the teach-back method. Afterward, the clinic manager asks those clinicians to use the teach-back method for one patient that day. At the end of the day, the clinic manager plans to ask the clinicians if the tool was useful, if using it was too onerous or time-consuming, and if they plan to use it again in the future.

- Do: The five clinicians agree to try using the teach-back method with at least one patient that clinic day.

SYSTEMS SOLUTION: KOTTER'S EIGHT-STEP CHANGE MODEL

The first phase of the Kotter's Eight-Step Change Model, collectively referred to as "creating a climate for change," involves three steps useful for planning an intervention. These three steps can be summarized as follows:

Step one: Establishing a sense of urgency. This step acknowledges that successful change requires the active participation of people throughout an organization. Part of planning a change within an organization includes creating a sense of urgency to inspire people's intrinsic motivation to participate in change. To do this, a leader within the organization needs to communicate the need for change to the broader organization, whether it be due to emergence of new competition, poor or declining financial or quality performance, the occurrence of a major error, or some other driver.

The leader must then have an honest discussion with other members of the organization highlighting where the organization is currently falling short, and framing the need for change in a way where it seems less risky than maintaining the status quo. Kotter believed that an adequate sense of urgency is achieved when 75% of an organization's management is convinced that not changing is unacceptable. Failure to achieve this step—or not establishing a great enough sense of urgency—could make getting any change off the ground unlikely.

Step two: Creating a powerful guiding coalition. In this step, Kotter acknowledged that while transformational change efforts may start with just one or two people, a critical mass of people must buy into the notion that change is needed for any change efforts to move forward. Part of planning a change, therefore, includes building a coalition that includes an array of people including those who are in leadership positions, who are respected within the organization, who have strong relationships inside and outside the organization, and who have expertise related to the change being undertaken.

Although senior leaders should be in the coalition, it should not consist solely of senior management. The change coalition also typically operates outside of the typical hierarchical structure of the overall organization. Failure to achieve this step—or not creating a powerful enough guiding coalition—might not hinder an organization's ability to make initial change. However, it could make overcoming any inevitable opposition to change more challenging.

Step three: Creating a vision. Once built, the guiding coalition must develop a vision of what the future would be like once transformational change is implemented and the overall direction in which the organization should move. The guiding coalition may take several months to plan the overall vision and a strategy for achieving it. Kotter's rule of thumb: One should be able to communicate the vision in 5 minutes or less, and that the listener must understand and be interested in the vision for it to be successful. Failure to achieve this step—or lacking a vision—could result in a transformational change effort devolving into disparate interventions without a clear direction, interventions heading in a different direction than originally intended, or members of the organization becoming confused and uninspired.

The second phase of the Kotter's Eight-Step Change Model, referred to as "engaging and enabling the whole organization," can guide organizations through change implementation and can be summarized as follows:

Step four: Communicating the vision. Once a vision is created, the next step is appropriate quantity and quality communication of that vision. Examples of poor communication of the vision include having just a single meeting to share the vision, having just the head of the organization communicate the vision (no matter how many times they communicate it), or having senior members of the organizations visibly act in a way contrary to the communicated vision.

Instead, effective communication requires regular communication by multiple members of the team, as well as incorporation of the vision into regular organizational communication and activities. In addition, organizations should communicate the vision through larger scale efforts. For example, organizations can include exciting articles about change activities in newsletters, host quarterly all-organization meetings focused on updates on the transformation change or organize trainings that build skills needed for achieving the vision.

Another critical component to communicating the vision includes the implicit communication of senior leaders "walking the walk" of the vision and change. This communicates authenticity to other members of an organization. Failure to achieve this step—or undercommunicating the vision by a factor of 10—could lead to an organizational change effort failing to capture the buy-in of other members of the organization.

Step five: Empowering others to act on the vision. If a vision is effectively communicated, members of the organization outside the guiding coalition may be motivated to participate. To encourage ongoing buy-in, organizations should empower their members to act on the vision and remove obstacles. For example, in some circumstances, a performance evaluation system that does not reward change-related activities might be an obstacle. In such situations, while people may want to pursue activities that advance the overall vision, they may instead devote their efforts to activities that are valued by the preexisting performance evaluation system. In this example, empowering others to act on the vision may mean adjusting the performance evaluation system to explicitly reward activities that advance the organization's vision.

In other circumstances, an obstacle may be a particular supervisor who resists change and makes demands contrary to the overall vision. In this example, senior leadership reinforcing the importance of the change with that supervisor is needed. Failure to achieve this step—or not removing obstacles to the new vision—could prevent people from getting and staying involved in the change.

Step six: *Planning for and creating short-term wins*. Transformational change can take time, and this step recognizes the challenge of maintaining people's interest in long-term change without evidence of early successes. In this step, organizations should actively look for ways to identify clear and achievable performance objectives related to the overarching vision (eg, product development, performance improvement).

Once identified, organizations can establish performance objectives as goals in yearly or quarterly planning processes, and publicly reward people for achieving those objectives. By identifying, achieving, and celebrating short-term wins, organizations can maintain interest and a sense of urgency related to the overall vision. Failure to achieve this step—or not systematically planning for and creating short-term wins—may result in people giving up on transformational change or actively opposing it.

The last phase of the Kotter model, referred to as "implementing and sustaining change," includes these final two steps:

Step seven: *Consolidating improvements and producing still more change*. This step acknowledges that in some cases, organizations may be inclined to claim success for the whole vision after achieving just a first small win. Instead of indulging this inclination, organizations should build on the credibility gained by a short-term win to focus on addressing an even bigger challenge related to the overall vision.

For example, organizations can take on projects that are larger in scope than the initial short-term win, refocus hiring and promotion strategies, and redesign company-wide policies to align with the vision. Failure to achieve this step—or declaring victory too soon—could result in the progress of a short-term win fizzling out or lead to change opponents claiming that the change cycle is over.

Step eight: *Institutionalizing new approaches*. This step focuses on engraining transformational change in the overall organizational structure. Kotter believed that two strategies are especially important in institutionalizing change. First, organization leaders should explicitly show people how the transformational change improved the overall organization, rather than assume members of the organization will otherwise see a connection between change and results. This strategy requires frequent and consistent communication connecting results with the implemented change. If this strategy is not undertaken, members of an organization may attribute positive results to other factors (eg, the charisma of a particular leader) rather than the transformational change. Second, organizations should ensure that the subsequent generation of management adopts and embodies institutionalized change. This embodiment includes incorporating principles of the vision into hiring and promotion. Failure to achieve this step—or not anchoring changes in the corporation's culture—can result in the breakdown of some or all the progress made by the transformational change efforts.

Since its introduction, Kotter's Eight-Step Change Model has been utilized by numerous organizations aiming to make transformational change. Indeed, the Model has been used domestically and internationally across sectors (eg, government, private corporations) and industries (eg, energy, health care, manufacturing, education).

Applying the Kotter Eight-Step Change Model: Launching I-PASS

Kotter's Eight-Step Change Model was used in the campaign that helped plan and launch a handoff tool called the Illness Severity, Patient Summary, Action List, Situational Awareness and Contingency Planning, and Synthesis by Receiver (I-PASS). Now widely used in medical care organizations, I-PASS was first launched and studied by a group called the I-PASS Campaign Committee, which first implemented the tool in non–intensive care medical-surgical units at nine North American pediatrics residency programs.

The I-PASS Campaign Committee used the first three steps in Kotter's Eight-Step Change Model to plan the I-PASS tool's launch, which can be summarized in the following way:

Step one: Establishing a sense of urgency. The I-PASS Campaign Committee created a sense of urgency by sharing data on gaps in care created and medical errors that occur during handoffs. The Committee also shared handoff tool pilot information that showed that positive change was possible. To create this sense of urgency, information was shared in meetings with leaders and presented at participating organizations.

Step two: Creating a powerful guiding coalition. To build a coalition across the multiple sites, the I-PASS Campaign Committee identified a champion for each site who led training and implementation efforts. The Committee also engaged senior leaders at participating organizations (eg, chief executive officers, patient safety officers, department chairs, residency program directors). Appreciating the role and influence of Chief Residents, the Committee also engaged them into the coalition by inviting them to provide feedback on the tool, highlight potential implementation barriers, and design a national branding strategy for the campaign. Faculty champions were also included in the guiding coalition, participating in early trainings and offering feedback to residents on I-PASS use.

Step three: Creating a vision. The Committee worked on creating a vision in preparation for its branding campaign, hiring a graphic designer to create a logo that communicated a vision that sharing patient care is a continuous process. Other components of the branding campaign included posters, pocket cards, and lanyards intended to reinforce the principles of I-PASS. In addition, the Committee created education modules, published daily tips on using I-PASS, and created I-PASS-themed fortune cookies.

After the first steps, the I-PASS Committee proceeded to Kotter's implementation-oriented steps, which can be summarized in the following way:

Step four: Communicating the vision. The Committee held a formal I-PASS launch event at participating sites. Appreciating that I-PASS might not stick without the buy-in of residents and participating organizations, the launch included departmental presentations highlighting early evidence of I-PASS, trainings on how to use I-PASS, meetings with faculty champions and frontline clinicians, and the distribution of campaign materials.

Step five: Empowering others to act on the vision. To empower residents to use I-PASS, the Committee worked with informatics teams at each organization to embed I-PASS into the electronic health record to incorporate the tool into usual workflows.

Step six: Planning for and creating short-term wins. The Committee celebrated short-term wins by publishing "shout-outs" for residents who were particularly adept at using I-PASS, and by giving prizes to teams with particularly strong I-PASS performance. One of the nine residency sites also threw a party to recognize the 1-year anniversary of I-PASS use.

Step seven: Consolidating improvements and producing still more change. After implementing I-PASS within pediatrics residencies, champions at participating sites aimed to produce still more change by spreading I-PASS to other units in their organizations, including within obstetrics and gynecology and internal medicine teams. The tool was also applied to nursing handoffs and transfers between hospital units.

Step eight: Institutionalizing new approaches. To institutionalize I-PASS for subsequent generations, participating sites required annual I-PASS training and observed handoffs for new residents. The Committee presented the curriculum at national conferences to expand the use of I-PASS beyond the original participating sites.

SYSTEMS SOLUTION: THE DOUBLE DIAMOND MODEL

The Double Diamond (DD) model—a concept adopted from a preceding divergence-convergence model—represents a structured and iterative four-step method. The first two steps of the DD model can help teams plan interventions to address complex problems, and the third step can help teams implement those interventions. First, in the Discover step, teams deeply explore and understand the multifaceted nature of the problem, including patient needs, system constraints, and best practices. In a subsequent Define step, the problem scope is clearly delineated, objectives are set, and key stakeholders are identified. Afterward, in the Develop step, teams ideate for prototypes and test them with end users.

Discover. In this step, teams work to better understand the problem (Figure 11.6). The Discover step is considered divergent in the sense that teams widen their perspective and aim to examine all possible ideas and information. Potential tools include field research, journey maps, and personas.

Define. Using insights gathered from the Discover step, teams work to define the problem (Figure 11.7). This step is considered convergent insomuch as teams aim to focus in and organize ideas to reach a clear definition (eg, problem statement). Potential tools include How Might We questions, pain/gain maps, and affinity diagrams.

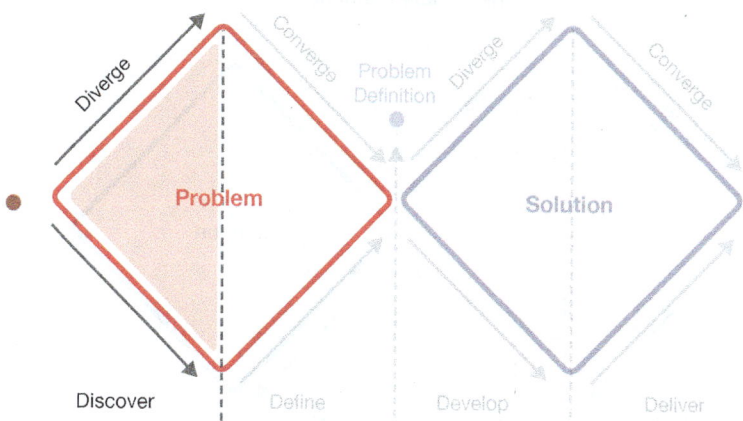

The Double Diamond

Figure 11.6 Discover Step of the Double Diamond Model. (Source: Reproduced with permission from Sobrinho R. UX process: the double diamond. Hi Interactive. July 13, 2023. Accessed May 7, 2024. https://www.hi-interactive.com/blog/ux-process-the-double-diamond/)

The Double Diamond

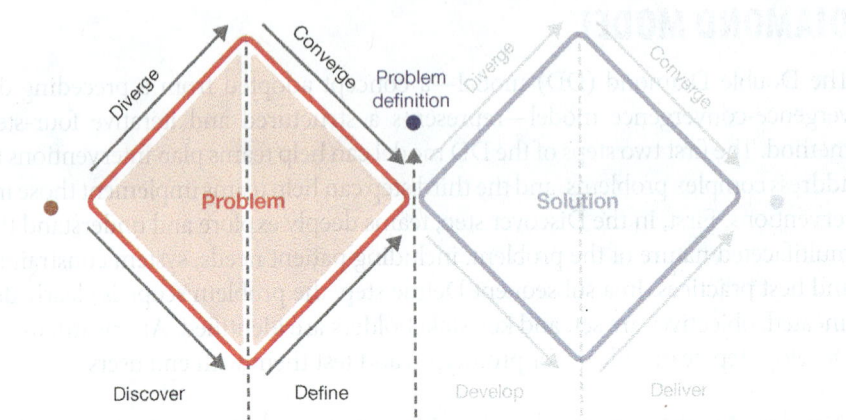

Figure 11.7 Define Step of the Double Diamond Model. (Source: Reproduced with permission from Sobrinho R. UX process: the double diamond. Hi Interactive. July 13, 2023. Accessed May 7, 2024. https://www.hi-interactive.com/blog/ux-process-the-double-diamond/)

Develop. In this step, teams ideate, create, and test prototypes with end users—divergent activities given the desire to generate multiple ideas and prototypes that could solve the problem (Figure 11.8). Tools that can be used in this step include brainstorming, rapid prototyping, and journey maps.

Deliver. Discussed in Chapter 12: Evaluating the Solutions

The Double Diamond

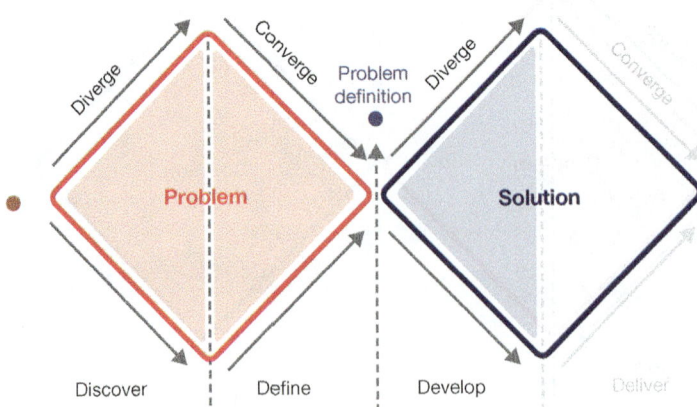

Figure 11.8 Develop Step of the Double Diamond Model. (Source: Reproduced with permission from Sobrinho R. UX process: the double diamond. Hi Interactive. July 13, 2023. Accessed May 7, 2024. https://www.hi-interactive.com/blog/ux-process-the-double-diamond/)

Applying the Discover, Define, and Develop Steps of the Double Diamond Model: Breastfeeding in the Neonatal Intensive Care Unit

The DD model has been used alongside other solutions such as the PDSA cycle to improve breastfeeding support for mothers in the neonatal intensive care unit (NICU). At a large US medical care organization, NICU clinicians received feedback that some mothers were dissatisfied about not meeting breastfeeding goals—surprising feedback given clinicians' understanding that mothers were well supported in breast milk pumping. In response to the feedback, the medical care organization formed an interdisciplinary team to better plan and implement interventions that could improve NICU breastfeeding practices.

Discover. The interdisciplinary team conducted human-centered design interviews with the mothers, clinicians, and other caregivers. Gathering the information from the interviews, the team created journey maps as well as value stream maps outlining the NICU's breastfeeding workflow and an Ishikawa diagram to identify root causes of maternal dissatisfaction with not meeting NICU breastfeeding goals.

Reviewing all the information from interviews, maps, and their diagram, the team discovered that NICU clinicians and mothers had different goals with respect to NICU breastfeeding practices. The clinicians' goals were for the infants to receive breast milk, regardless of whether the infants were fed at the breast or received pumped milk. In contrast, the mothers' goals were for the infants to be fed at the breast as much as possible and to be able to bond with their infants.

Define. The team subsequently created a new problem statement. Instead of defining the problem as an issue of infants receiving breast milk, the team reframed the issue around mothers' breastfeeding experiences: "How might we better support a mother's breastfeeding experience in the NICU?" In concert, the team created the following aim statement for their PDSA cycle: "We aim to increase the rate of feeding at the breast among first time mothers in the NICU from 33 percent to 50 percent within six months of starting the project."

Develop. The team hosted multiple brainstorming sessions with mothers, clinicians, and other caregivers to ideate interventions. Eventually, the team decided on the idea of prototyping, or quickly testing, a team of NICU nurses with dedicated time to assist mothers with feeding at the breast during each shift. Over the course of 6 months, the team developed multiple prototype iterations in line with PDSA cycles.

Back to the Clinical Case

In this case, the clinician and her team could adopt any of the three health system solutions to plan for and implement clinic expanded hours. Using the PDSA cycle, the team could use the Plan step to define the objective of having expanded hours and articulate what the expansion will be, who will staff the expanded hours, and when it will be carried out. Then, in the Do step, the team can engage the staff to carry out the implementation of expanded hours, ideally on a small scale via a pilot a few days per week, while documenting observed problems.

Alternatively, using the Kotter Eight-Step Change Model, the clinician could begin planning with establishing a sense of urgency, highlighting the presence of competition, declining patient satisfaction, frequent emergency room and urgent care center visits, and other drivers. The clinician can then proceed to create a powerful guiding coalition, which includes senior clinicians and clinic leaders, who buy into the notion of expanded clinic hours. Subsequently, the clinician and her coalition can create a vision of the transformational change that would occur were the clinic to implement expanded hours. After communicating this vision and empowering others to act on this vision, the clinician can focus on planning for and creating short-term wins, such as preventing emergency room and urgent care center visits, as a way of maintaining staff and patient long-term interest in expanded clinic hours. Finally, the clinician can consolidate and institutionalize expanded hours.

Lastly, using the DD model, the clinician could begin with the Discover step to create journey and value stream maps to envision what it would look like to plan and implement an expanded hours clinic to bring value to patients. Then, in the Define step, the clinician could evaluate the pains and gains that would be felt by the staff in operating expanded clinic hours. Finally, in the Develop step, the team could prototype and quickly test operating expanded clinic hours for a few days per week.

TAKEAWAYS

Planning

- The Plan step of the PDSA cycle enables teams to prepare an intervention as part of a systematic approach to iterative change.
- The first phase of Kotter's Eight-Step Change Model, referred to as "creating a climate for change" and consisting of three steps, can be used to help plan for change.
- The first two steps of the DD model—Discover and Define—can be used by teams to identify issues and define a problem in ways that help plan for interventions.

Implementing
- The Do step of the PDSA cycle enables teams to implement an intervention as part of a systematic approach to iterative change.
- The second and third phases of Kotter's Eight-Step Change Model, referred to as "engaging and enabling the whole organization" and "implementing and sustaining change," can be used to help implement an intervention in an organization.
- The third step of the DD Model—Develop—can be used by teams to implement interventions.

Multiple-Choice Questions

1. Nancy is a pharmacist who wants to reduce emergency room medication errors due to similarly named medications. She examines the emergency room medication dispenser and notices that medications are organized alphabetically. She creates an idea for an intervention where medications would instead be grouped by indication. This work falls under which step of the PDSA cycle?

    A. Plan
    B. Do
    C. Study
    D. Act

2. A hospital administrator adopts the Kotter Eight-Step Change Model to address high hospital infection rates. Recognizing areas of early opportunity, the hospital administrator initially targets reducing catheter-associated urinary tract infections by incorporating electronic health record reminders to evaluate the necessity of urinary catheters 3 days after they are placed. Seven months into the effort, the hospital experiences a 20% reduction in catheter-associated urinary tract infections. What step of the model does this achievement represent?
    A. Communicating the vision
    B. Empowering others to act on the vision
    C. Planning for and creating short-term wins
    D. Institutionalizing new approaches

3. An interdisciplinary team at a primary care clinic is engaged in the Discover step of the DD model to improve care for their patients. Which of the following is not a tool that the team would use?

A. Field research

B. Personas

C. Ishikawa diagrams

D. Journey maps

Answers

1. The correct answer is A. Nancy is defining the objective of her intervention and what her intervention will entail, which are components of the Plan step of the PDSA cycle.

2. The correct answer is C. This achievement of reducing catheter-associated urinary tract infections is an example of planning for and creating short-term wins.

3. The correct answer is C. The Ishikawa diagram is not a tool associated with the DD model.

Bibliography

Agency for Healthcare Research and Quality. Health literacy universal precautions toolkit, 3rd edition: plan-do-study-act (PDSA) directions and examples. https://www.ahrq.gov/health-literacy/improve/precautions/tool2b.html

American Society for Quality. Walter A. Shewhart: father of statistical quality control. https://asq.org/about-asq/honorary-members/shewhart

Best M, Neuhauser D. Walter A Shewhart, 1924, and the Hawthorne factory. *Qual Saf Health Care*. 2006;15(2):142-143.

Bodenheimer T. A 63-year-old man with multiple cardiovascular risk factors and poor adherence to treatment plans. *JAMA*. 2007;298(17):2048-2055.

Chapman CR. The Shewhart cycle. The Digestible Deming. Published November 12, 2021. https://digestibledeming.substack.com/p/the-shewhart-cycle

Crowe B, Gaulton JS, Minor N, et al. To improve quality, leverage design. *BMJ Qual Saf*. 2022;31(1):70-74.

Design Council. Framework for innovation. https://www.designcouncil.org.uk/our-resources/framework-for-innovation/

Gearon M. 4 phases of the double diamond model. Krystal. https://mgearon.com/ux/double-diamond-model/

Gökce K. Successful organizational transformation—Kotter's 8-steps change model. Evolutionizer. Published February 12, 2014. https://www.evolutionizer.com/en-blog/kotter-change-management-8-steps-model

Institute for Healthcare Improvement. How to improve: model for improvement. https://www
.ihi.org/resources/how-to-improve

Kotter JP. Leading change: why transformation efforts fail. Harvard Business Review. Published
May-June 1995. https://hbr.org/1995/05/leading-change-why-transformation-efforts-fail-2

Kotter JP. *Leading Change.* Harvard Business School Press; 1996.

Kotter. What we do. https://www.kotterinc.com/what-we-do/

Moen RD. Foundation and history of the PDSA cycle. The W. Edwards Deming Institute.
https://deming.org/wp-content/uploads/2020/06/PDSA_History_Ron_Moen.pdf

Moen RD, Norman CL. Circling back: clearing up methods about the Deming cycle and seeing
how it keeps evolving. *Basic Quality.* Published November 2010. https://deming.org/
wp-content/uploads/2020/06/circling-back.pdf

Oh EG, Lee JY, Lee HJ, Oh S. Effects of discharge education using teach-back methods in
patients with heart failure: a randomized controlled trial. *Int J Nurs Stud.* 2023;140:104453.

Rosenbluth G, Destino LA, Starmer AJ, et al. I-PASS Handoff Program: use of a campaign to
effect transformational change. *Pediatr Qual Saf.* 2018;3(4):e088.

Shewhart WA. Statistical Method from the Viewpoint of Quality Control: USDA Miscella-
neous *327285.* United States Department of Agriculture; 1939.

Sobrinho R. UX process: the double diamond. Hi Interactive. Published July 13, 2023. https://
www.hi-interactive.com/blog/ux-process-the-double-diamond

University of Cambridge. Deming Cycle—PDCA. https://www.ifm.eng.cam.ac.uk/research/
dstools/pdca/

Wang Q, Zou H, Wang Q. The effectiveness of multimedia combined with teach-back method
on the level of knowledge, confidence and behavior of professional caregivers in preventing
falls in elderly patients: a randomized non-blind controlled clinical study. *Medicine
(Baltimore).* 2022;101(39):e30869.

12

Evaluating the Solutions

Clinical Case

Dr Jackson and colleagues plan for and expand clinic hours. Three months into this change, they want to determine whether the intervention has been effective and whether certain elements should be retained or changed. Dr Jackson and her team hope to conduct an evaluation that would answer these questions as part of determining the clinic's long-term policies for hours of operation.

This situation, where a clinician and their team hope to evaluate the effectiveness of an intervention, is widespread in health care. Information that teams may want to obtain through evaluations include whether a particular intervention was effective, for whom it was effective, and which components were effective. This information can inform efforts to continue an intervention unchanged or adjust versus sunset it. Several health systems solutions—Plan-Do-Study-Act (PDSA) cycle, the Double Diamond (DD) model, the Reach, Efficacy/Effectiveness, Adoption, Implementation, and Maintenance (RE-AIM) Framework, and Consolidated Framework for Implementation Research (CFIR) of implementation science—can support efforts in evaluating interventions.

SYSTEMS SOLUTION: PLAN-DO-STUDY-ACT CYCLE AND THE MODEL FOR IMPROVEMENT

As an iterative process for change, the PDSA cycle encompasses efforts to evaluate interventions with the intention of implementing subsequent action. These efforts occur in the Study and Act steps, which follow the Plan and Do steps and can be summarized in the following way:

- Plan: Discussed in Chapter 11: Planning and Implementing the Solutions
- Do: Discussed in Chapter 11: Planning and Implementing the Solutions

- Study: Teams assess what they learned from the implemented intervention, determining what went right and what went wrong. Teams complete their data analysis during this step, compare observed data to initial predictions, and summarize key lessons.

- Act: Teams decide to adopt the change, abandon the change, or restart the cycle. If they choose to restart the cycle, teams will decide what type of change(s) they should make next.

Applying the Study and Act Steps of the Plan-Do-Study-Act Cycle: Teach-Back Method in Primary Care

In an example described in Chapter 11: Planning and Implementing the Solutions, a clinic manager planned for and implemented a teach-back method in a primary care clinic. In particular, she started with the three questions in the Model for Improvement, as well as the Plan and Do steps.

Plan-Do-Study-Act Cycle One

- What are we trying to accomplish?

  To increase clinician use of the teach-back method

- How will we know that a change is an improvement?

  Clinicians who try the method will affirm its usefulness and plan to use it in the future without finding teach-back to be too time-consuming or onerous.

- What change can we make that will result in an improvement?

  Train clinicians who may not be aware of the teach-back method and ask them to utilize it.

- Plan: The clinic manager showed five clinicians a video explaining the teach-back method.

- Do: The five clinicians agreed to try using teach-back for one patient.

To evaluate the intervention, the clinic manager completed the Study and Act steps of the PDSA cycle by observing clinicians as they were using teach-back, which can be described in the following way:

- Study: The clinic manager observed that four of the five clinicians used the method with a patient. The four clinicians who used the method reported that it was useful without being onerous and that they planned to use the method again in the future. The one clinician who did not use the teach-back method reported he was not sure how to integrate the method into his clinic visits.

■ Act: The clinic manager enacted a number of efforts in the Act step, including providing additional educational resources to the clinician who did not know how to integrate the teach-back method into visits. In addition, since the other four clinicians found the method useful and did not identify undue burden, the clinic manager decided to introduce the method to all clinicians in the group.

The clinic team completed two additional PDSA cycles over the ensuing 3 weeks, starting with the following three questions in the Model for Improvement.

Plan-Do-Study-Act Cycle Two

■ What are we trying to accomplish?

  To increase sustained clinician use of the teach-back method

■ How will we know that a change is an improvement?

  If all five clinicians use the teach-back method for at least three patients per day.

■ What change can we make that will result in an improvement?

  Provide additional training tools to the one clinician who struggled with the teach-back method, and then ask them to use the method.

■ Plan: The clinic manager planned to ask the same five clinicians how many patients they used the teach-back method with, and whether they still found it useful, too onerous or time-consuming.

■ Do: The clinic manager found that only three of the five clinicians used the tool with three or more patients a day. However, all the clinicians who used the teach-back method felt it was a worthwhile tool and not too onerous or time-consuming.

■ Study: Simultaneous to the Do step, the clinic manager observed that of the two clinicians who did not meet the improvement goal, one used teach-back with one patient and the other did not with any. On further discussion, these two clinicians said they needed help with remembering to use the tool and needed to practice using it more.

■ Act: The clinic manager concluded that teach-back was being used with lower uptake than the improvement goal. The clinic manager resolved to consider putting up reminder signs to use the teach-back method in the clinic rooms as a change to implement in subsequent PDSA cycles.

Plan-Do-Study-Act Cycle Three

■ What are we trying to accomplish?

  To increase consistent and sustained clinician use of the teach-back method

- How will we know that a change is an improvement?

   If all five clinicians use the teach-back method for at least half of their patients.
- What change can we make that will result in an improvement?

   Post reminder signs in the clinic rooms to use the teach-back method.
- Plan: The clinic manager put up reminder signs on computer monitors in clinic rooms that read "teach it back." The clinic manager asked the same five clinicians if they noticed the signs and with how many patients they used the teach-back method.
- Do: The clinic manager observed that some nurses commented that the "teach it back" signs sometimes obscured the computer monitor.
- Study: The clinic manager noted that four of the five clinicians noticed the signs, and one did not. Four of the five clinicians used the teach-back method for half or more of their patients, and the other used the method for just one patient.
- Act: The clinic manager concluded that even after an initial training, a visible reminder could be useful to increase uptake of the teach-back method with patients, and decided to leave the signs on the computer monitors in clinic rooms.

SYSTEMS SOLUTION: THE DOUBLE DIAMOND MODEL

The DD model offers a structured and iterative approach for teams to effectively evaluate solutions. Following the Discover, Define, and Develop steps (discussed in Chapter 11: Planning and Implementing the Solutions), the last step—Deliver—focuses on work to refine and validate interventions through user testing and feedback (Figure 12.1). Teams use feedback to improve iterative versions of the intervention through tools such as powerful questions, user experience surveys, and user shadowing.

Applying the Deliver Step of the Double Diamond Model: Breastfeeding in the Neonatal Intensive Care Unit

As described in Chapter 11: Planning and Implementing the Solutions, the DD model has been used alongside other solutions such as the PDSA cycle to improve breastfeeding support for mothers in the NICU. A medical care organization formed an interdisciplinary team to better plan and implement interventions that could improve NICU breastfeeding practices, which can be summarized as follows:

Discover. The team created journey and value stream maps to outline the NICU's breastfeeding workflow and an Ishikawa diagram to identify root causes of maternal dissatisfaction with not meeting NICU breastfeeding goals.

Define. The team reframed the mothers' breastfeeding experiences to "how might we better support a mother's breastfeeding experience in the NICU?" and created an aim statement "to increase the rate of feeding at the breast among first-time mothers in the NICU from 33 percent to 50 percent within six months of starting the project."

Develop. In line with PDSA cycles, the team prototyped multiple versions of a team of NICU nurses dedicated to assisting mothers with feeding at the breast.

Lastly, the interdisciplinary team evaluated the prototypes that could improve NICU breastfeeding practices.

Deliver. The team used powerful questions to guide prototype (ie, a team of NICU nurses) refinement and elicit feedback from patients and clinicians over the course of 6 months. The team gathered data such as process, outcome, and balancing measures commonly used in the Model for Improvement and tracked the team's progress toward their aim statement. At the end of 6 months, the team observed a statistically significant increase in rates of feeding at the breast among mothers in the NICU.

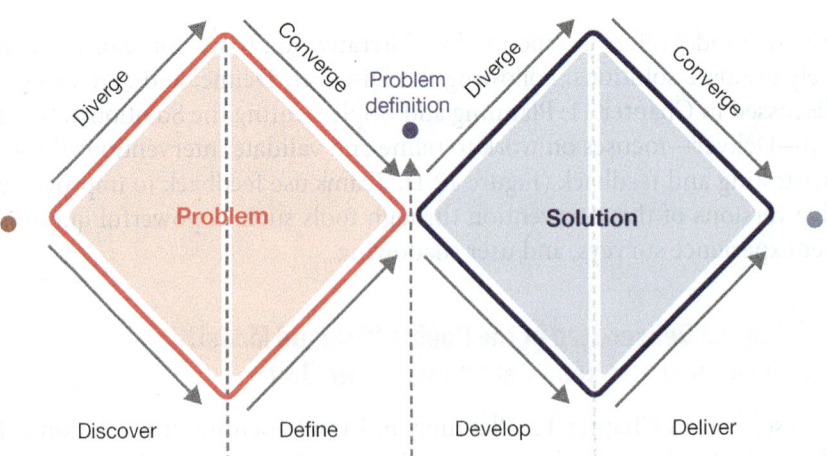

The Double Diamond

Figure 12.1 Deliver Step of the Double Diamond (DD) Model. (Source: Reproduced with permission from Sobrinho R. UX process: the double diamond. Hi Interactive. July 13, 2023. Accessed May 7, 2024. https://www.hi-interactive.com/blog/ux-process-the-double-diamond/)

SYSTEMS SOLUTION: RE-AIM FRAMEWORK

The RE-AIM framework was originally developed in 1999 by researchers to improve the study of public health and community-based interventions. They argued that existing evaluation methods focused too much on whether a particular intervention was efficacious—that is, impactful when tested via strict adherence to protocol, controlled environments, and specifically defined populations. The researchers believed that the existing "efficacy paradigm" failed to account for how interventions would work in real-world environments and settings in which factors could not be closely managed via protocols.

The researchers articulated RE-AIM as a framework for evaluating the effectiveness of an intervention grounded in implementation science, a field that emerged to bridge the gap between evidence-based practice and subsequent incorporation in real-world settings. Among such implementation science frameworks, RE-AIM has become foundational and commonly used in public health, medical care, education, and other contexts.

The RE-AIM framework guides its users through five domains (Figure 12.2):

Reach. This domain of the framework is focused on who participated in an intervention and who was impacted by it. One component of Reach is related to the scope of the intervention (eg, did it impact one clinic within a medical care organization or the whole medical care organization). An additional component of Reach is related to the characteristics of individuals who were impacted by an intervention, such as their demographic information, medical history, and social circumstances. Although it may be difficult to collect this information, it is important to understand the composition of who was impacted by an intervention because this information provides insights into whether the results of the intervention are representative of the true population of interest. For example, if the intent of an intervention was to increase exercise among people who do not already exercise, but the intervention was implemented only in clinics whose patients already exercise, the Reach of that intervention may not be as it was intended.

Efficacy/Effectiveness. In the original article outlining RE-AIM, the authors emphasized this domain as efficacy in real-world settings, which can be also understood as effectiveness. In this domain, teams should use a broad construct of what it means for an intervention to work. First, teams evaluate both positive and negative consequences of a given intervention when reporting Effectiveness. For example, instead of strictly studying whether an intervention improved a particular outcome, teams should also evaluate whether the intervention had any unintended harms, or whether the positive effects were experienced disproportionately by certain subgroups.

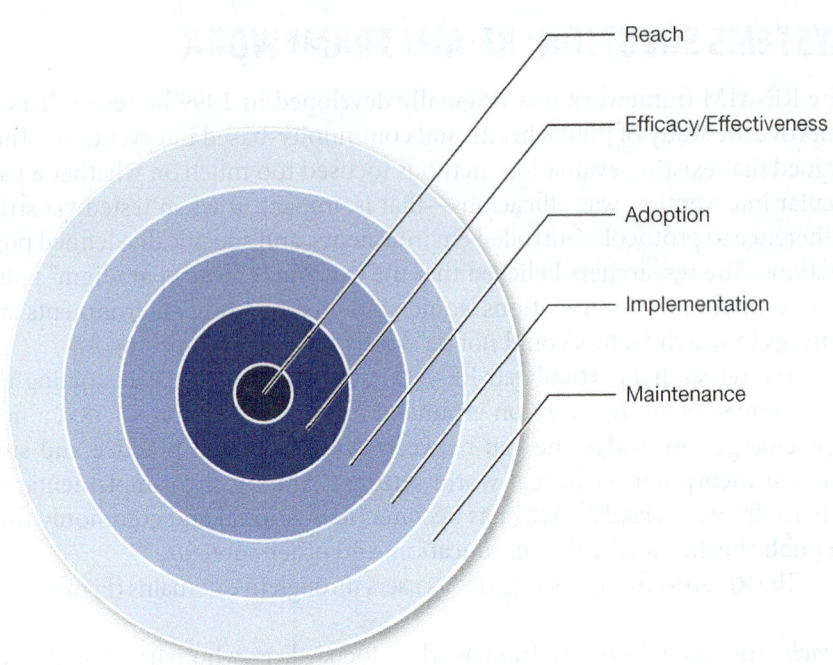

Figure 12.2 The Reach, Efficacy/Effectiveness, Adoption, Implementation, and Maintenance (RE-AIM) Framework. (Data from Glasgow RE, Vogt TM, Boles SM. Evaluating the public health impact of health promotion interventions: the RE-AIM framework. *Am J Public Health.* 1999;89(9):1322-1327.)

In addition, instead of solely measuring a biologic endpoint (eg, body mass index), teams should also study behavioral outcomes for recipients of the intervention (eg, eating and exercise habits), for staff who delivered the intervention (eg, whether staff felt comfortable approaching patients about a topic, number of follow-up calls made to patients), and for payers of an intervention (eg, whether the payer changed a reimbursement policy). Lastly, teams also measure outcomes from a patient-centered quality-of-life perspective, including measures of patient functioning, patient satisfaction with the intervention, or indicators of mental health status.

Adoption. This domain refers to the proportion of settings where an intervention was tested that actually end up using it, and whether those settings were representative of the true population of interest. The RE-AIM framework acknowledges that some settings may adopt an intervention at different times than others, and encourages teams to evaluate adoption by direct observation over time, interviews, and surveys. Teams examine barriers that may have influenced certain settings to not adopt a particular intervention.

Implementation. This domain evaluates the extent to which a tested intervention was actually administered as intended. This intervention administration can be evaluated at the individual level (eg, how frequently a patient adhered to the instructions of a given intervention) and at the setting level (eg, how consistently staff performed the intervention according to protocol). This domain can help teams differentiate if an intervention was hindered by patient factors, setting factors, or a combination. Implementation of an intervention should take place at least over the course of 6 months to 1 year.

Maintenance. This domain is intended to address the fact that while an intervention may be implemented during a research period, its continued use in a given context long term is not guaranteed. Therefore, to assess Maintenance, teams evaluate the extent to which a particular intervention was utilized by individuals long term, and the extent to which the intervention became part of a particular setting's usual practice. Maintenance should be followed for at least 2 years after the intervention's initial implementation.

Applying the RE-AIM Framework: Hypertension and Weight Self-Management Program

The RE-AIM framework was used to evaluate the effectiveness of "Be Fit, Be Well," a hypertension and weight self-management program that was implemented in three Boston-based community health center primary care clinics caring for low-income communities over the course of 2 years. The intervention was designed for individuals with a body mass index between 30 and 50, who received medication treatment for hypertension, who were older than age 21, and who spoke either English or Spanish. The intervention included individually tailored behavioral goals, behavior self-monitoring, and support from the research and clinical teams. Patients were randomized to either receive usual care or the intervention. The results of the "Be Fit, Be Well" are as follows:

Reach. The intervention enrolled approximately 60% of eligible patients. The most common reasons patients were not included were that they did not speak English or Spanish or were taking medications that might have interfered with the weight loss component of the intervention. Of the eligible patients who could be reached by telephone, nearly 85% agreed to participate, and 60% of those patients actually participated in the randomized evaluation. Eligible patients who did participate, on average, were younger and had a higher body mass index than patients who chose not to participate. There were no statistically significant differences in gender or diabetes status between eligible patients who did versus did not participate.

Efficacy/Effectiveness. Patients who received the intervention had, on average, a modestly larger amount of weight loss than the control group over the

2-year course of the intervention. The intervention group lost a larger percentage of their total body weight 2 years into the evaluation compared with the control group. The intervention group also had lower systolic blood pressure than the control group for the entirety of the 2-year intervention. The intervention group had higher levels of medication adherence at 6 and 12 months into the intervention, but not at 18 or 24 months. There was no difference in quality-of-life measures between the two groups at 12 and 24 months into the intervention.

Adoption. All three of the community health center primary care clinics that were invited chose to participate in the intervention. Within these clinics, 95% of participating primary care clinicians referred their patients to the intervention. Four community health center primary care clinics were considered for the intervention but ultimately were not included because they did not have the necessary electronic health record or scheduling systems for large-scale patient recruitment.

Implementation. More than 60% of patients participated in at least 70% of their assigned counseling calls related to the intervention. There was no difference in this call participation rate based on the patient's primary care clinic or preferred language. However, patients whose income was more than $10 000 per year had a higher call participation rate (73%) than patients who had a lower annual income (62%). Patients who spoke English and whose income was more than $10 000 per year were more likely to have their health goals, barriers, and strategies evaluated by clinics than other patients. In addition, English-speaking patients had a higher self-monitoring rate than Spanish-speaking patients.

Maintenance. There were no differences in patient-level Maintenance of behaviors and blood pressure control by race, education, gender, or income. For clinic-level Maintenance, staff interviews revealed that there was some interest in adapting some of the blood pressure control components of the intervention, but none of the clinics actually adopted the intervention after it ended. Some of the primary care clinics added walking fitness programs after the intervention ended but it was not clear if they were organic or inspired by the intervention.

SYSTEMS SOLUTION: CONSOLIDATED FRAMEWORK FOR IMPLEMENTATION RESEARCH

CFIR was first described in 2009 by researchers at the Veterans Health Administration (VHA) who noted that while implementation science had grown in prominence over time, the field was beset by two challenges. First, although helpful, multiple published theories could inadvertently create diffuseness and impede unified or comprehensive frameworks. Second, terms were inconsistent across theories, thereby limiting shared implementation science language. CFIR emerged to address these issues as a product of efforts to widely review and synthesize existing theories into a unifying framework with uniform terminology.

CFIR includes five domains: intervention characteristics, outer setting, inner setting, characteristics of individuals, and process (Figure 12.3). Each offers a different lens from which teams can evaluate an intervention's success, as well as any associated barriers or facilitators. Each domain includes multiple constructs and/or subconstructs that can be used to focus and conduct analyses most appropriate to the desired context. CFIR's 39 constructs or subconstructs (Table 12.1) are intended to provide a comprehensive way—and in turn, uniform terminology—for evaluating the impact of interventions.

An evaluation using CFIR does not need to include constructs from all five domains. Rather, teams using CFIR select constructs based on the type of intervention being tested, the context in which it is tested, and the lessons desired from their evaluation. The five domains comprising CFIR, and some example constructs or subconstructs, can be summarized in the following way:

Intervention characteristics. This domain focuses on the nature of the intervention itself and how it might be implemented in a given context. This domain acknowledges that an evidence-based intervention may need to be adapted in order to be successfully implemented in a particular setting.

When considering how to adapt an intervention to a new context, an intervention can be broken down into "core components" (critical intervention elements that need to be incorporated in any implementation) and "adaptable periphery" (other intervention elements that can be reasonably

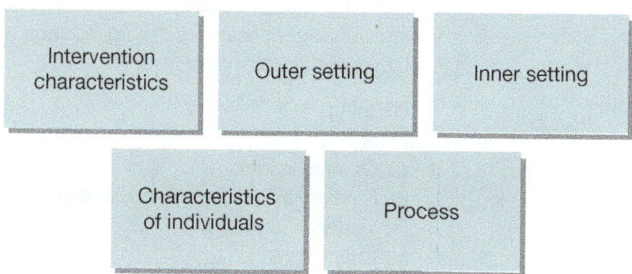

Figure 12.3 Consolidated Framework for Implementation Research (CFIR) Domains. (Source: Data from Damschroder LJ, Aron DC, Keith RE, Kirsh SR, Alexander JA, Lowery JC. Fostering implementation of health services research findings into practice: a consolidated framework for advancing implementation science. *Implement Sci.* 2009;4:50.)

Table 12.1   CFIR Domains, Constructs, and Subconstructs

Domains	Constructs and Subconstructs
Intervention characteristics	Intervention source Evidence strength and quality Relative advantage Adaptability Trialability Complexity Design quality and packaging Cost
Outer setting	Patient needs and resources Cosmopolitanism Peer pressure External policies and incentives
Inner setting	Structural characteristics Networks and communications Culture Implementation climate ■ Tension for change ■ Compatibility ■ Relative priority ■ Organizational incentives and rewards ■ Goals and feedback ■ Learning climate Readiness for implementation ■ Leadership engagement ■ Available resources ■ Access to knowledge and information
Characteristics of individuals	Knowledge and beliefs about the intervention Self-efficacy Individual stage of change Individual identification with organization Other personal attributes
Process	Planning Engaging ■ Opinion leaders ■ Formally appointed internal implementation leaders ■ Champions ■ External change agents Executing Reflecting and evaluating

Source: Data from Alexander JA, Lowery JC. Fostering implementation of health services research findings into practice: a consolidated framework for advancing implementation science. *Implement Sci.* 2009;4:50.

adjusted in a given implementation). Several constructs within Intervention Characteristics can be described as follows:

Intervention source. This construct examines the perception that individuals within an organization have regarding the legitimacy of an intervention. For example, this construct suggests that individuals may be more inclined to view an intervention as legitimate if they believe it is developed internally to address a problem within the organization, rather than developed by an external group that does not understand their organization's context.

Evidence strength and quality. This construct examines how individuals within an organization perceive the strength of supporting evidence for a particular intervention. For example, this construct suggests that individuals may feel differently about data from published literature, guidelines, or anecdotes from respected colleagues as opposed to unfamiliar sources.

Complexity. This construct examines the perception that individuals within an organization have regarding the difficulty of implementing an intervention. The perceived difficulty of an intervention can reflect how long the implementation is expected to take, how detailed the steps of an intervention are, or how disruptive the intervention might be to the usual flow of the organization.

Cost. This construct examines the initial and ongoing financial investment, supplies, and opportunity costs related to implementing an intervention.

Relative advantage. This construct examines how individuals within an organization perceive the merit of implementing a particular intervention compared to available alternatives.

Outer setting and inner setting. These two domains are closely related, and sometimes it may be difficult to determine where Outer Setting ends and Inner Setting begins. In general, Outer Setting refers to the economic, political, and social circumstances of the community (eg, a city) where an organization is implementing an intervention. In contrast, Inner Setting refers to the economic, political, and social circumstances within the organization (eg, a hospital) that is implementing the intervention. Changes to the Outer Setting may influence an intervention's implementation by virtue of influencing circumstances in the Inner Setting.

Representative constructs within Outer Setting can be summarized in the following way:

Cosmopolitanism. This construct examines whether an organization implementing an intervention has relationships with outside organizations that can offer support, as well as the quality and depth of those relationships.

External policies and incentives. This construct examines the policies that can influence an organization's motivation to implement an intervention (eg, reporting requirements, financial incentives).

Peer pressure. This construct examines the sense of urgency felt within an organization to implement an intervention, such as situations where an organization may want to obtain a competitive advantage over others or wants to catch up to other organizations that have already implemented a given intervention.

Representative constructs and subconstructs within Inner Setting can be described in the following way:

Culture. This construct evaluates the norms and values of an organization, and how a particular intervention succeeds or fails based on whether it is in line with those norms and values. In contrast to implementation climate (see subsequent text), culture is generally considered to be a stable and subconscious characteristic of a whole organization.

Implementation climate. This construct examines an organization's readiness to change and implement an intervention. In contrast to culture (see preceding text), climate is generally viewed as variable across teams within an organization, and less consistent over time. Factors to consider when examining implementation climate include whether individuals in the organization view the status quo as in need of a change; whether individuals view the intervention as compatible with their own values and interests; whether individuals feel the intervention is important for the organization's success; whether individual-level incentives are embedded in the intervention; whether the goals of the intervention and feedback on performance are clearly communicated; and whether an organization's leaders authentically solicit staff feedback and allow them to safely test new approaches.

Networks and communications. This construct examines social networks and formal and informal communication practices. For example, this construct can examine the communication between units in a hospital or the camaraderie of staff within a particular hospital unit. Overall, this construct emphasizes that the nature of relationships within an organization can strongly influence an intervention's implementation.

Compatibility. This subconstruct examines the extent to which an intervention fits within an organization's existing workflows, suggesting that if individuals in an organization perceive an intervention to be compatible, then the intervention is more likely to be successful.

Available resources. This subconstruct evaluates the amount and nature of resources (eg, money, training, time, space) that are available and specifically allocated to an intervention's initial and ongoing needs.

Access to knowledge and information. This subconstruct examines the information provided about an intervention, as well as how accessible, comprehensible, and applicable that information is to the actual work of implementing the intervention. Information can be provided in several ways including by access to experts, trainings, or through computer systems.

Characteristics of individuals. This domain focuses on traits of the recipients of a particular intervention, acknowledging that their decisions can be influenced by cultural or professional backgrounds, preexisting mindsets, or biases. This domain also acknowledges that individuals experiencing an intervention can influence others, which can subsequently impact the broader implementation effort. Representative constructs included in this domain can be summarized in the following way:

Knowledge and beliefs about the intervention. This construct evaluates an individual's familiarity with an intervention and overall opinion of it. This construct recognizes that the opinions of respected colleagues about an intervention, whether positive or negative, can significantly influence an individual's buy-in and ultimately the intervention's implementation.

Self-efficacy. This construct examines an individual's confidence in their own ability to carry out an intervention in their context. This construct recognizes that individuals with higher confidence, or self-efficacy, are more likely to try an intervention and navigate any unexpected barriers.

Individual stage of change. This construct examines an individual's openness to change and adopt a new intervention long term. This construct can be applied using a variety of behavior change models (eg, Prochaska's model which includes precontemplation, contemplation, preparation, action, and maintenance as the stages of change).

Process. This domain focuses on the steps taken to implement an intervention, underscoring that successful implementation requires a purposeful change process. Representative constructs included in this domain can be summarized in the following way:

Planning. This construct examines the steps taken to plot out an intervention prior to its implementation. According to this construct, implementation plans can be evaluated based on whether they consider relevant individuals' needs and perspectives; whether they tailor strategies for relevant subgroups of the intervention population; whether they track progress toward intervention goals; and whether they identify strategies to simplify implementation.

Executing. This construct examines whether an intervention's implementation occurs as planned. The construct defines high-quality execution as implementation that aligns with the initial plan, engages members of the organization, and includes intervention tasks that are carried out efficiently.

Reflecting and evaluating. This construct examines whether members of an organization are able to provide feedback about how interventions are implemented. This feedback can be provided via reports, graphs, or individual anecdotes with the intent of facilitating shared learning across the organization to improve implementation.

Applying Consolidated Framework for Implementation Research: Implementing Patient Aligned Care Teams

CFIR has been applied to a patient-centered medical home model called Patient Aligned Care Teams (PACT) within the VHA. Implemented in 2010, PACT was deployed in 900 primary clinics across the country, including 120 VHA primary care clinics that were part of academically affiliated medical centers. At the center of PACT was the unit of the teamlet, which consisted of one registered nurse care manager, one licensed practical nurse, one clerk, and one primary care clinician working in a coordinated manner to care for panels of patients.

At the time that PACT was implemented, patient-centered medical home models were mostly implemented in practices not affiliated with academic medical centers. Therefore, researchers used CFIR to evaluate early experiences with PACT implementation in one academic primary care clinic. The evaluation involved the following:

- Interviews with more than 20 participants in PACT, including clinic leadership, clinicians, and staff
- Direct observations of 30 nurse care manager staff meetings
- Quantitative analysis of the growth in number of clinicians, staff, and patients at the clinic

The evaluation included findings from five CFIR constructs from two domains (one from Intervention Characteristics, four from Inner Setting):

Intervention characteristics. In this domain, the researchers used the complexity construct.

Complexity. Using this construct, researchers learned that clinic leadership found PACT to be "phenomenally complicated." Clinic leaders noted that implementing PACT required core changes to the way a clinic was structured, its usual flow, and the roles that clinicians and other staff took. Clinic leadership identified that the clinic was generally understaffed and did not have the necessary foundational resources to create PACT teamlets. Without a PACT teamlet structure, clinic leadership relied on redesigning existing processes and roles to fill gaps. Clinic staff had the perception that successful implementation of PACT was unlikely.

Inner setting. In this domain, researchers used the compatibility, available resources, networks and communication, and access to knowledge and information constructs and subconstructs.

Compatibility. This subconstruct revealed that PACT was incompatible with the clinic's prior workflows in several ways. Prior to PACT's implementation, the clinic was organized into four large teams, each of which included approximately 15 clinicians, 2 registered nurse care managers, 2 licensed practical nurses, and 1 clerk. Transitioning to a teamlet structure required a major clinic reorganization, including a doubling of the amount of staff. In addition, the teamlet structure relied on the idea of a full-time clinician, which was not compatible with the reality that many of the clinicians in the academic clinic worked part-time. Due to this incompatibility, it took nearly a full year into the intervention's implementation for clinicians and staff to be given teamlet assignments.

Available resources. This subconstruct revealed that the slow process of hiring new nurses and high levels of turnover of existing nurses were barriers to staffing the clinic at required levels. This shortage and high turnover resulted in changing workloads for existing teamlets. Clinic leadership also experienced difficulty finding new space to accommodate teamlets working in a shared location.

Networks and communication. Using this construct, researchers learned that limited space impacted communication. For example, staff members often did not work in the same physical place each day and, consequently, did not have consistent phone numbers where they can be reached. Communicating with resident primary care clinicians was also a challenge, as they were often on different clinical rotations.

Access to knowledge and information. This subconstruct elucidated the difficulty with sharing PACT principles with part-time clinicians. Information about PACT was typically shared during all staff meetings. Part-time clinicians were often unable to attend these meetings and did not subsequently learn the information discussed.

Researchers also identified challenges with educating staff. To address this issue, clinic leadership decided to designate a PACT nurse trainer who would be responsible for teaching PACT principles to all new staff. However, since not all existing staff had been fully trained on PACT principles, this inconsistency in teaching new versus existing staff created confusion about appropriate processes.

Based on lessons gleaned from this CFIR evaluation, researchers recommended potential adjustments to PACT for future implementation efforts to VHA academic primary care clinics.

Back to the Clinical Case

In this case, the clinician and the team can adopt any of the four health systems solutions. Using the Study and Act steps of the PDSA cycle and the Deliver step of the DD model, the team can ensure that an evaluation of expanded hours can focus on patients and inform future cycles of iterative change.

Using the RE-AIM framework, the team can evaluate whether expanded hours reached the intended patients, whether it was implemented as intended, whether it was effective at reducing emergency room and urgent care center visits, and whether it was offered by the primary care clinic and used by patients long term.

Using CFIR, the team can evaluate barriers and facilitators of expanded hours, including those related to the intervention, the inner setting of the clinic, the outer setting of the community where the clinic is located, and the characteristics of patients. The team can use these health system solutions alone or in combination with one another.

TAKEAWAYS

- The Study and Act steps of the PDSA cycle encompass efforts to evaluate interventions with the intention of implementing subsequent action as part of an iterative process for change.
- In the last step of the DD model—Deliver—teams work to refine and validate interventions through testing and user feedback.
- RE-AIM is a framework grounded in implementation science that is focused on evaluating how well an intervention works in real-world environments and settings in which factors cannot be closely managed via protocols.
- CFIR is another implementation science evaluation framework consisting of five domains, each of which offers a different lens from which teams can evaluate an intervention's success, as well as any associated barriers or facilitators.

Multiple-Choice Questions

1. James is a hospital charge nurse who wants to reduce postoperative infections in his ward by improving hand sanitization processes. He counts the percentage of clinicians who used hand sanitizer before entering a patient's room the day before and the day after he places a sign on the

door that reads, "Bacteria Travel on Your Hands, Please Sanitize Before Entering." He observes that 30% of clinicians sanitized their hands the day before the sign was placed, and that 45% of clinicians sanitized their hands the day afterward. This work falls under which step of the PDSA cycle?

A. Plan

B. Do

C. Study

D. Act

2. Which of the following is not a tool commonly used in the Deliver step in the DD model?

A. User surveys

B. Shadowing

C. Affinity diagrams

D. Powerful questions

3. A school nurse used CFIR to evaluate the implementation of a school-based influenza vaccine intervention, where he performed daily rounds of all classrooms to see if any student wanted and had parental permission for a flu vaccine. As part of the analysis, the nurse interviewed teachers about how daily rounds fit in the overall flow of the classroom. Which domain and construct or subconstruct did the nurse use for this part of the analysis?

A. Intervention characteristics domain, intervention source construct

B. Outer setting domain, peer pressure construct

C. Inner setting domain, compatibility subconstruct

D. Characteristics of individuals domain, self-efficacy construct

4. A primary care clinic's medical director uses the RE-AIM framework to evaluate the effectiveness of implementing an evidence-based intervention to improve tobacco cessation rates in their primary care clinic. Two years after the intervention, the medical director measures the percentage of patients who have sustained tobacco cessation and the percentage of primary care clinicians who still use the intervention. What domain of RE-AIM does this component of the evaluation represent?

A. Reach

B. Adoption

C. Efficacy

D. Maintenance

Answers

1. The correct answer is C. James is studying the initial impact of his intervention, which reflects work corresponding to the "Study" step of the PDSA cycle.

2. The correct answer is C. Affinity diagrams are tools generally used in the Discover and/or Define steps, not the Deliver step, within the DD model.

3. The correct answer is C. The nurse is using the Inner Setting domain and compatibility subconstruct, which examine how the intervention fits within an organization's existing workflows and values.

4. The correct answer is D. The medical director is engaging in Maintenance by evaluating whether individual patients follow the intervention long term and the extent to which the intervention has become part of the primary care clinic's usual practice.

Bibliography

Agency for Healthcare Research and Quality. Health literacy universal precautions toolkit, 2nd edition: plan-do-study-act (PDSA) directions and examples. https://www.ahrq.gov/health-literacy/improve/precautions/tool2b.html

Boulton R, Sandall J, Sevdalis N. The cultural politics of 'implementation science'. *J Med Humanit.* 2020;41:379-394.

Crowe B, Gaulton JS, Minor N, et al. To improve quality, leverage design. *BMJ Qual Saf.* 2022;31(1):70-74.

Damschroder LJ, Aron DC, Keith RE, Kirsh SR, Alexander JA, Lowery JC. Fostering implementation of health services research findings into practice: a consolidated framework for advancing implementation science. *Implement Sci.* 2009;4:50.

Design Council. Framework for innovation. https://www.designcouncil.org.uk/our-resources/framework-for-innovation/

Forman J, Harrod M, Robinson C, et al. First things first: foundational requirements for a medical home in an academic medical center. *J Gen Intern Med.* 2014;29(suppl 2):S640-S648.

Frambach RT, Schillewaert N. Organizational innovation adoption: a multi-level framework of determinants and opportunities for future research. *J Bus Res.* 2001;55:163-176.

Gearon M. 4 phases of the double diamond model. Krystal. https://mgearon.com/ux/double-diamond-model/

Glasgow RE, Askew S, Purcell P, et al. Use of RE-AIM to address health inequities: application in a low-income community health center based weight loss and hypertension self-management program. *Transl Behav Med.* 2013;3(2):200-210.

Glasgow RE, Vogt TM, Boles SM. Evaluating the public health impact of health promotion interventions: the RE-AIM framework. *Am J Public Health.* 1999;89(9):1322-1327.

Godin G, Belanger-Gravel A, Eccles M, Grimshaw J. Healthcare professionals' intentions and behaviours: a systematic review of studies based on social cognitive theories. *Implement Sci.* 2008;3:36.

Greenhalgh T, Robert G, Macfarlane F, Bate P, Kyriakidou O. Diffusion of innovations in service organizations: systematic review and recommendations. *Milbank Q.* 2004;82:581-629.

Institute for Healthcare Improvement. How to improve: model for improvement. https://www.ihi.org/resources/how-to-improve

Kirk MA, Kelley C, Yankey N, et al. A systematic review of the use of the Consolidated Framework for Implementation Research. *Implement Sci.* 2015;11:72.

Mendel P, Meredith LS, Schoenbaum M, Sherbourne CD, Wells KB. Interventions in organizational and community context: a framework for building evidence on dissemination and implementation in health services research. *Adm Policy Ment Health.* 2008;35:21-37.

Moen RD, Norman CL. Circling back: clearing up methods about the Deming cycle and seeing how it keeps evolving. Basic Quality. Published November 2010. https://deming.org/wp-content/uploads/2020/06/circling-back.pdf

Prochaska JO, Velicer WF. The transtheoretical model of health behavior change. *Am J Health Promot.* 1997;12:38-48.

Sobrinho R. UX process: the double diamond. UX design. Published July 13, 2023. https://www.hi-interactive.com/blog/ux-process-the-double-diamond

Index